This report contains the collective views of an international group of experts and does not necessarily represent the decisions or the stated policy of the United Nations Environment Programme, the International Labour Organization or the World Health Organization.

Environmental Health Criteria 237

PRINCIPLES FOR EVALUATING HEALTH RISKS IN CHILDREN ASSOCIATED WITH EXPOSURE TO CHEMICALS

First drafts prepared by Dr Germaine Buck Louis, Bethesda, USA; Dr Terri Damstra, Research Triangle Park, USA; Dr Fernando Díaz-Barriga, San Luis Potosi, Mexico; Dr Elaine Faustman, Washington, USA; Dr Ulla Hass, Soborg, Denmark; Dr Robert Kavlock, Research Triangle Park, USA; Dr Carole Kimmel, Washington, USA; Dr Gary Kimmel, Silver Spring, USA; Dr Kannan Krishnan, Montreal, Canada; Dr Ulrike Luderer, Irvine, USA; and Dr Linda Sheldon, Research Triangle Park, USA

Published under the joint sponsorship of the United Nations Environment Programme, the International Labour Organization and the World Health Organization, and produced within the framework of the Inter-Organization Programme for the Sound Management of Chemicals.

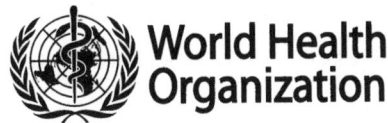

The **International Programme on Chemical Safety (IPCS)**, established in 1980, is a joint venture of the United Nations Environment Programme (UNEP), the International Labour Organization (ILO) and the World Health Organization (WHO). The overall objectives of the IPCS are to establish the scientific basis for assessment of the risk to human health and the environment from exposure to chemicals, through international peer review processes, as a prerequisite for the promotion of chemical safety, and to provide technical assistance in strengthening national capacities for the sound management of chemicals.

The **Inter-Organization Programme for the Sound Management of Chemicals (IOMC)** was established in 1995 by UNEP, ILO, the Food and Agriculture Organization of the United Nations, WHO, the United Nations Industrial Development Organization, the United Nations Institute for Training and Research and the Organisation for Economic Co-operation and Development (Participating Organizations), following recommendations made by the 1992 UN Conference on Environment and Development to strengthen cooperation and increase coordination in the field of chemical safety. The purpose of the IOMC is to promote coordination of the policies and activities pursued by the Participating Organizations, jointly or separately, to achieve the sound management of chemicals in relation to human health and the environment.

WHO Library Cataloguing-in-Publication Data

Principles for evaluating health risks in children associated with exposure to chemicals
(Environmental health criteria ; 237)

"First drafts prepared by Dr Germaine Buck Louis ... [et al.]."

1.Environmental health. 2.Risk assessment. 3.Child. 4.Organic chemicals - adverse effects. 5.Inorganic chemicals - adverse effects. 6.Environmental exposure. I.Louis, Germaine Buck. II.World Health Organization. III.Inter-Organization Programme for the Sound Management of Chemicals. IV.Series.

ISBN 92 4 157237 X   (NLM classification: WA 30.5)
ISBN 978 92 4 157237 8
ISSN 0250-863X

©World Health Organization 2006

All rights reserved. Publications of the World Health Organization can be obtained from WHO Press, World Health Organization, 20 Avenue Appia, 1211 Geneva 27, Switzerland (tel: +41 22 791 3264; fax: +41 22 791 4857; e-mail: bookorders@who.int). Requests for permission to reproduce or translate WHO publications — whether for sale or for noncommercial distribution — should be addressed to WHO Press, at the above address (fax: +41 22 791 4806; e-mail: permissions@who.int).

The designations employed and the presentation of the material in this publication do not imply the expression of any opinion whatsoever on the part of the World Health Organization concerning the legal status of any country, territory, city or area or of its authorities, or concerning the delimitation of its frontiers or boundaries. Dotted lines on maps represent approximate border lines for which there may not yet be full agreement.

The mention of specific companies or of certain manufacturers' products does not imply that they are endorsed or recommended by the World Health Organization in preference to others of a similar nature that are not mentioned. Errors and omissions excepted, the names of proprietary products are distinguished by initial capital letters.

All reasonable precautions have been taken by WHO to verify the information contained in this publication. However, the published material is being distributed without warranty of any kind, either express or implied. The responsibility for the interpretation and use of the material lies with the reader. In no event shall the World Health Organization be liable for damages arising from its use.

The named authors alone are responsible for the views expressed in this publication.

This document was technically and linguistically edited by Marla Sheffer, Ottawa, Canada, and printed by Wissenschaftliche Verlagsgesellschaft mbH, Stuttgart, Germany.

CONTENTS

ENVIRONMENTAL HEALTH CRITERIA ON PRINCIPLES FOR EVALUATING HEALTH RISKS IN CHILDREN ASSOCIATED WITH EXPOSURE TO CHEMICALS

PREAMBLE	xi
PREFACE	xvii
ACRONYMS AND ABBREVIATIONS	xix

1. SUMMARY, CONCLUSIONS, AND RECOMMENDATIONS   1

    1.1 Summary   1
    1.2 Conclusions and recommendations   4

2. INTRODUCTION AND BACKGROUND   7

    2.1 Introduction   7
    2.2 Purpose and scope of document   9
    2.3 Global burden of disease in children   12
    2.4 Major environmental threats to children   14
        2.4.1 Economic and nutritional factors   15
        2.4.2 Social, cultural, demographic, and lifestyle factors   16
        2.4.3 Chemical hazards   17
    2.5 Intrinsic factors   19
    2.6 The significance of a developmental stage approach   20
    2.7 Summary and conclusions   21

3. UNIQUE BIOLOGICAL CHARACTERISTICS OF CHILDREN   22

    3.1 General physical growth of children   22
        3.1.1 Body weight and height   22
        3.1.2 Organ weights/volumes   23
        3.1.3 Skin   25
    3.2 Anatomical and functional characteristics   25
    3.3 Physiological characteristics   26

		3.3.1 Breathing rate	26
		3.3.2 Cardiac output	26
		3.3.3 Blood flow to organs	27
		3.3.4 Body composition	28
		3.3.5 Tissue composition	29
		3.3.6 Bone growth and composition	29
	3.4	Metabolic characteristics	29
	3.5	Toxicokinetics	31
		3.5.1 Absorption, distribution, metabolism, and elimination	31
		3.5.2 Physiological changes in mothers and their influence on toxicokinetics	33
		3.5.2.1 Pregnancy	33
		3.5.2.2 Lactation and breast milk	35
		3.5.3 Dose to target	36
	3.6	Normal development	39
		3.6.1 Basic principles of normal development	39
		3.6.2 Nervous system	40
		3.6.3 Reproductive system	42
		3.6.4 Endocrine system	44
		3.6.4.1 Hypothalamic–pituitary axis	44
		3.6.4.2 Thyroid gland	46
		3.6.4.3 Adrenal glands	47
		3.6.4.4 Gonads	48
		3.6.4.5 Somatotropin (growth hormone), calcium homeostasis, and bone development	48
		3.6.4.6 Pancreas	48
		3.6.5 Cardiovascular system	49
		3.6.6 Immune system	49
		3.6.7 Respiratory system	50
		3.6.8 Kidney	52
	3.7	Summary and conclusions	53
4.		DEVELOPMENTAL STAGE–SPECIFIC SUSCEPTIBILITIES AND OUTCOMES IN CHILDREN	55
	4.1	Introduction	55
	4.2	Mortality, growth restriction, and birth defects	60
		4.2.1 Mortality	60
		4.2.2 Growth restriction	63
		4.2.3 Birth defects (structural malformations)	64

		4.2.3.1 Etiology	66
		4.2.3.2 Functional developmental toxicity	67
4.3	Specific organ systems		68
	4.3.1 Nervous system		68
		4.3.1.1 Periods of susceptibility and consequences of exposures	69
		4.3.1.2 Specific examples	72
	4.3.2 Reproductive system		78
		4.3.2.1 Periods of susceptibility	79
		4.3.2.2 Consequences of exposures	80
	4.3.3 Endocrine system		85
		4.3.3.1 Periods of susceptibility	85
		4.3.3.2 Consequences of exposures	92
	4.3.4 Cardiovascular system		95
		4.3.4.1 Periods of susceptibility	96
		4.3.4.2 Consequences of exposures	96
	4.3.5 Immune system		97
		4.3.5.1 Periods of susceptibility	98
		4.3.5.2 Consequences of exposures	101
	4.3.6 Respiratory system		105
		4.3.6.1 Periods of susceptibility	105
		4.3.6.2 Consequences of exposures	106
	4.3.7 Kidney		113
		4.3.7.1 Periods of susceptibility	113
		4.3.7.2 Consequences of exposures	114
4.4	Cancer		115
	4.4.1 Childhood cancers that may have environmental causes		116
		4.4.1.1 Lymphoid tissues	116
		4.4.1.2 Liver	118
		4.4.1.3 Thyroid	118
		4.4.1.4 Brain and nervous system	119
		4.4.1.5 Other organ sites	119
	4.4.2 Adult cancers related to childhood exposures		120
		4.4.2.1 Brain and nervous system	120
		4.4.2.2 Thyroid	121
		4.4.2.3 Female breast	122
		4.4.2.4 Female reproductive tract	122
		4.4.2.5 Integument	122
		4.4.2.6 Other organ sites	123

		4.4.3 Chemical exposures of special concern	123
	4.5	Summary and conclusions	126

5. **EXPOSURE ASSESSMENT OF CHILDREN** — 129

	5.1	Introduction	129
	5.2	General principles of exposure assessments	129
	5.3	Methods for conducting exposure assessments	133
		5.3.1 Direct methods	133
		5.3.2 Biomarkers of exposure	136
		5.3.3 Modelling	137
	5.4	Unique characteristics of children that affect exposure	139
	5.5	Exposure as it relates to children around the world	144
		5.5.1 Sources/geographical location	144
		5.5.2 Pathways of exposure	145
		5.5.2.1 Ambient air exposure pathway	145
		5.5.2.2 Indoor exposure pathways	150
		5.5.2.3 Water exposure pathway	152
		5.5.2.4 Soil exposure pathway	153
		5.5.2.5 Food-chain exposure pathway	154
		5.5.2.6 Human to human exposure pathways	155
		5.5.3 Settings/microenvironments	156
		5.5.3.1 Residential	157
		5.5.3.2 School	157
		5.5.3.3 Child-care centres	157
		5.5.3.4 Recreational	158
		5.5.3.5 Special settings	159
		5.5.4 Environmental equity factors (vulnerable communities)	161
	5.6	Special considerations for children's exposure: case-studies	162
		5.6.1 Influence of activities	162
		5.6.1.1 Arsenic	162
		5.6.1.2 Insecticides	162
		5.6.1.3 Environmental tobacco smoke (ETS)	162
		5.6.1.4 Lead	163
		5.6.2 Hazardous waste sites	163
		5.6.3 Aggregate exposure	164
		5.6.3.1 Chlorpyrifos	164

		5.6.3.2	Smelter areas	165
		5.6.3.3	Malarious areas	165
	5.6.4	Cumulative exposure		165
5.7	Summary and conclusions			166

6. **METHODOLOGIES TO ASSESS HEALTH OUTCOMES IN CHILDREN** — 168

- 6.1 Introduction — 168
  - 6.1.1 Methodological approaches for children's health studies — 168
    - 6.1.1.1 Epidemiological methods — 171
    - 6.1.1.2 Comparison of study designs — 171
    - 6.1.1.3 Descriptive designs — 176
    - 6.1.1.4 Analytic designs — 178
    - 6.1.1.5 Unique methodological considerations — 180
  - 6.1.2 Methodological approaches for animal studies — 181
    - 6.1.2.1 Developmental stage susceptibility, dosing periods, and assessment of effects — 184
    - 6.1.2.2 Dosing of fetuses and pups — 190
- 6.2 Growth and development — 190
  - 6.2.1 Human studies — 190
    - 6.2.1.1 Puberty — 194
    - 6.2.1.2 Birth defects — 195
  - 6.2.2 Animal studies — 195
    - 6.2.2.1 Body weight and postnatal growth — 195
    - 6.2.2.2 Pre-, peri-, and postnatal death — 196
    - 6.2.2.3 Physical and functional developmental landmarks — 196
    - 6.2.2.4 Birth defects and malformations — 198
- 6.3 Reproductive development and function — 198
  - 6.3.1 Human studies — 198
  - 6.3.2 Animal studies — 202
    - 6.3.2.1 Malformations of reproductive organs — 202
    - 6.3.2.2 Anogenital distance — 203
    - 6.3.2.3 Nipple/areola retention — 204
    - 6.3.2.4 Sexual maturation and puberty — 204

		6.3.2.5 Fertility	204
		6.3.2.6 Histopathology of reproductive organs	206
		6.3.2.7 Sperm quality and estrous cyclicity	207
6.4	Neurological and behavioural effects		207
	6.4.1 Human studies		207
	6.4.2 Animal studies		208
		6.4.2.1 Motor activity	208
		6.4.2.2 Motor and sensory functions	209
		6.4.2.3 Learning and memory	209
		6.4.2.4 Evaluation of effects	210
6.5	Cancer		211
	6.5.1 Human studies		211
	6.5.2 Animal studies		212
6.6	Immune system effects		212
	6.6.1 Human studies		212
	6.6.2 Animal studies		213
6.7	Respiratory system effects		213
	6.7.1 Human studies		213
	6.7.2 Animal studies		213
6.8	Haematopoietic/cardiovascular, hepatic/renal, skin/musculoskeletal, and metabolic/endocrine system effects		214
	6.8.1 Human studies		214
	6.8.2 Animal studies		214
6.9	Summary and conclusions		214

7. **IMPLICATIONS AND STRATEGIES FOR RISK ASSESSMENT FOR CHILDREN** — 217

7.1	Introduction	217
7.2	Problem formulation	220
7.3	Hazard identification	221
	7.3.1 End-points and critical periods of exposure	223
	7.3.2 Human studies	224
	7.3.3 Relevance of animal studies for assessing potential hazards to children	225
	7.3.4 Reversibility and latency	229
	7.3.5 Characterization of the health-related database	230
7.4	Dose–response assessment	230
	7.4.1 Application of health outcome data	232

		7.4.2	Quantitative evaluation	233
			7.4.2.1 Tolerable daily intake (TDI) and reference dose (RfD)/reference concentration (RfC) approaches	233
			7.4.2.2 Benchmark dose (BMD)/benchmark concentration (BMC) approach	236
			7.4.2.3 Biologically based dose–response models	236
			7.4.2.4 Duration adjustment	237
			7.4.2.5 Toxicokinetics	237
	7.5	Exposure assessment		238
		7.5.1	Age-specific exposures	238
		7.5.2	Assessment methods	240
	7.6	Risk characterization		242
	7.7	Summary and conclusions		244

REFERENCES	247
ANNEX 1: WORKING DEFINITIONS OF KEY TERMS	310
RESUME, CONCLUSIONS ET RECOMMANDATIONS	315
RESUMEN, CONCLUSIONES Y RECOMENDACIONES	323

NOTE TO READERS OF THE CRITERIA MONOGRAPHS

Every effort has been made to present information in the criteria monographs as accurately as possible without unduly delaying their publication. In the interest of all users of the Environmental Health Criteria monographs, readers are requested to communicate any errors that may have occurred to the Director of the International Programme on Chemical Safety, World Health Organization, Geneva, Switzerland, in order that they may be included in corrigenda.

Environmental Health Criteria

PREAMBLE

Objectives

In 1973, the WHO Environmental Health Criteria Programme was initiated with the following objectives:

(i) to assess information on the relationship between exposure to environmental pollutants and human health, and to provide guidelines for setting exposure limits;
(ii) to identify new or potential pollutants;
(iii) to identify gaps in knowledge concerning the health effects of pollutants;
(iv) to promote the harmonization of toxicological and epidemiological methods in order to have internationally comparable results.

The first Environmental Health Criteria (EHC) monograph, on mercury, was published in 1976, and since that time an ever-increasing number of assessments of chemicals and of physical effects have been produced. In addition, many EHC monographs have been devoted to evaluating toxicological methodology, e.g. for genetic, neurotoxic, teratogenic, and nephrotoxic effects. Other publications have been concerned with epidemiological guidelines, evaluation of short-term tests for carcinogens, biomarkers, effects on the elderly, and so forth.

Since its inauguration, the EHC Programme has widened its scope, and the importance of environmental effects, in addition to health effects, has been increasingly emphasized in the total evaluation of chemicals.

The original impetus for the Programme came from World Health Assembly resolutions and the recommendations of the 1972 UN Conference on the Human Environment. Subsequently, the work became an integral part of the International Programme on Chemical Safety (IPCS), a cooperative programme of WHO, ILO, and UNEP. In this manner, with the strong support of the new partners, the importance of occupational health and environmental effects was fully recognized. The EHC monographs have become widely established, used, and recognized throughout the world.

The recommendations of the 1992 UN Conference on Environment and Development and the subsequent establishment of the Intergovernmental Forum on Chemical Safety with the priorities for action in the six programme areas of Chapter 19, Agenda 21, all lend further weight to the need for EHC assessments of the risks of chemicals.

Scope

Two different types of EHC documents are available: 1) on specific chemicals or groups of related chemicals; and 2) on risk assessment methodologies. The criteria monographs are intended to provide critical reviews on the effect on human health and the environment of chemicals and of combinations of chemicals and physical and biological agents and risk assessment methodologies. As such, they include and review studies that are of direct relevance for evaluations. However, they do not describe *every* study carried out. Worldwide data are used and are quoted from original studies, not from abstracts or reviews. Both published and unpublished reports are considered, and it is incumbent on the authors to assess all the articles cited in the references. Preference is always given to published data. Unpublished data are used only when relevant published data are absent or when they are pivotal to the risk assessment. A detailed policy statement is available that describes the procedures used for unpublished proprietary data so that this information can be used in the evaluation without compromising its confidential nature (WHO (1990) Revised Guidelines for the Preparation of Environmental Health Criteria Monographs. PCS/90.69, Geneva, World Health Organization).

In the evaluation of human health risks, sound human data, whenever available, are preferred to animal data. Animal and in vitro studies provide support and are used mainly to supply evidence missing from human studies. It is mandatory that research on human subjects is conducted in full accord with ethical principles, including the provisions of the Helsinki Declaration.

Preamble

The EHC monographs are intended to assist national and international authorities in making risk assessments and subsequent risk management decisions. They represent a thorough evaluation of risks and are not, in any sense, recommendations for regulation or standard setting. These latter are the exclusive purview of national and regional governments.

Procedures

The following procedures were followed in the development and publication of this EHC. A designated IPCS Staff Member (Dr T. Damstra), responsible for the scientific content of the document, serves as the Responsible Officer (RO). The IPCS editor is responsible for layout and language.

An advisory group of scientific experts was convened by the RO to provide oversight, expertise, and guidance for the project and to ensure its scientific accuracy and objectivity. This advisory group met in Gex, France (22–23 October 2002), to develop and evaluate the structure and content of this EHC document and designate chapter coordinators and contributors of text. Initial drafts of the document were prepared by chapter coordinators (Dr Germaine Buck Louis, Bethesda, Maryland, USA; Dr Terri Damstra, Research Triangle Park, North Carolina, USA; Dr Fernando Díaz-Barriga, San Luis Potosi, Mexico; Dr Elaine Faustman, Washington, D.C., USA; Dr Ulla Hass, Soborg, Denmark; Dr Robert Kavlock, Research Triangle Park, North Carolina, USA; Dr Carole Kimmel, Washington, D.C., USA; Dr Gary Kimmel, Silver Spring, Maryland, USA; Dr Kannan Krishnan, Montreal, Quebec, Canada; Dr Ulrike Luderer, Irvine, California, USA; Dr Linda Sheldon, Research Triangle Park, North Carolina, USA) with input from the following experts who contributed text for various sections of the document: Tom Burbacher, Department of Environmental and Occupational Health Sciences, University of Washington, Seattle, Washington, USA; George Daston, Procter & Gamble Company, Cincinnati, Ohio, USA; Rodney Dietert, Department of Microbiology and Immunology, College of Veterinary Medicine, Cornell University, Ithaca, New York, USA; Agneta Falk-Filipsson, Karolinska Institutet, Stockholm, Sweden; Fernando Froes, USP School of Medicine, Sao Paulo, Brazil; Gonzalo Gerardo Garcia Vargas, Universidad Juárez del Estado de Durango, Gómez Palacio, Mexico;

Kimberly Grant, University of Washington, Seattle, Washington, USA; Tony Myres, Ottawa, Ontario, Canada; Asher Ornoy, Hebrew University, Jerusalem, Israel; Susan Ozanne, University of Cambridge, Cambridge, United Kingdom; Jerry Rice, Washington, D.C., USA; Peter Sly, Department of Pediatrics and Physiology, Telethon Institute; and Jorma Toppari, University of Turku, Turku, Finland.

The advisory group members, chapter coordinators, and contributors of text serve as individual scientists, not as representatives of any organization, government, or industry. All individuals who as authors, consultants, or advisers participating in the preparation of EHC monographs must, in addition to serving in their personal capacity as scientists, inform the RO if at any time a conflict of interest, whether actual or potential, could be perceived in their work. They are required to sign a conflict of interest statement. Such a procedure ensures the transparency of the process. The composition of the advisory group is dictated by the range of expertise required for the subject of the meeting and, where possible, by the need for a balanced geographical distribution.

The chapter coordinators met over a three-year period to evaluate and revise various drafts of the document. Once the RO found the unedited final draft acceptable, it was sent to over 100 contact points throughout the world for review and comment. The unedited draft was also made available on the IPCS web site for external review and comment for a period of two months. These comments were peer-reviewed by the RO and chapter coordinators, and additions and revisions to the draft document were made if necessary. A file of all comments received and revisions made on the draft is available from the RO. When the RO was satisfied as to the scientific correctness and completeness of the document, it was forwarded to an IPCS editor for language editing, reference checking, and preparation of camera-ready copy. After approval by the Director, IPCS, the manuscript was submitted to the WHO Office of Publications for printing. It will also be available on the IPCS web site.

WHO TASK GROUP ON ENVIRONMENTAL HEALTH CRITERIA ON PRINCIPLES FOR EVALUATING HEALTH RISKS IN CHILDREN ASSOCIATED WITH EXPOSURE TO CHEMICALS

Dr T. Damstra, IPCS, served as the Responsible Officer and was responsible for the preparation of the final document and for its overall scientific content. Marla Sheffer, Ottawa, Canada, was the IPCS editor responsible for layout and language.

* * *

Risk assessment activities of IPCS are supported financially by the Department of Health and Department for Environment, Food & Rural Affairs, United Kingdom; Environmental Protection Agency, Food and Drug Administration, and National Institute of Environmental Health Sciences, USA; European Commission; German Federal Ministry of Environment, Nature Conservation and Nuclear Safety; Health Canada; Japanese Ministry of Health, Labour and Welfare; and Swiss Agency for Environment, Forests and Landscape.

* * *

Advisory group members

Dr Patric Amcoff, Organisation for Economic Co-operation and Development, Paris, France

Dr Bingheng Chen, Environmental Health, Fudan University School of Public Health, Shanghai, People's Republic of China

Dr Thea De Wet, Department of Anthropology and Developmental Studies, Rand Afrikaans University, Auckland Park, South Africa

Dr Agneta Falk-Filipsson, Utredningssekretariatet, Institutet för miljömedicin (IMM), Karolinska Institutet, Stockholm, Sweden

Dr Elaine Faustman, Pediatric Environmental Health Research Center, University of Washington, Seattle, Washington, USA

Dr Ryuichi Hasegawa, Division of Medicinal Safety Science, National Institute of Health Sciences, Tokyo, Japan

Dr Carole Kimmel, Office of Research and Development, National Center for Environmental Assessment, Environmental Protection Agency, Washington, D.C., USA

Dr Kannan Krishnan, University of Montreal, Montreal, Quebec, Canada

Dr Irma Makalinao, National Poisons Control & Information Service, Philippines General Hospital, Manila, Philippines

Dr Mathuros Ruchirawat, Chulabhorn Research Institute, Bangkok, Thailand

Dr Radim J. Srám, Institute of Experimental Medicine, Academy of Sciences of the Czech Republic, Prague, Czech Republic

Dr William Suk, Division of Extramural Research and Training, National Institute of Environmental Health Sciences, Department of Health and Human Services, Research Triangle Park, North Carolina, USA

Dr Jan E. Zejda, Department of Epidemiology, Medical University of Silesia, Katowice, Poland

Secretariat

Dr Terri Damstra, International Programme on Chemical Safety, World Health Organization, Research Triangle Park, North Carolina, USA

PREFACE

The International Programme on Chemical Safety (IPCS) was initiated in 1980 as a collaborative programme of the United Nations Environment Programme (UNEP), the International Labour Organization (ILO), and the World Health Organization (WHO). One of the major objectives of IPCS is to improve scientific methodologies for assessing the effects of chemicals on human health and the environment. As part of this effort, IPCS publishes a series of monographs, called Environmental Health Criteria (EHC) documents, that evaluate the scientific principles underlying methodologies and strategies to assess risks from exposure to chemicals.

Since its inception, IPCS has been concerned about the effects of chemical exposures on susceptible populations, including children. Past EHC publications addressing methodologies for risk assessment in children include EHC 30, *Principles for Evaluating Health Risks to Progeny Associated with Exposure to Chemicals during Pregnancy* (IPCS, 1984), and EHC 59, *Principles for Evaluating Health Risks from Chemicals during Infancy and Early Childhood: The Need for a Special Approach* (IPCS, 1986b). EHC 30 focused on the use of short-term tests and in vivo animal tests to assess prenatal toxicity and postnatal alterations in reproduction, development, and behaviour following chemical exposure during gestation, and EHC 59 focused on methods to detect impaired reproductive and neurobehavioural development in infants and children who were exposed during the prenatal and early postnatal periods. Since these monographs were published in the 1980s, new data and methodologies have emerged, indicating that children are a vulnerable population subgroup with special susceptibilities and unique exposures to environmental factors that have important implications for public health practices and risk assessment approaches. In recognition of this new scientific knowledge, IPCS was asked to provide an up-to-date EHC on scientific principles and approaches to assessing risks in children associated with exposures to environmental chemicals.

IPCS is producing this monograph as a tool for use by public health officials, research and regulatory scientists, and risk assessors. It is intended to complement the monographs, reviews, and test guidelines on reproductive and developmental toxicity currently available. However, this document does not provide specific guidelines or protocols for the application of risk assessment strategies or the conduct of specific tests. Specific testing guidelines for assessing reproductive toxicity from exposure to chemicals have been developed by the Organisation for Economic Co-operation and Development (OECD) and national governments.

The efforts of all who helped in the preparation, review, and finalization of the monograph are gratefully acknowledged. Special thanks are due to the United States Environmental Protection Agency (USEPA) and the United States National Institute of Environmental Health Sciences/National Institutes of Health for their financial support of the planning and review group meetings.

ACRONYMS AND ABBREVIATIONS

ACE	angiotensin converting enzyme
ACTH	adrenocorticotropic hormone
AGD	anogenital distance
AIDS	acquired immunodeficiency syndrome
APEX	Air Pollutants Exposure
AT_2	angiotensin II
BMC	benchmark concentration
BMCL	a statistical lower confidence limit on the BMC
BMD	benchmark dose
BMDL	a statistical lower confidence limit on the BMD
CI	confidence interval
CNS	central nervous system
CYP	cytochrome P450
DDE	dichlorodiphenyldichloroethene
DDT	dichlorodiphenyltrichloroethane
DEPM	Dietary Exposure Potential Model
DES	diethylstilbestrol
DHEA	dehydroepiandrosterone
DHT	dihydrotestosterone
DNA	deoxyribonucleic acid
EDSTAC	Endocrine Disruptor Screening and Testing Advisory Committee
EHC	Environmental Health Criteria
EPA	Environmental Protection Agency (USA)
ETS	environmental tobacco smoke
EU	European Union
FEF	forced expiratory flow
FEV	forced expiratory volume
FSH	follicle stimulating hormone

GD	gestation day
GH	growth hormone
GnRH	gonadotropin releasing hormone
GST	glutathione-S-transferase
HAPEM	Hazardous Air Pollutant Exposure Model
hCG	human chorionic gonadotropin
HIV	human immunodeficiency virus
HPG	hypothalamic–pituitary–gonadal
IAQX	Indoor Air Quality and Inhalation Exposure
IEUBK	Integrated Exposure Uptake Biokinetic
IGF	insulin-like growth factor
ILO	International Labour Organization
IPCS	International Programme on Chemical Safety
IQ	intelligence quotient
IUGR	intrauterine growth restriction
LH	luteinizing hormone
LOAEL	lowest-observed-adverse-effect level
MOE	margin of exposure
NDMA	N-nitrosodimethylamine
NOAEL	no-observed-adverse-effect level
OECD	Organisation for Economic Co-operation and Development
OR	odds ratio
PAH	polycyclic aromatic hydrocarbon
PBB	polybrominated biphenyl
PBPK	physiologically based pharmacokinetic
PCB	polychlorinated biphenyl
PCDD	polychlorinated dibenzo-p-dioxin
PCDF	polychlorinated dibenzofuran
pH	relative hydrogen ion concentration
$PM_{2.5}$	particulate matter less than 2.5 µm in diameter

PM_{10}	particulate matter less than 10 µm in diameter
PND	postnatal day
PNS	peripheral nervous system
p.o.	per oral (by mouth)
POP	persistent organic pollutant
PRL	prolactin
RfC	reference concentration
RfD	reference dose
RNA	ribonucleic acid
RO	Responsible Officer
s.c.	subcutaneous
SCALE	**S**cience, **C**hildren, **A**wareness, EU **L**egislation, and Continuous **E**valuation
SF-1	steroidogenic factor 1
SHEDS	Stochastic Human Exposure and Dose Simulation
T3	triiodothyronine
T4	thyroxine (tetraiodothyronine)
TCDD	2,3,7,8-tetrachlorodibenzo-*p*-dioxin
TCP	3,5,6-trichloro-2-pyridinol
TDI	tolerable daily intake
TERIS	Teratogen Information System
TG	Test Guideline
TGF-α	transforming growth factor-alpha
TGF-β	transforming growth factor-beta
Th1	T helper 1
Th2	T helper 2
TSH	thyroid stimulating hormone
UN	United Nations
UNEP	United Nations Environment Programme
USA	United States of America

EHC 237: Principles for Evaluating Health Risks in Children

USEPA	United States Environmental Protection Agency
VOC	volatile organic compound
WHO	World Health Organization

1. SUMMARY, CONCLUSIONS, AND RECOMMENDATIONS

1.1 Summary

Environmental factors play a major role in determining the health and well-being of children.[1] Accumulating evidence indicates that children, who comprise over one third of the world's population, are among the most vulnerable of the world's population and that environmental factors can affect children's health quite differently from adults' health. Poor, neglected, and malnourished children suffer the most. These children often live in unhealthy housing, lack clean water and sanitation services, and have limited access to health care and education. One in five children in the poorest parts of the world will not live to their fifth birthday, mainly because of environment-related diseases. The World Health Organization (WHO) estimates that over 30% of the global burden of disease in children can be attributed to environmental factors.

Health is determined by a variety of factors. In addition to the physical environment, genetics, and biology, social, economic, and cultural factors play major roles. Although it is critical to understand the various driving forces during childhood that shape health and behaviour throughout life, the emphasis of this document is specifically on exposure to environmental chemicals. This document evaluates the scientific principles to be considered in assessing health risks in children from exposures to environmental chemicals during distinct developmental stages and provides information for public health officials, research and regulatory scientists, and other experts responsible for protecting children's health. The central focus of this document is on the developmental stage rather than on a specific environmental chemical or a specific disease or outcome. Developmental stage–specific periods of susceptibility have been referred to as "critical windows for exposure" or "critical windows of development". These distinct life stages are defined by relevant dynamic processes occurring at the molecular, cellular, organ

---

[1] The terms "children" and "child" as used in this document include the stages of development from conception through adolescence.

system, and organism level. It is the differences in these life stages along with exposures that will define the nature and severity of environmental impacts.

Children have different susceptibilities during different life stages owing to their dynamic growth and developmental processes as well as physiological, metabolic, and behavioural differences. From conception through adolescence, rapid growth and developmental processes occur that can be disrupted by exposures to environmental chemicals. These include anatomical, physiological, metabolic, functional, toxicokinetic, and toxicodynamic processes. Exposure pathways and exposure patterns may also be different in different stages of childhood. Exposure can occur in utero through transplacental transfer of environmental agents from mother to fetus or in nursing infants via breast milk. Children consume more food and beverages per kilogram of body weight than do adults, and their dietary patterns are different and often less variable during different developmental stages. They have a higher inhalation rate and a higher body surface area to body weight ratio, which may lead to increased exposures. Children's normal behaviours, such as crawling on the ground and putting their hands in their mouths, can result in exposures not faced by adults. Children's metabolic pathways may differ from those of adults. Children have more years of future life and thus more time to develop chronic diseases that take decades to appear and that may be triggered by early environmental exposures. They are often unaware of environmental risks and generally have no voice in decision-making.

The accumulating knowledge that children may be at increased risk at different developmental stages, with respect to both biological susceptibility and exposure, has raised awareness that new risk assessment approaches may be necessary in order to adequately protect children. Traditional risk assessment approaches and environmental health policies have focused mainly on adults and adult exposure patterns, utilizing data from adult humans or adult animals. There is a need to expand risk assessment paradigms to evaluate exposures relevant to children from preconception to adolescence, taking into account the specific susceptibilities at each developmental stage. The full spectrum of effects from childhood exposures cannot be predicted from adult data. Risk assessment approaches for exposures in children must be linked to life stages.

Summary, Conclusions, and Recommendations

A broad spectrum of diseases in children are known (or suspected) to be associated with unhealthy environments. For much of the world, traditional environmental health hazards continue to remain the primary source of ill-health. These include lack of adequate nutrition, poor sanitation, contaminated water, rampant disease vectors (e.g. mosquitoes and malaria), and unsafe waste disposal. In addition, rapid globalization and industrialization coupled with unsustainable patterns of production and consumption have released large quantities of chemical substances into the environment. Although the term "environmental exposure" can encompass a variety of factors, the focus of this document is specifically on environmental chemical exposures. Most of these substances have not been assessed for potential toxicity to children, nor have the most vulnerable subpopulations of children been identified. The incidence of a number of important paediatric diseases and disorders (e.g. asthma, neurobehavioural impairment) is increasing in several parts of the world. Although a variety of factors are likely to be involved, this may be due, in part, to the quality of the environment in which children live, grow, and play.

Establishing causal links between specific environmental exposures and complex, multifactorial health outcomes is difficult and challenging, particularly in children. For children, the stage in their development when the exposure occurs may be just as important as the magnitude of exposure. Very few studies have characterized exposures during different developmental stages. Examples have shown that exposures to the same environmental chemical can result in very different health outcomes in children compared with adults. Some of these outcomes have been shown to be irreversible and persist throughout life. Furthermore, different organ systems mature at different rates, and the same dose of an agent during different periods of development can have very different consequences. There may also be a long latency period between exposure and effects, with some outcomes not apparent until later in life. Some examples of health effects resulting from developmental exposures include those observed prenatally and at birth (e.g. miscarriage, stillbirth, low birth weight, birth defects), in young children (e.g. infant mortality, asthma, neurobehavioural and immune impairment), and in adolescents (e.g. precocious or delayed puberty). Emerging evidence suggests that an increased risk of certain diseases in adults (e.g.

cancer, heart disease) can result in part from exposures to certain environmental chemicals during childhood.

While research has addressed the impact of environmental chemicals on children's health, typically investigators have focused on exposure to a particular environmental chemical, such as heavy metals or pesticides, and a particular organ system or end-point. Noticeably absent are prospective longitudinal studies capturing exposures over key developmental windows or life stages. Virtually no studies have captured periconceptional exposures either alone or in addition to other life stage exposures. Advancing technology and new methodologies now offer promise for capturing exposures during these critical windows. This will enable investigators to detect conceptions early and estimate the potential competing risk of early embryonic mortality when considering children's health outcomes that are conditional upon survival during the embryonic and fetal periods.

The special vulnerability of children should form the basis for development of child-protective policies and risk assessment approaches. A lack of full proof for causal associations should not prevent efforts to reduce exposures or implement intervention and prevention strategies.

1.2 Conclusions and recommendations

While substantial knowledge has been gained on the effects of exposure to environmental agents on children's health, much remains to be learned. Child-protective risk assessment approaches must be based on a better understanding of the interactions of exposures, biological susceptibility, and socioeconomic and cultural (including nutritional) factors at each stage of development. In order to gain a better understanding, further research is needed in the following areas:

- Design and implement prospective cohort studies of pregnant women, infants, and children with longitudinal capture of exposures at critical windows and sensitive health end-points along the continuum of human development. Efforts to recruit couples prior to conception are needed to address critical data regarding periconceptional exposures and children's health.

Summary, Conclusions, and Recommendations

- Continue to develop and enhance population-based surveillance systems for the real-time capture of sentinel health end-points. This includes current surveillance systems such as vital registration for birth size and gestation and birth defects registries for capture of major malformations. Consideration of emerging sentinel end-points such as fecundability, as measured by time to pregnancy and sex ratios, should receive added research consideration.

- Strengthen exposure monitoring efforts in children during different developmental stages, including efforts to assess aggregate and cumulative exposures.

- Strengthen exposure monitoring efforts in developing countries.

- Identify subpopulations with the highest exposure levels.

- Develop validated, sensitive, and cost-effective biomarkers of exposure, susceptibility, and effects, particularly during early developmental stages.

- Improve characterization of the differences in toxicokinetic and toxicodynamic properties of xenobiotics at different developmental stages. Develop databases of developmental stage–specific physiological and pharmacokinetic parameters in both human and animal studies.

- Conduct studies focusing on mechanisms of action during different developmental stages by which exposures may cause adverse outcomes.

- Develop end-points that can be used to assess organ system functions in both humans and animal species and to identify analogous periods of development across species.

- Examine the utility of newer molecular and imaging technologies to assess causal associations between exposure and effect at different developmental stages.

- Improve characterization of the windows of susceptibility of different organ systems in relation to structural and functional end-points.

- Develop and validate biological models and animal testing guidelines that can address health outcomes at different developmental stages.

- Determine which exposure reductions will have the greatest overall impact on children's health.

The development of risk assessment strategies that address the developmental life stages through which all future generations must pass is essential to any public health strategy. Protection of children is at the core of the sustainability of the human species. It should be a priority of all countries and international and national organizations to provide safe environments for all children and reduce exposure to environmental hazards through promotion of healthy behaviours, education, and awareness raising at all levels, including the community, family, and child. In order to better accomplish this, research on the effectiveness of risk reduction and intervention practices, including the most effective means to educate and communicate the need for child-protective public health policies, legislation, and safety standards, is needed. The active participation of all sectors of society plays an important role in promoting safe and healthy environments for all.

2. INTRODUCTION AND BACKGROUND

2.1 Introduction

Although the last three decades have witnessed a significant decline in childhood mortality and morbidity, these gains have not been apparent everywhere, and in some countries mortality and morbidity are increasing (WHO, 2005a). Exposure to environmental hazards is a major reason for ill-health in children,[1] particularly in children who are impoverished and malnourished. Yet because of their increased susceptibility, these children are the very group that can least afford to be exposed to other environmental hazards. The heightened susceptibility of children to several environmental pollutants derives primarily from the unique biological and physiological features that characterize the various stages of development from conception through adolescence (see chapter 3), as well as certain behavioural characteristics and external factors that may result in increased exposure levels (see chapter 5).

The increased awareness about the special vulnerability of children has led to a number of new research programmes, international agreements, and international alliances that specifically address and promote healthy environments for children (UNICEF, 1990, 2001a; WHO, 1997, 2002a; Suk, 2002; Suk et al., 2003). A few key international activities are cited below:

- In 1989, the **United Nations Convention on the Rights of the Child** laid down the basic standards for the protection of children, taking into consideration the dangers of environmental pollution, and declared that children are entitled to special care and assistance.

- In 1990, the **World Summit for Children** adopted a declaration on the survival, protection, and development of children in which the signatories agreed to work together to protect the

---

[1] The terms "children" and "child" as used in this document include the stages of development from conception through adolescence.

environment so that all children could enjoy a safer and healthier future.

- In 1992, the **United Nations Conference on Environment and Development** (the Earth Summit) declared that the health of children is more severely affected by unhealthy environments than that of any other population group, that children are highly vulnerable to the effects of environmental degradation, and that their special susceptibilities need to be fully taken into account.

- In 1997, the **Declaration of the Environment Leaders of the Eight on Children's Environmental Health** acknowledged the special vulnerability of children and committed their countries to take action on several specific environmental health issues, such as chronic lead poisoning, microbiologically contaminated drinking-water, endocrine disrupting chemicals, environmental tobacco smoke (ETS), and poor air quality.

- In 2002, WHO launched the **Healthy Environments for Children Alliance**, which seeks to mobilize support and intensify global action to provide healthy environments for children.

- In 2002, the Bangkok Statement (adopted by over 400 participants) at the **WHO International Conference on Environmental Threats to Children: Hazards and Vulnerability**, in Bangkok, Thailand, identified the need for improved risk assessment methodologies in children.

- In 2005, the **Second International Conference of Environmental Threats to Children**, in Buenos Aires, Argentina, assessed major environmental threats to children in Central and Latin American countries and identified priority areas for research collaboration.

Many countries have also established specific regulations to protect children from exposure to certain environmental hazards, including toxic chemicals. Examples include banning of heavy metals in toys, strict limit setting for persistent toxic substances in baby foods, and the setting of environmental limit values derived on the basis of infants' sensitivities (e.g. nitrates in drinking-water). In the United States, concerns about children's special vulnerabilities resulted in the Food Quality Protection Act (USFDA, 1996), which directs the United States Environmental Protection Agency (USEPA) to use an additional 10-fold safety factor in assessing the risks of exposure of infants and children to pesticides, particularly when there are limited toxicology and exposure data. In Europe, an action plan is being developed to evaluate risks through SCALE, which focuses on **S**cience, **C**hildren, **A**wareness, European Union (EU) **L**egislation, and Continuous **E**valuation (see http://www.environmentandhealth.org).

In the past, approaches to assessing risks from chemicals were based largely on adult exposures, toxicities, and default factors. The publication in 1993 of the United States National Academy of Sciences' report on *Pesticides in the Diets of Infants and Children* (NRC, 1993) was critical in raising awareness of the importance of considering the vulnerable life stages of children when conducting risk assessments of exposure in children. In 2001, the International Life Sciences Institute convened a number of scientific experts to develop a conceptual framework for conducting risk assessments from chemical exposures in children, which takes into consideration their unique characteristics and special vulnerabilities (ILSI, 2003; Olin & Sonawane, 2003; Daston et al., 2004). This document builds on these previous activities and takes into account the availability of updated test guidelines, new technologies, and revised models for exposure assessment in order to evaluate the scientific knowledge base that underlies a "child-centred" risk assessment strategy (see chapters 6 and 7).

2.2 Purpose and scope of document

The primary purpose of this document is to provide a systematic analysis of the scientific principles to be considered in assessing health risks in children from exposures to environmental agents during distinct stages of development. The developmental stages used throughout this document are defined in Table 1 and are considered temporal intervals with distinct anatomical, physiological, behavioural, or functional characteristics that contribute to potential differences in vulnerability to environmental exposures. Exposure before conception (maternal and/or paternal) may also affect health outcomes during later stages of development. Adverse health effects may be detected during the same life stage as when the exposure occurred, or they may not be expressed until later in life. The central focus of this document is on *the child* rather than on a specific environmental agent, target organ, or disease. Thus, it addresses the difficult task of integrating all that is known about exposure, toxicity, and health outcomes at different life stages, which is especially challenging when data are limited for particular life stages (e.g. exposure levels during pregnancy).

Table 1. Working definitions for stages in human development

Developmental stage/ event	Time period
Preconception	Prefertilization
Preimplantation embryo	Conception to implantation
Postimplantation embryo	Implantation to 8 weeks of pregnancy
Fetus	8 weeks of pregnancy to birth
Preterm birth	24–37 weeks of pregnancy
Normal-term birth	40 ± 2 weeks of pregnancy
Perinatal stage	29 weeks of pregnancy to 7 days after birth
Neonate	Birth to 28 days of age
Infant	28 days of age to 1 year
Child	
- Young child	1–4 years of age
- Toddler	2–3 years of age
- Older child	5–12 years of age
Adolescent	Beginning with the appearance of secondary sexual characteristics to achievement of full maturity (usually 12–18 years of age)

Although the term "environmental exposures" includes a variety of factors, the focus in this document is specifically on environmental chemical exposures. Other factors, such as dietary, behavioural, and lifestyle factors and use of pharmaceuticals, are also considered environmentally related, but fall beyond the scope of this document, except when they interact with environmental exposures.

Similarly, the document is not intended to be a comprehensive review of the literature on the effects of exposures to all environmental pollutants on the health of children. Rather, the effects of illustrative pollutants are described to demonstrate how exposure

Introduction and Background

patterns, susceptibilities, and mechanisms of toxicity change at different life stages and how these changes can impact risk assessment. References are provided throughout the document for more detailed information on environmental threats to children. A list of WHO web sites relevant to children's health is provided in Box 1. These WHO web sites also provide links to other sites relevant to children's health.

Box 1. WHO web site resources relevant to children's health

WHO Child and Adolescent Health and Development:
http://www.who.int/child-adolescent-health/

WHO Children's Environmental Health: http://www.who.int/ceh

WHO Global Database on Child Growth and Malnutrition:
http://www.who.int/nutgrowthdb

WHO Data on Global Burden of Disease by Country, Age, Sex: available from http://www3.who.int/whosis/menu

WHO Food Safety: http://www.who.int/foodsafety/en/

WHO Global Environmental Change: http://www.who.int/globalchange/en/

WHO International Programme on Chemical Safety:
http://www.who.int/ipcs

WHO Maternal and Newborn Health: http://www.who.int/reproductive-health/MNBH/index.htm

WHO Health in the Millennium Development Goals:
http://www.who.int/mdg/publications/mdg_report/en/

WHO Nutrition: http://www.who.int/nut/

WHO Quantifying Environmental Health Impacts:
http://www.who.int/quantifying_ehimpacts/en/

WHO School Health and Youth Health Promotion:
http://www.who.int/school_youth_health/en/

WHO Water, Sanitation & Health:
http://www.who.int/water_sanitation_health/en/

WHO World Health Reports: http://www.who.int/whr

WHO World Health Statistics: http://www.who.int/healthinfo/statistics

---

This document is intended to be used as a tool for use by public health officials, research and regulatory scientists, and risk assessors. It does not provide practical advice, guidelines, or protocols for the conduct of specific tests and studies. In addition to the documents cited in the introduction to this chapter, it builds on two previous

EHCs addressing methodologies for assessing risks in children: EHC 30, *Principles for Evaluating Health Risks to Progeny Associated with Exposure to Chemicals during Pregnancy* (IPCS, 1984), and EHC 59, *Principles for Evaluating Health Risks from Chemicals during Infancy and Early Childhood: The Need for a Special Approach* (IPCS, 1986b). EHC 30 focused on the use of short-term tests and in vivo animal tests to assess prenatal toxicity and postnatal alterations in reproduction, development, and behaviour following chemical exposure during gestation, and EHC 59 focused on methods to detect impaired reproductive and neurobehavioural development in infants and children who were exposed during the prenatal and early postnatal periods.

2.3 Global burden of disease in children

Scientific, medical, and public health advances, expanded access, and receipt of primary health care and basic social services have significantly improved the health and well-being of children. Nevertheless, at the beginning of the 21st century, nearly 11 million children (29 000 per day) under five years of age will die annually from causes that are largely preventable. Among these yearly deaths are four million babies who will not survive the first month of life. A similar number will be stillborn (WHO, 2005a). Most of these deaths will occur in developing countries, particularly in the African and South-east Asian regions of the world.

At the global level, an analysis of the WHO database on burden of disease (http://www.who.int/evidence) shows that most of these deaths result from a handful of causes (WHO, 2005a). Figure 1 shows the major causes of death in children under five years of age. Estimates from the 2000–2003 database attribute 37% of these deaths to neonatal causes, 19% to pneumonia, 17% to diarrhoea, 20% to "other" — including injuries, measles, and human immunodeficiency virus (HIV)/acquired immunodeficiency syndrome (AIDS) — and 8% to malaria.

Figure 1 also shows the major causes of neonatal deaths (birth to 28 days). The largest fraction of deaths (28%) is attributed to preterm births, which may also result in long-term adverse health consequences (see chapter 4). Thus, the perinatal and neonatal developmental stages can be considered particularly vulnerable periods.

Introduction and Background

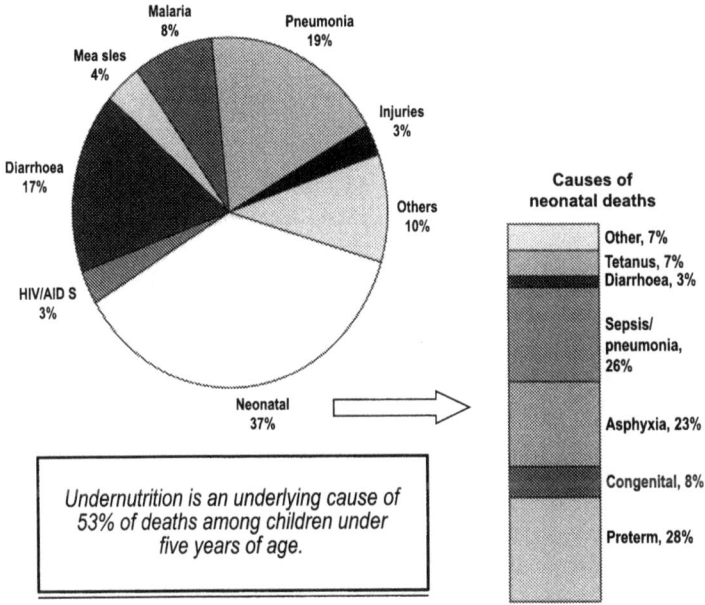

Fig. 1. Estimated distribution of major causes of death among children under five years of age and neonates in the world, 2000–2003 (from WHO, 2005a).

The estimates in Figure 1 are at the global level and will differ significantly among various regions of the world and among countries within a given region. For example, in a number of African countries, the surge of HIV/AIDS in recent years is now becoming one of the top killers of children (WHO, 2003a). Many diseases are also largely diseases of the developing world rather than diseases of the developed world.

Numerous risk factors contribute to the global burden of disease. Genetics, economics, social, lifestyle, and nutritional factors, as well as environmental chemical exposures, play large roles and are discussed in the following sections.

2.4 Major environmental threats to children

In its broadest sense, the environment encompasses all factors that are external to the human host, and children may be exposed to numerous environmental hazards from multiple sources and in a variety of settings.

WHO estimates that over 30% of the global burden of disease can be attributed to environmental factors and that 40% of this burden falls on children under five years of age, who account for only 10% of the world's population (WHO, 2004a). At least three million children under five years of age die annually due to environment-related illnesses. Environmental risk factors act in concert and are exacerbated by adverse social and economic conditions, particularly poverty and malnutrition.

It should also be noted that millions of children suffer from unsafe environments, abuse, and neglect due to armed conflict, natural disasters (e.g. hurricanes and earthquakes), and human-made disasters. Many of these children become refugees and/or orphans and are engaged in forced, hazardous, and exploitative labour. These "marginalized" children suffer from the very beginning of their lives. Many are "invisible", and over 36% of all births go unregistered, mainly in developing countries (UNICEF, 2006).

In 2003, there were an estimated 143 million orphans under the age of 18 in 93 developing countries (UNICEF, 2005a). The precise number of refugee children, street children, and children caught up in armed conflict is difficult to quantify, but estimates are in the millions (UNICEF, 2006). The estimated number of children affected by natural disasters is in the hundreds of thousands, including several thousand children orphaned following the December 2004 tsunami in Asia (UNICEF, 2005a). These vulnerable groups of children are also the ones who suffer from extreme poverty, malnutrition, undernutrition, and lack of health care and, thus, live in the most hazardous environments, with often devastating, irreversible health consequences.

For the majority of the world's population, the primary environmental threats continue to be the following "traditional" risks: (1) unsafe drinking-water, (2) poor sanitation, (3) indoor air pollution from household solid fuel use, (4) diarrhoeal, infectious, and vector-borne diseases, and (5) contaminated food supplies. However, in both developing and developed countries, "emerging" and "modern" risks pose an increasing threat to children's health. These include exposure to natural or human-made toxic substances in air, water, soil, and the food-chain, inadequate toxic waste disposal, injuries and poisonings, urbanization, and environmental degradation associated with unsustainable patterns of consumption and development. More recently, emerging environmental hazards, such as transboundary contamination by persistent toxic substances, ozone depletion, global climate change, and exposure to chemicals that disrupt endocrine function, have been identified as potential risks to children's health globally. In both developing countries and countries in transition, "emerging" and "modern" hazards can compound the effects of the "traditional" hazards, and children from all socioeconomic backgrounds are vulnerable to all these hazards. WHO projects that the burden of chronic diseases (e.g. cancer, cardiovascular) in developing countries is becoming relatively more important and will outweigh the burden of infectious disease by 2025 (WHO, 2003a).

2.4.1 Economic and nutritional factors

Poverty is one of the major driving forces for unhealthy environmental conditions and ill-health in children. Over 1.2 billion people struggle to survive on less than one US dollar per day; at least half of these are children (UN, 2001a). Even in the world's richest countries, one in six children lives below the poverty line, mainly in urban centres (UN, 2001a). Patterns of unsustainable development, globalization, and urbanization are major driving forces influencing poverty and directly impacting children.

Poverty is also intricately linked to malnutrition, which, in turn, is a major contributor to children's mortality and morbidity. It is estimated that over 50% of all deaths of children under five years of age globally are associated with malnutrition (see Figure 1). The devastating effects of poverty and malnutrition on health, particularly children's health, were recognized by representatives from 189 countries at the Millennium Summit in 2000 (http://www.un.org/millenniumgoals), where eight Millennium Development Goals were established. The first goal agreed upon by all United Nations Member States was to reduce poverty and hunger by 50% by 2015.

The effects of general undernutrition (reduced caloric intake and protein deficiency) are frequently compounded by deficiencies in important micronutrients, such as iodine, vitamin A, iron, zinc, and folate. Protein malnutrition in pregnant women results in anaemia, which can severely impact fetal growth and development, resulting in diminished birth size or infant and child morbidity. Low-birth-weight infants are more likely to have developmental and learning deficits throughout childhood (see chapter 4). Chronic undernutrition during the first two to three years of life may result in similarly delayed growth and learning disabilities. Underweight children may also have impaired immune systems and thus be more prone to infections. Iron deficiency is a major cause of anaemia and affects over two billion people worldwide (WHO, 2002b). About one fifth of perinatal mortality is attributed to iron deficiency, and there is a growing body of evidence that iron deficiency anaemia in early childhood reduces intelligence in mid-childhood (Stoltzfus et al., 2001). Iron deficiency has also been associated with increased susceptibility to lead exposure (Gulson et al., 1999). Other examples of micronutrient deficiencies that have a major impact on the global health of children include vitamin A, vitamin B, and folic acid. Vitamin A deficiency is the leading cause of preventable blindness in children (WHO, 2002b). Inadequate folic acid prior to conception and during early pregnancy has been associated with birth defects, including neural tube defects (see section 4.2.3.1). The incidence of these serious birth defects varies from country to country, but a large percentage of them can be prevented by periconceptional folate supplementation. Unfortunately, to date, fewer than 40 countries have initiated such supplementation programmes (Oakley, 2004). WHO maintains a database that indicates the status of micronutrient deficiencies in a number of countries (http://www3.who.int/whosis/micronutrient/).

At the other end of the nutrition scale, obesity in children is becoming a health threat, mainly in developed countries, but increasingly in developing countries (de Onis et al., 2004; Koplan et al., 2005). Poor maternal nutrition has been linked to adverse health outcomes in affected offspring later in life (see section 4.3.3).

2.4.2 Social, cultural, demographic, and lifestyle factors

Social, cultural, demographic, and lifestyle factors also play significant roles in influencing the exposure of children to environmental threats and, consequently, their health (see chapter 5). For example, these factors can determine dietary habits and, thus, the nature and extent of exposures of children to chemicals via the food-chain. They also impact whether and for how long infants are breastfed. Other examples determined largely by cultural factors include the use of toys and medicines (e.g. folk medicines and herbs). Lifestyle factors will influence the extent of concomitant exposures such as alcohol and tobacco smoke, and demographic factors (including climate) will determine certain exposures such as indoor air pollutants from wood-burning stoves. Rural versus urban settings may determine the extent and nature of children's exposure to pesticides. Another example of a particularly susceptible subpopulation of children is children whose families (e.g. indigenous peoples) rely on marine mammals and fish, which may be heavily contaminated with persistent organic pollutants (POPs) or heavy metals, for subsistence food (Damstra, 2002; Barr et al., 2006; Debes et al., 2006).

WHO considers social, cultural, and economic factors to be major determinants of ill-health, the "causes behind the causes" of morbidity and mortality. In 2004, WHO established a high-level commission, the Commission on Social Determinants of Health, to develop plans that address key social determinants of health, including the health of children (see http://www.who.int/social_ determinants).

2.4.3 Chemical hazards

The production and use of toxic chemicals pose potentially significant environmental threats to the health of children and are the major focus of this document. Global industrialization, urbanization, and intensified agriculture, along with increasing patterns of unsustainable consumption and environmental degradation, have released large amounts of toxic substances into the air, water, and soil. In addition, children may be exposed to naturally occurring hazardous chemicals, such as arsenic and fluoride in groundwater (IPCS, 2001c,d; WHO, 2001). An estimated 50 000 children die annually as a result of accidental or intentional ingestion of toxic substances (Pronczuk de Garbino, 2002). The global burden of disease in children attributed to environmental chemical exposures is largely unknown and has only recently begun to be investigated (see http://www.who.int/quantifying_ehimpacts/global/en/). Some estimates of the global burden of disease in children due to environmental risks have been reviewed by Valent et al. (2004), Tamburlini et al. (2002), and Gordon et al. (2004).

Although estimates of the burden of disease in children due to environmental chemicals are generally not available, there is clear scientific evidence that exposure to environmental chemicals during different developmental stages can result in a number of adverse outcomes in children and have resulted in an increased incidence of certain childhood diseases (see chapter 4). A wide range of chemicals can affect children's health, but a few chemical classes are of particular concern. These include heavy metals, POPs, pesticides, and air pollutants. Heavy metals and lipophilic POPs cross the placenta and also favour transfer into breast milk, usually the primary source of food for neonates. Heavy metals and POPs are known to interfere with the normal growth and development of children (Damstra et al., 2002; Coccini et al., 2006). Because of the persistence and toxicity of these chemicals, an international global treaty (the Stockholm Convention on Persistent Organic Pollutants) was ratified in 2004, which called for the elimination or phase-out of 12 initial POPs (UNEP, 2004).

Neonates and infants are also exposed to toxic chemicals (e.g. organochlorine pesticides, heavy metals) through breast milk. As infants are weaned from breast milk, they become exposed to a greater range of toxic chemicals via formula, drinking-water, and solid foods. They may also be heavily exposed to air pollutants, particularly indoor air pollutants such as carbon monoxide and polycyclic aromatic hydrocarbons (PAHs). In households dependent on biomass fuel for cooking and heating (2.5 billion people worldwide), infants are at particular risk while resting on the backs of mothers as they tend fires. In addition, mouthing or play behaviour of infants can lead to the ingestion of toxic chemicals that accumulate on surfaces (e.g. toys) or in soil.

The younger child and toddler are susceptible to exposure from chemicals in solid food (e.g. pesticides) and air (e.g. particulate matter) and through dermal exposure (e.g. heavy metals in soil). As children are introduced to day care and schools, potential new sources of exposure to certain chemicals (e.g. cleaning agents) may occur. Older children continue to be exposed to chemicals present in

Introduction and Background

school and/or day-care environments. In addition, exploratory behaviours may result in exposure to chemicals present in outdoor environments and dangerous settings (e.g. hazardous waste sites).

Exposure to organophosphate pesticides typically occurs in older children and adolescents in rural areas through agricultural work or as bystanders during agricultural pest control. Adolescents may also be exposed occupationally to other chemicals, such as solvents. Puberty is associated with growth spurts and hormone fluctuations, and the effects of chemical exposure during puberty are largely unknown. A more comprehensive list of chemical hazards and their effects can be found in a number of reviews (Tamburlini et al., 2002; WHO, 2002c, 2004b; Etzel, 2003; ECETOC, 2005).

2.5 Intrinsic factors

In addition to some of the extrinsic factors addressed in section 2.3, intrinsic (e.g. genetic) factors that control the dynamics of development play a key role in determining the susceptibility of children to environmental exposures at different life stages (see also section 3.6).

The outcome of developmental exposure is influenced significantly by the genetics of the organism. The basis for these differences is due to complex and multiple mechanisms, which have been discussed in a number of recent reviews (Faustman et al., 2000; NRC, 2000a). Recent advances in genomics have also provided valuable information on gene–environment interactions (Ottman, 1996; Christiani et al., 2001; Cummings & Kavlock, 2004; Nebert, 2005). Most studies of gene–environment interactions have focused on adults, but studies are becoming available demonstrating the existence of genetic polymorphisms for developmentally important genes that may enhance the susceptibility of children. The most frequent genetic polymorphisms that have been examined involve differences in the capacity to metabolize toxic agents over the course of various developmental stages.

One example of a gene–environment interaction affecting children is the association between heavy maternal cigarette smoking (more than 10 cigarettes per day) and cleft lip and/or palate in the offspring. This association is only marginally significant unless an allelic variant for transforming growth factor-alpha (TGF-α) is present. The combination of smoking and the uncommon variant of the gene raises the odds ratio to a highly significant level (Hwang et al., 1995). Another example is the gene–environment interactions that mediate the effects of organophosphate pesticides (Costa et al., 2005). Two genes are known to increase susceptibility to organophosphate pesticides: acetylcholinesterase and paraoxonase. About 4% of the population carries a gene that results in lower levels of acetylcholinesterase, the target enzyme of organophosphates (which, in turn, increases the vulnerability of the developing brain to organophosphate pesticides; Costa et al., 2003). Another family of genetically determined enzymes, paraoxonase, further modifies an individual's susceptibility to organophosphate pesticide toxicity. For example, individuals can vary 11-fold in the ability to inactivate the organophosphate pesticide parathion, depending on which gene for this enzyme they carry (Brophy et al., 2001).

2.6 The significance of a developmental stage approach

The stages of "childhood" can be viewed from a variety of perspectives (e.g. chronological, developmental, legal, educational). This document focuses on age-specific developmental stages (see Table 1) that may exhibit unique susceptibility and vulnerability to environmental influences. Susceptibility is determined by intrinsic factors (e.g. genetics) that can modify the effect of a specific exposure, whereas vulnerability is used to describe the capacity for higher risk due to the combined effects of susceptibility and differences in exposure. Age-specific periods of susceptibility have been termed "critical windows of exposure". Data on various developmental stages and their corresponding critical windows of exposure have been summarized in a number of recent reviews (Dietert et al., 2000; Rice & Barone, 2000; Selevan et al., 2000; Zoetis & Hurtt, 2003a; Daston et al., 2004; Landrigan et al., 2004).

Adverse effects in children may result from exposure prior to conception (paternal and/or maternal), during prenatal development, or postnatally to the time of full maturity. Even within a given developmental stage, shorter intervals of exposure may determine susceptibility for particular outcomes. Different organ systems develop at different rates, but it has been shown that for each developmental stage, there are both broad windows of susceptibility and more specific periods of susceptibility (Faustman et al., 2000;

Selevan et al., 2000). This has been worked out in some detail for certain systems and agents (e.g. central nervous system development and radiation exposure); in most cases, however, the exact time when organ systems are susceptible to the actions of toxic chemicals is unknown. Limited data are available on susceptibility during the adolescent period, but with the current greater interest in the effects of hormonally active agents, more information is becoming available.

As indicated previously, adverse health outcomes from early exposures may become apparent at any point in the lifespan. In some instances, they may be apparent only after long latency periods. Chapter 6 addresses the various methodologies that can be used to assess health outcomes. Studies have shown that the effects of toxic exposures on developmental processes may result from different mechanisms of action, and the toxic exposures may produce different health outcomes compared with the same exposures in adults. Some examples of health effects resulting from developmental exposures include those observed prenatally and at birth (e.g. miscarriage, stillbirth, low birth weight, birth defects), in young children (e.g. asthma, neurobehavioural and immune impairment), in adolescents (e.g. precocious or delayed puberty), and in adults (e.g. diabetes and heart disease).

2.7 Summary and conclusions

Environmental threats to the health of today's children result from a complex interaction of influences in children's biological, social, behavioural, physical, and economic environments. Attempts to partition the global burden of disease by causative risk factors are admittedly oversimplified and difficult owing to the inadequacies of the database and the multifactorial nature of most diseases. Notwithstanding these difficulties, it is clear that 1) environmental exposures play a significant role in the production of adverse health outcomes in children and that this is a serious public health concern, 2) due to health, wealth, or opportunity, many children are disadvantaged from the time of conception, 3) the health of the "child" at each stage of development will set the stage for and affect future health, and 4) current risk assessment paradigms need to address more directly the dynamic interactions of intrinsic and extrinsic factors over different developmental stages of childhood.

3. UNIQUE BIOLOGICAL CHARACTERISTICS OF CHILDREN

This chapter summarizes the distinct characteristics of children across life stages that contribute to unique differences in their susceptibility to environmental exposures. These include anatomical, physiological, metabolic, functional, toxicokinetic, and toxicodynamic characteristics. The normal development of various organ systems is also addressed. Differences in exposure pathways and behavioural characteristics will be addressed in chapter 5. Different organ systems develop at different rates, and comparison across life stages will allow for identification of specific systems that are at risk during specific stages of development.

3.1 General physical growth of children

3.1.1 Body weight and height

Human beings grow more slowly than many other species. Birth weight is increased by about 18 times over the first 20 years. Infants gain weight more rapidly during the first four to six months than during the rest of their lives. At the age of two years, a boy is about half his adult height, whereas a girl is slightly more than half her adult height (Lowrey, 1973). By six years of age, children in general are about 70% of their adult height. The height and weight of children of any given age group are highly variable, reflecting the complex influence of genetic, cultural, dietary/nutritional, and other environmental factors.

The records of physical change over time (i.e. growth curves) show how far and how fast the child has grown. In utero, specific periods of growth spurts usually coincide with the last two trimesters. Postnatally, six growth spurts have been named according to the developmental periods in which peak velocity of growth is reached: neonatal, infantile, early childhood, middle childhood, late childhood, and pubertal period (Walker & Walker, 2000). Such growth curves have been developed using growth data from a variety of international studies. Empirical mathematical models describing these developmental growth curves have also been developed

(USEPA, 2000). Most growth charts have been developed using data from industrialized countries. Less information is available on the growth curves of children (by developmental stages) from developing countries.

For children under five years of age, WHO maintains the WHO Global Database on Child Growth and Malnutrition (http://www.who.int/nutgrowthdb/en/), which provides anthropometric data on 90% of the world's children. The anthropometric indices in the WHO database for assessing child growth status include height-for-age, which can reveal characteristics of linear growth, and age- and height-specific growth, for assessing children's proportionality.

An analysis of the WHO database indicates that childhood malnutrition resulting in stunted growth remains a global problem. The prevalence of underweight children (de Onis & Blössner, 2003) continues to be a major contributor to ill-health in children, particularly in developing countries (WHO, 2005a). By contrast, in developed countries, there is concern about the increasing prevalence of obesity in children (Koplan et al., 2005). A person is considered obese if he or she has a body mass index (weight in kilograms divided by height in metres squared) of 30 or greater. Little information is available about the prevalence of obesity in children in developing countries, although some developing countries (particularly Latin American countries) are reporting increasing numbers of obese children (de Onis & Blössner, 2000).

3.1.2 Organ weights/volumes

From birth to adulthood, physical changes, including the size of body parts and organs, occur at an uneven rate (see Figure 2). At any time during infancy and early childhood, different organ systems grow at different rates. This asynchrony is typical of how humans grow before and after birth. Vital organs grow at different rates because their cells divide and grow at different rates. The absolute brain weight, for example, does not change much with age, but the brain to body weight ratio decreases with age. In contrast, the absolute weights of kidney and liver increase with age, whereas the relative kidney and liver weights show minimal change. Even though there is a general increase in muscle and adipose tissue volumes as a function of age, the rate of their relative increase is somewhat different at the early ages. For example, between two and six months of age, the increase in the volume of adipose tissue is more than twice as great as the increase in the volume of muscle. Between 6 and 12 months of age, however, the increase in muscle volume is slightly more rapid than that of adipose tissue. Quantitative relationships for computing organ weights from age, body weight, and height have been developed (ICRP, 1975; Haddad et al., 2001; K. Price et al., 2003; P.S. Price et al., 2003).

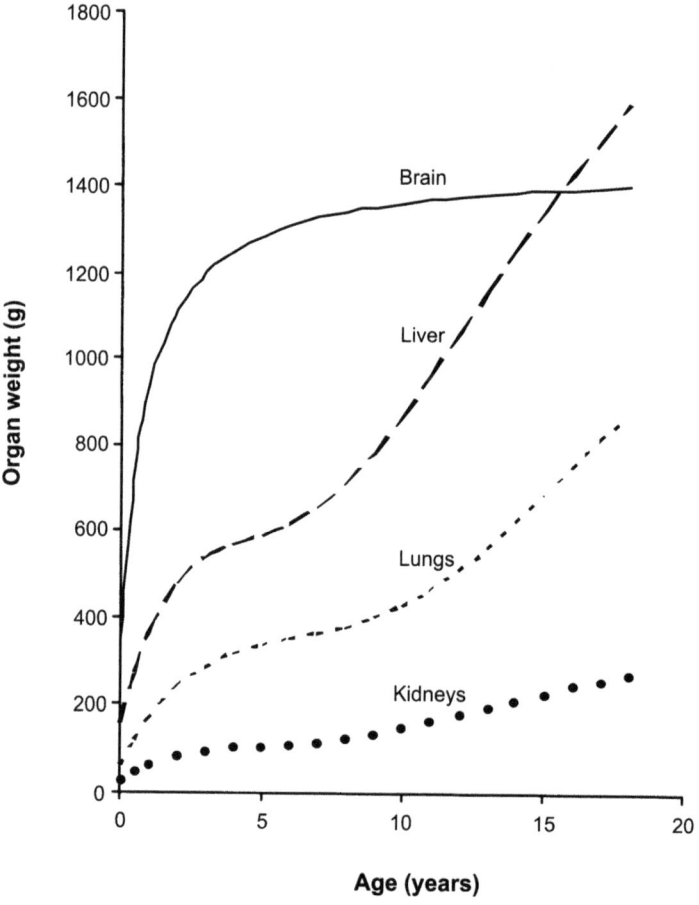

Fig. 2. Organ weight from birth to adolescence in boys (based on Haddad et al., 2001).

3.1.3 Skin

A baby at full term has a mature skin with barrier properties similar to those of older children and adults. However, the hydration state of the epidermis is greater in neonates than in older children, suggesting the potential for some hydrophilic chemicals to be absorbed more efficiently and hydrophobic chemicals less efficiently. In preterm infants, the epidermal barrier is poorly developed, resulting in increased percutaneous absorption of chemical agents. The preterm infant represents a special case, since studies of the development of the stratum corneum in fetal life have suggested that the permeability barrier is incomplete until just before term (Singer et al., 1971). There have been reports of greater blood concentrations of chemicals in preterm newborns than in full-term newborns when both are bathed in the same solution (Greaves et al., 1975). Neonates and infants in general have larger surface area relative to body weight than do adults.

3.2 Anatomical and functional characteristics

Most organs and organ systems lack structural or functional maturity at birth. The blood–brain barrier is immature at birth, and the development of this barrier and the nervous system in general continues in postnatal life. Much of the myelination of the brain takes place after birth and continues until adolescence (Hoar & Monie, 1981). The structural development of the lung also continues postnatally in terms of the alveolar surface area (Langston, 1983). Components of the immune system are not fully developed at birth, resulting in enhanced susceptibility of newborns to certain bacterial infections (Andersson et al., 1981). The gastrointestinal, endocrine, and reproductive systems are all immature at birth. A number of factors influencing gastrointestinal absorption of drugs and chemicals undergo maturational changes during the first 2 years of life (gastric acidity, gastrointestinal motility, enzymatic activity, bacterial flora), and less is known about these changes in such parameters between 2 and 18 years of age. These factors contribute to higher gastric pH in children and increased gastric and intestinal motility compared with adults.

Although the full-term neonate is born with kidneys containing essentially the same number of nephrons as the adult, overall renal function is reduced compared with that in older children or adults (Stewart & Hampton, 1987). Therefore, neonates are less able than older children and adults to eliminate many xenobiotics and endogenous chemicals renally. The function of the renal tubules is less mature at birth than in adulthood, and this persists until six months of age (Schwartz et al., 1976). The glomerular filtration rate increases after birth in humans (Gomez et al., 1999). These changes are attributed to vascular factors such as blood pressure and vascular resistance within the kidney. In rats, the glomerular filtration barrier and proximal tubule resorption become mature about seven days after birth (Gomez et al., 1999). It takes about a week after birth for the infant to start making concentrated urine; concentrating ability largely matures by one year of age (Gomez et al., 1999). In the rat, the concentrating ability is not mature until two to three weeks after birth (Kavlock & Gray, 1982; Zoetis & Hurtt, 2003b).

Another difference between adults and infants is that most of the cells are smaller in infants than in adults. Small cells have greater surface area in relation to mass compared with larger cells. This may have important implications for chemicals that come in contact with the cells in target organs (NRC, 1993).

3.3 Physiological characteristics

3.3.1 Breathing rate

Compared with adults, neonates have fewer alveoli and a faster breathing rate. Emery & Mithal (1960) suggested that the number of alveoli in the terminal respiratory branches of infants shows a rapid rise during the first year and a gradual increase up to age 12, by which time there are nine times as many alveoli as were present at birth. The breathing rate relative to body weight is greater in infants than in adults. For example, the volume of air passing through the lungs of a resting infant is twice that of a resting adult per unit body weight, which implies that twice the amount of chemical is taken up by the infant than by the adult under identical exposures. The breathing rate decreases steadily during growth in both boys and girls.

3.3.2 Cardiac output

Heart rate and cardiac output are greater in newborns than in older children and adults (Cayler et al., 1963; Sholler et al., 1987;

Brown et al., 1997). This is in line with the general notion that animals with a smaller body size have a faster heart rate. The circulation time (between any two points of the body) is shorter in infants and children than in adults, owing to small body size coupled with faster heart rate. Heart rate falls gradually as a function of age between birth and adolescence (Shock, 1944; Iliff & Lee, 1952), with no apparent sex difference until the age of 10. Quantitative descriptions of the relationship between cardiac output and body surface area and body height have been established for infants, children, and adults (Cayler et al., 1963; Krovetz et al., 1969).

3.3.3 Blood flow to organs

The rate of blood flow to organs changes with age and is not always proportional to changes in organ weights. For example, liver blood flow rates measured in children 4–8, 9–12, and 13–15 years of age corresponded to 325, 665, and 915 ml/min, respectively (Szantay et al., 1974). These values are smaller than the reference adult value (1612 ml/min) and remain so even when expressed on the basis of liver weight (Arms & Travis, 1988). Regional cerebral blood flow is lower in neonates than in adults; it increases until five to six years of age to values 50–85% higher than those for adults and decreases thereafter, reaching adult levels in the late teen years. Ogawa et al. (1989) reported that there was a marked decrease in blood flow with age in grey matter where neurons are located, but they did not observe any age-related change in white matter. In general, cognitive development of children seems to be related to changes in blood flow to corresponding brain regions (Chiron et al., 1992).

Renal blood flow increases with age as a result of the reduction of peripheral vascular resistance. The kidneys of neonates receive only 5–6% of total cardiac output, compared with 15–25% for adults (Hook & Baillie, 1979). The blood flow to kidney normalized to tissue weight, however, remains fairly constant after about the age of one year (Grunert et al., 1990). This is somewhat consistent with reports that renal maturity is attained during the second year of life. No significant difference in muscle blood flow rate, compared with adults, is reported for children aged 5–17 years (Goetzova et al., 1977). However, blood flow normalized to muscle weight decreases as a function of age (Lindbjerg, 1966; Amery et al., 1969).

3.3.4 Body composition

The body composition changes from birth to adulthood. Water content, expressed as a percentage of body weight, decreases rapidly between birth and six months of age and then remains fairly constant (Figure 3). Body water content is about 80–90% in neonates and decreases to 55–60% in adulthood, with most of the excess water in neonates being extracellular (Widdowson & Dickerson, 1964). The percent fat in the body, however, increases rapidly up to 6 months and then decreases, accounting for similar percentages of body weight at ages 4 and 12 months. Whole-body analysis suggests that fat comprises about 0.5% body weight at five months of gestation, increasing to 11–16% at birth and over 20% in adults. Protein content of the body also increases from birth to adulthood, mainly due to the growth of muscular tissue, which is proportionally much higher in the adult body (Figure 3).

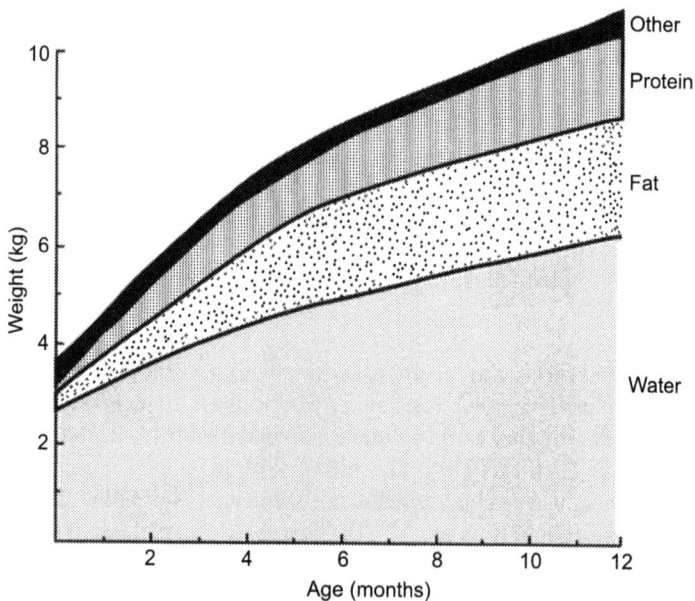

Fig. 3. Weights of water, fat, protein, and other components as a function of age, from birth to one year of age. [Figure reproduced from Fomon (1966) with permission from W.B. Saunders Co.]

3.3.5 Tissue composition

The lipid, water, and protein contents of certain tissues vary markedly as a function of age. For example, the adipose tissues of neonates contain about 55% water and 35% lipids, whereas the corresponding figures for the adult are about 25% and 70%, respectively (Friis-Hansen, 1971). The proportion of water in skin falls as a function of age, due to an increase in collagen. The water contents of liver, brain, and kidneys decrease from birth to adulthood by 5–15%. The decrease in water contents of liver and kidneys is primarily due to an increase in protein, whereas this change in the brain is due to an increase in myelin. The overall composition of muscle in terms of lipid and water does not seem to vary with age (Dickerson & Widdowson, 1960).

3.3.6 Bone growth and composition

Bone formation begins during fetal life with cartilage, which then calcifies into bone. Whole-body mineral content triples between weeks 32–33 and 40–41 of gestation in humans (Salle et al., 2000). Despite this dramatic mineralization, the bones of infants contain more water and less fat, protein, and minerals than adult bones. The chemical maturation of bone, as evidenced by a decrease in the percentage of water and an increase in calcification, takes place after one to two years. Linear growth occurs at the metaphyses, the body of cartilage that separates the diaphysis (body of bone) and epiphysis (the end of the bone). Linear growth ceases around age 16 years in girls and 18 years in boys, but epiphyseal closure of some bones (e.g. posterior spinous processes) does not occur until 25 years of age.

3.4 Metabolic characteristics

Metabolism, in the present context, refers to the elimination or transformation of specific functional groups of chemicals (Phase I) and conjugation of chemicals and their metabolites with endogenous cofactors (e.g. glucuronide, sulfate, glutathione; Phase II). Neonates and young children may be better or less able than adults to deal with toxic substances, owing to differences in metabolic capacity (Spielberg, 1992; NRC, 1993; Dorne et al., 2005). Studies have indicated that the sometimes increased sensitivity of neonates may be related to their very low, or at times unmeasurable, metabolizing capacity.

Phase I reactions are predominantly catalysed by cytochrome P450 (CYP)–dependent monooxygenases, which exist in more than 20 isoforms, as well as flavin-dependent monooxygenases. Even though the liver is the major site of Phase I reactions, the P450 isozymes are also present in all other tissues except red blood cells, albeit at lower levels. The total P450 content of human liver microsomes remains fairly stable at about one third of the adult value during fetal life (second and third trimesters of gestation) and the first year following birth (Treluyer et al., 1996). It is suggested that P450 isoforms develop independently and are regulated during the perinatal period by multiple mechanisms and elements (Cresteil, 1998). Altogether, three groups of P450s can be described: a first group expressed in the fetal liver, including CYP3A7 and CYP4A1; a second group, including CYP2D6 and CYP2E1, which surges within hours after birth, although the protein levels associated with these isozymes cannot always be detected in all fetal samples; and a third group that develops during the months following birth (CYP3A4, CYP2C, and CYP1A2) (Figure 4).

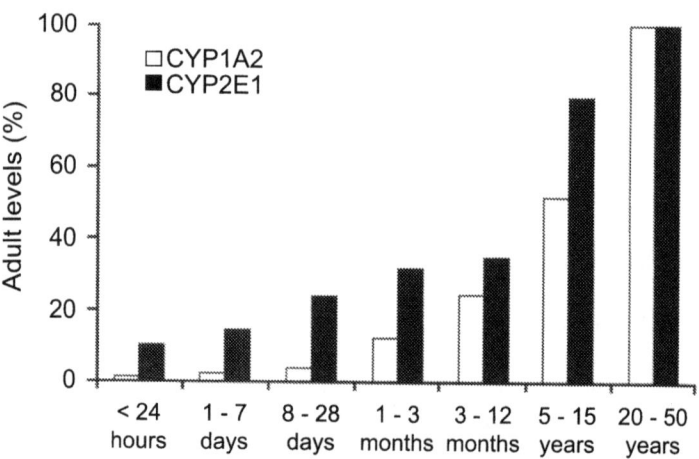

Fig. 4. Hepatic cytochrome CYP1A2 and CYP2E1 in children of various age groups as a percentage of adult weights (from Cresteil, 1998).

Limited data are available regarding the ontogeny of Phase II enzymes in human tissues. Epoxide hydrolase is active in the fetal liver and accounts for 50% of the adult activity, but it is extremely low in the fetal lung (Cresteil, 1998). Glutathione-*S*-transferases (GSTs) exist as multiple isoforms; of these, GSTπ has been reported to be responsible for 50% of glutathione conjugation in fetal liver, but it regresses at birth and is not expressed in adults. Other classes of GST, including GSTμ and GSTα, are present in the fetal liver at low levels and increase after birth (Cresteil et al., 1982; Strange et al., 1989). Conjugation with glucuronic acid is significantly lower at birth than in adults, although the capability for conjugation with sulfate is well developed in neonates (Levy et al., 1975). The levels of conjugation to glycine in newborns are comparable to those of adults (Dutton, 1978).

In general, most of the metabolizing enzyme systems would appear to develop from the middle of gestation until a few months after birth. Enzyme activities related to oxidation/hydroxylation and reduction are developed early after birth and reach adult levels at approximately six months of age. Oxidative demethylation, on the other hand, is not expressed until several months after birth, and the adult capacity will not be reached until one to two years after birth.

3.5 Toxicokinetics

3.5.1 Absorption, distribution, metabolism, and elimination

Absorption of chemicals may occur by a variety of routes, such as oral, dermal, and pulmonary. Since the functional determinants of these uptake processes vary as a function of age, the uptake of chemicals is also likely to vary between children and adults. For example, the respiratory ventilation rate in infants is significantly larger relative to lung surface (133 ml/min per kilogram of body weight per square metre) compared with adults (2 ml/min per kilogram of body weight per square metre). Therefore, infants potentially receive a greater exposure of lung surface to airborne compounds on a body weight basis (Bennett et al., 1996). Ginsberg et al. (2005) indicated that the particle dose in the pulmonary region is also likely to be two to four times higher in three-month-old children than in adults, particularly for submicrometre-size particles. The skin surface area relative to body weight is greater in children than in adults, such that the potential dose received following dermal exposure is likely to be about three times greater in infants than in adults (Clewell et al., 2002). The permeability of the epidermal barrier is poorly developed in the preterm infant, resulting in greater percutaneous absorption of chemical agents.

Gastric pH is higher in newborns (pH 6–8) than in adults (pH 1–3), thus causing differences in ionization and absorption of certain chemicals (Radde, 1985). Adult levels of gastric acid production are reached at about two years of age. The alkaline gastric pH in newborns and infants may lead to enhanced bioavailability of weakly basic compounds but reduced bioavailability of weakly acidic compounds (Alcorn & McNamara, 2003).

The physiological distribution volume for chemicals may vary between children and adults because of the differences in water and lipid content as a function of age. For example, the relatively larger extracellular fluid volume of the infant means somewhat greater dilution of water-soluble chemicals (Friis-Hansen, 1971; Rylance, 1988; Kearns et al., 2003). However, the lipid-soluble substances would be distributed in a smaller volume of fat in infants relative to adults (Alcorn & McNamara, 2003). The volume distribution of chemicals is also determined by plasma protein concentrations. Even though the total plasma protein concentrations do not seem to change dramatically with age, the concentrations of the specific binding proteins, such as steroid hormone binding protein, albumin, α1-acid glycoprotein, and serum lipoproteins, do vary with age. The concentration of albumin in the plasma of neonates, for example, is low, and hence the number of binding sites is low. Moreover, these binding sites are occupied by endogenous substances, such as fatty acids, steroids, and bilirubin. Therefore, newborn infants have a lower capacity for binding exogenous chemicals to plasma albumin. The binding affinity may also be different in neonates and adults. The neonate–adult difference in albumin binding affinity for many drugs is likely related to the differences in the form of protein as well as the amino acid content of albumin (Alcorn & McNamara, 2003).

The difference in volume of distribution between adults and children may not always lead to corresponding differences in blood or tissue concentrations. This is particularly likely to be the case during continuous exposures to chemicals that lead to a steady-state situation. At steady state, the adult–child differences in toxicokinetics are influenced by the rates of absorption, metabolism, and elimination processes.

Metabolism and elimination rates are generally lower in neonates than in adults. The elimination half-lives of substances used as indicators of liver function (e.g. bromosulfthalein, bilirubin), for example, are longer in newborns than in adults. Renal clearance has been shown to be lower in neonates than in older children and adults, for all chemical classes: lipophilic, hydrophilic, and organic ions (Clewell et al., 2002). Glomerular filtration rate at normal-term birth is about one third of the adult value when expressed on the basis of body surface area and matures in about six months. On the other hand, the tubular reabsorption process reaches adult levels within a few days after birth.

A systematic comparison of the available information on age-dependent maturation of metabolic and elimination processes as well as the toxicokinetics of chemicals in developing neonatal and young animals with that in infants and children can be found elsewhere (Gladtke, 1973; Stewart & Hampton, 1987; Crom, 1994; Renwick, 1998; Clewell et al., 2002; Alcorn & McNamara, 2003; Kearns et al., 2003; de Zwart et al., 2004; Ginsberg et al., 2004c). Table 2 summarizes the age dependency of toxicokinetic processes and determinants in children compared with adults.

3.5.2 *Physiological changes in mothers and their influence on toxicokinetics*

3.5.2.1 *Pregnancy*

During pregnancy, many physiological changes occur in the maternal organ system as a consequence of, and in order to support, the growing fetus. These changes may influence the uptake, absorption, distribution, metabolism, and excretion of xenobiotics, not only in the mother, but also in the developing fetus (Hytten, 1984; Krauer, 1987; Mattison et al., 1991). For example, the gastric emptying time increases and the intestinal motility decreases during pregnancy, which may result in longer retention of ingested xenobiotics in the upper intestinal tract, leading to the possibility for increased absorption of xenobiotics and increased exposure of the fetus (Klaassen, 1996). Cardiac output and peripheral blood flow increase by approximately 30% during the first trimester of gestation. The net respiratory volume is raised by about 50% as a result of increased tidal volume, while the pulmonary ventilation rate is not changed. Thus, volatile and airborne chemicals tend to be absorbed more readily. However, faster elimination of volatile compounds from the body may also occur. Thus, depending on the characteristics of chemicals, the change in net respiratory volume of the mother could result in either higher or lower exposure of the fetus. The renal blood flow and glomerular filtration rate are increased during pregnancy, which may result in enhanced renal clearance of certain xenobiotics, thus protecting the fetus from exposure to chemicals in the systemic circulation.

Table 2. Summary of the age dependency of the determinants of toxicokinetics in children in comparison with normal adults[a]

	Age of child				
	Newborn preterm	Term (0–4 weeks)	Infancy	1–4 years	5–12 years
Oral absorption	↓	↔	↔	↔	↔
Distribution:					
- Body water	↑↑↑	↑↑	↑	↑	↑
- Body fat	↓↓	↓	↓ (Slight)	↔	↔
- Plasma albumin	↓	↓	↓ (Slight)	↔	↔
Biotransformation:					
- Oxidation/ hydrolysis	↓↓↓	↓↓	↑↑ (After some weeks)	↑	↑ (Slight)
- N-Demethylation	↓↓↓	↓	↑↑	↑	↔
- Acetylation	↓	↓	↑	↑	↔
- Conjugation– glucuronidation	↓↓	↓	↑	↑	↔
Renal excretion:					
- Glomerular filtration	↓↓	↓	↓	↔	↔
- Tubular secretion	↓↓	↓	↓ (Slight to 6 months)	↔	↔

[a] Based on Rylance (1988). ↑ = increased, ↓ = decreased, ↔ = unaltered.

Changes in the blood concentrations of lipids, free fatty acids, and hormones during pregnancy may also influence the distribution of xenobiotics in the body. By the end of pregnancy, the total body water content has increased by up to 30%, and often fat deposits have been formed. The albumin concentration in plasma decreases to about two thirds of the normal level. This may lead to a higher amount of free unbound xenobiotics in the blood during dynamic exposure scenarios. These conditions may influence the distribution of xenobiotics between the mother and the conceptus. In addition to maternal physiology, the limited evidence available suggests that relative rates of drug metabolizing enzymes also change during pregnancy (Juchau, 1981; Juchau & Faustman-Watts, 1983). In experimental animals, the hepatic metabolism of xenobiotics is altered during pregnancy. In the rat, decreases in hepatic monooxygenase and glucuronidase activities have been observed, and there seems to be an overall decrease in hepatic xenobiotic biotransformation during pregnancy. However, this decrease is accompanied by an increase in liver weight of 40% during pregnancy. A similar change in liver weight has not been reported in humans.

3.5.2.2 *Lactation and breast milk*

Breastfeeding plays a critical role in human infant development, since it provides not only essential nutrition but also protection against infection and other immunological disorders (Lawrence, 1989). Unfortunately, the nursing mother can also serve as a source of infant exposure to drugs and chemicals. Unlike drug therapy, which can be terminated in most cases, environmental exposures may be continuous and chronic in nature. However, based on the numerous advantages of breastfeeding, the benefits in the majority of cases by far exceed the potential risk (Kacew, 1992; Pronczuk et al., 2004).

Milk composition is not constant and is influenced by the timing of feeding and duration of nursing postpartum. Human milk contains about 2–3% fat and a large number of proteins. The pH of milk tends to be lower than that of plasma. Most water-soluble substances are excreted into the milk by simple diffusion, and lipid-soluble compounds are transported along with lipid molecules from plasma into the mammary gland. The amount of a certain substance transferred to the milk depends on the physicochemical properties of the substance, the milk composition, maternal factors, such as dose, frequency, and route of exposure, and infant-related factors, such as the amount, duration, and frequency of feeding. A number of mathematical models for predicting the transfer of chemicals and drugs into human milk have been developed (Corley et al., 2003; Fleishaker, 2003).

3.5.3 Dose to target

The dose to target tissue, a key determinant of the ensuing toxicity, is determined by toxicokinetics or the rate and extent of the absorption, distribution, metabolism, and excretion of chemicals. When neonates and adults are exposed to the same concentration of atmospheric contaminants, the initial uptake rate is greater in neonates. This behaviour has been reported with several anaesthetics, such as halothane, cyclopropane, and nitrous oxide (Gregory et al., 1969; Salanitre & Rackow, 1969; Gallagher & Black, 1985). The greater rate of pulmonary uptake of these chemicals is the net result of a larger alveolar ventilation rate relative to body weight, greater perfusion rates, and lower fat content in neonates and infants (Cook, 1976). The steady-state blood concentration, however, is comparable in children of all age groups and adults, when the only critical determinant is the blood:air partition coefficient (reflective of blood solubility), which is fairly similar between adults and children (K. Price et al., 2003).

Following inhalation exposure to the same ambient concentrations, the peak blood concentrations of highly metabolized chemicals (e.g. furan) in children of age groups 6, 10, and 14 years have been computed to be greater than those in adults by a factor of 1.5 using a physiological modelling approach (K. Price et al., 2003). In the case of such highly extracted chemicals, the blood concentration is determined by the age-dependent tissue volumes, blood flow rates, breathing rate, and cardiac output. Based on such modelling studies, Sarangapani et al. (2003) concluded that adult to children differences in blood concentration would be <2 in the case of a number of inhaled gases and vapours (vinyl chloride, isopropanol, styrene, ozone, tetrachloroethene) as well. Recently, Nong et al. (2006), using subject-specific data on physiology and CYP2E1 protein content in physiologically based toxicokinetic models, reported that the interindividual differences in internal dose would be greater in neonates than in older children or adults. The greater variability of internal dose in neonates compared with adults was attributed to 1) interchild differences in the expression and maturation of CYP2E1 and 2) the adult–child difference in the limiting factor of hepatic metabolism (i.e. enzyme capacity in neonates versus liver blood flow rate in adults) (Nong et al., 2006).

The toxicokinetic difference between children and adults may also be evaluated by comparing certain parameters such as clearance (volume of blood from which chemical is eliminated per unit time) and half-life (time taken to reduce the initial concentration by 50%). Ginsberg et al. (2002) compiled these toxicokinetic parameters for children and adults for 45 drugs. Analysing these data, Hattis et al. (2003) reported that the half-lives of orally administered drugs in children of 2 months to 18 years were within a factor of 3.2 of the adult half-lives. However, 27% of the zero- to one-week age group and 19% of the one-week to two-month age group had half-lives that exceeded the adult values by more than a factor of 3.2 (Figure 5). It should be noted that most of the drugs evaluated by these authors have short half-lives (less than one day).

The toxicokinetic parameters and models, when available, can be useful in evaluating the half-lives and target tissue dose in infants and children following exposures. In the absence of such chemical-specific toxicokinetic data or models, dose adjustment based on body surface area appears to be a reasonable alternative. Crom (1994) suggested that for drugs such as antipyrine and indocyanine green (which are metabolized by microsomal enzymes and eliminated quickly), the dosages based on body weight will yield lower serum concentrations in younger children, while dosages based on body surface area are more likely to result in similar concentrations in children and adults. These authors also showed that the age-dependent differences in clearance correlate better with body surface area than with body weight.

Adjustment based on body surface area signifies that the oral dose for children (mg/kg of body weight per day) is likely to be greater than for adults by a factor of two or so (Renwick, 1998). Such a body surface area–based dose adjustment should result in blood or tissue concentrations of parent chemicals that are comparable between children and adults, provided the toxicokinetic determinants are all related to body surface area. When this is not the case, and when the toxic moiety is not the parent chemical (as is the case with a number of environmental contaminants), the default approaches of adult–child dose extrapolation are unlikely to be accurate. In such cases, physiological modelling approaches that take into account the quantitative changes in physiological and biochemical determinants may be used to evaluate the age-dependent change in target tissue dose of chemicals (Nong et al., 2006). The adult–child difference in susceptibility may be not only related to differences in target tissue dose but also due to toxicodynamics or the interaction between the toxic moiety and biological macromolecules in target tissues, resulting in the onset and progression of injury (Ginsberg et al., 2004c).

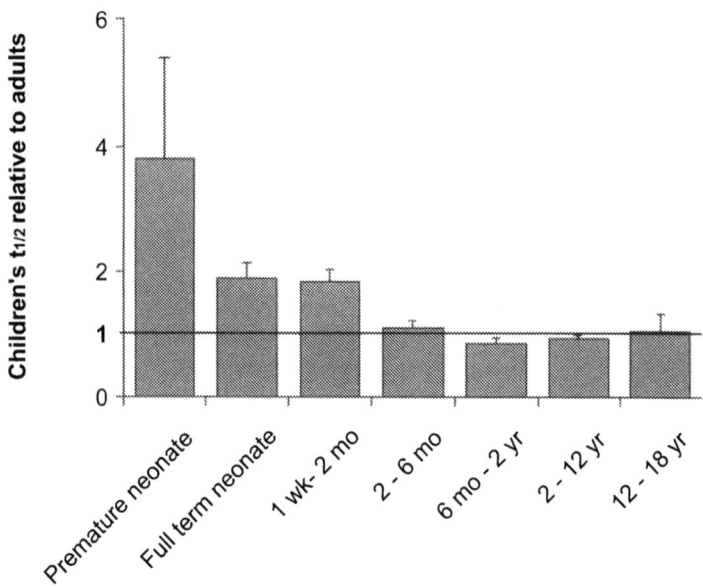

Fig. 5. Half-life results for 40 substrates in children relative to adults. A ratio of 1 indicates that the half-lives in adults and children are the same. Half-lives for the first three age groups are significantly different from those of adults. [Reprinted from Ginsberg et al. (2002), with permission from Oxford University Press.]

The following section provides an overview of the functional and structural development of various organ systems as well as the molecular determinants associated with these processes.

3.6 Normal development

3.6.1 Basic principles of normal development

Following fertilization and replication to the blastocyst stages, the body axes are determined and the three germ layers of the embryo are formed. Early organ development is largely defined by the complex orchestration of the critical processes: cell proliferation, differentiation, migration, and apoptosis (programmed cell death). Cell differentiation is the process by which undifferentiated cells increasingly take on characteristics of differentiated adult cells. These characterizations include stage-specific gene and protein expression, altered functional activities such as cell cycling, and altered physical characteristics such as shape or location. In the neocortex, for example, 11 cell cycles occur during neurogenesis before neuronal differentiation and migration from the pseudostratified ventricular epithelium to the periventricular zone (Olney et al., 2000; Gohlke et al., 2002).

In other brain regions such as the cerebellum, there are cells simultaneously undergoing proliferation, differentiation, migration, and apoptosis. Thus, the contribution of these basic cellular processes to organ development can vary temporally across organ regions and in relation to each other.

Apoptosis in development is extremely important for controlling physical development, as indicated by its role in limb and digit development, where cells programmed to die allow for digit separation. It is also important in neurodevelopment, where apoptosis plays a critical role in culling neurons that have not properly formed functioning synapses. Cell proliferation plays an important role in development by providing critical numbers and types of cells to differentiate or migrate. In general, less differentiated cells proliferate more, and, as differentiation proceeds, cells lose their ability to actively cycle.

The interactions between cells involved in these critical processes for organ development are of great importance and make them susceptible to perturbations by outside influences. Characteristics of these interactions include the need for sufficient populations of cells in proximity to each other and the need for sufficient functional capabilities of the cell populations to produce sufficient messages of developmental importance (e.g. inducers) at specific times and locations to influence other populations of cells (responders). The responding cells must then be functionally competent to be able to receive such signals (e.g. already expressing a receptor for the inducer substance to influence) (Daston et al., 2004).

A report by the United States National Academy of Sciences reviewed 17 cell signalling pathways that are evolutionarily conserved and that can explain how cells and cell populations can accomplish the complex and timed interactions outlined above (NRC, 2000a). As highlighted in this report, it has been postulated that these signalling pathways appear to be able to explain most, if not all, relevant signalling pathways necessary for development. A review of the data shows that disrupting these processes (either by using genetically sensitized animal models or by using agents that cause developmental toxicity) can have devastating impacts on development (NRC, 2000a). Interesting examples are the vinca alkaloids such as cyclopamine, which can inhibit the sonic hedgehog signalling pathway (NRC, 2000a). Many of the signalling pathways can exert overlapping functions, especially in mammalian species. This redundancy has contributed to the plasticity of developing organs to develop normally if challenged and has also emphasized the need to evaluate toxicological impacts in the broader context of in vivo development. For example, isolated reports that particular toxicants may impact apoptosis must be viewed in a temporal and toxicokinetic and toxicodynamic context to interpret the potential for overall impacts on in vivo development.

3.6.2 Nervous system

The central nervous system arises from a thickened area of the ectoderm called the neural plate on day 19 in the human embryo. This process is referred to as induction. The neural plate then differentiates into the neural tube (providing the origins for the brain and spinal cord) and the neural crest (forming the basis of the peripheral nervous system). The process by which the neural tube arises from the neural plate is referred to as neurulation. To form the neural tube, the neural plate changes shape and forms a pronounced groove, closing from the cranial end to the caudal end. The neural tube has openings on both ends that close on about day 25 and day 27, respectively.

The neural tube provides the basis for the entire central nervous system. The spinal cord, a tubular structure in the mature nervous system, retains the basic original shape of the neural tube. Early in histogenesis, the walls of the neural tube are made up of neuroepithelial cells that constitute the ventricular zone. A zone known as the marginal zone develops into the white matter of the spinal cord. In the ventricular zone, some cells differentiate into neurons called neuroblasts. Primitive supporting cells called glioblasts also differentiate from the neuroepithelial cells of the ventricular zone. Some glioblasts become astrocytes, and other glioblasts become oligodendrocytes. Neuroepithelial cells will ultimately give rise to all the neurons and microglial cells of the central nervous system. Many other important processes, such as the formation of the spinal ganglia, spinal meninges, and myelin sheaths, take place in the developing spinal cord over time. Myelination begins between the fifth and sixth months of fetal development in the cervical portion of the spinal cord and continues until well into adolescence and young adulthood. Corticospinal tracts begin to myelinate immediately prior to birth and are not fully myelinated until the second or third year of life (Hoar & Monie, 1981).

In contrast to the spinal cord, which retains the original shape of the neural tube, the brain undergoes a series of transformations that take place well into adolescence to reach the adult form of the human brain. Starting at the cranial end, the neural tube begins to close during the fourth week of embryonic life, and three brain primary vesicles are formed — the prosencephalon, the mesencephalon, and the rhombencephalon — by day 26. During the fifth week, the prosencephalon (forebrain) divides into the telencephalon (cerebral hemispheres) and the diencephalon (thalami, posterior lobe of the pituitary gland, pineal body, optic vesicles). At the same time, the rhombencephalon divides into the metencephalon (pons and cerebellum) and the myelencephalon (medulla oblongata). The end result of this developmental stage is the creation of five secondary brain vesicles that form the structural backdrop of the human brain.

During the fourth week of development, the brain is growing quickly and bends ventrally with the head fold to produce the midbrain flexure and the cervical flexure. The formation of the flexures allows for significant changes in the shape of the developing brain and the distribution of the grey and white matter. By day 30, rudimentary cerebral hemispheres are apparent in the embryo. Individual cerebral hemispheres grow in the shape of horseshoes, remaining in communication with the third ventricle in the diencephalon. As they expand, the hemispheres gradually cover the diencephalon, midbrain, and hindbrain and eventually meet in the midline. The corpus callosum, the largest cerebral commissure that connects the neocortical areas, is apparent by the 12th week and has reached its structural maturity by the 20th week of fetal development. Brain sulci (fissures) are present by the fifth month of prenatal development and are firmly in place at birth in human infants. In most animal species, with the exception of monkeys and the great apes, the brain hemispheres are smooth at birth and lack the sulci observed in newborn human infants. Because central nervous system development begins during the embryonic period and continues during the fetal period and postnatally, there are numerous periods of susceptibility, which are discussed in section 4.3.1 (Barone et al., 2000; Rice & Barone, 2000).

3.6.3 Reproductive system

The gonads are derived from the urogenital ridges, which are derivatives of the intermediate mesoderm. Also arising from the urogenital ridges are the Wolffian (male) and Müllerian (female) ducts, which are contained in the mesonephros. The embryonic germ cells migrate from the hindgut to the primitive, undifferentiated gonads. Male sex is determined by a Y chromosome genetically. Gonadal sex determination (i.e. decision as to whether a primordial gonad differentiates into a testis or an ovary) is initiated by the activation of the SRY (sex-determining region of the Y chromosome) gene located in the pseudoautosomal region of the short arm of the Y chromosome. SRY gene expression starts at 41–44 days after ovulation, peaks at day 44, and continues at low levels thereafter (Hanley et al., 2000). SRY activation initiates the testis-determining cascade by the transformation of pre-Sertoli cells to Sertoli cells, and SOX9 (SRY-related HMG BOX gene 9) is proposed to be a specific target of SRY (Bishop et al., 2000). The genetic pathways involved in gonadal development include the roles of SRY, the transcription factor WT-1, the orphan nuclear receptors steroidogenic factor 1 (SF-1) and DAX-1, and SOX9 (Park & Jameson, 2005). In the absence of SRY in females, the SOX9 gene remains silent, and Sertoli cells are not formed. However, this lack of testicular differentiation is not enough for ovarian development.

Active WNT-4 signalling is needed for normal ovarian development (Vainio et al., 1999; Biason-Lauber et al., 2004).

Hormones produced by the developing testis control differentiation of male genitalia. Ovaries remain hormonally inactive during development, and, in the absence of male reproductive hormones, female inner and outer genitalia are formed. Sertoli cells secrete anti-Müllerian hormone during weeks 8–10 of gestation, resulting in the regression of Müllerian ducts. In the absence of anti-Müllerian hormone (i.e. absence of the testis), Müllerian structures differentiate to oviducts, the uterus, and the upper part of the vagina. The testicular hormone testosterone is needed to stimulate Wolffian ducts to differentiate into the vas deferens, epididymis, and seminal vesicle. Leydig cells in the testis secrete testosterone and insulin-like hormone 3, which are needed for testicular descent. In the absence of androgens and insulin-like hormone 3, Wolffian ducts regress in the female, and the ovaries remain in the abdomen.

Testosterone is converted to dihydrotestosterone (DHT) by 5α-reductase type II enzyme in the prostate and outer genitalia. DHT is necessary for normal development of the scrotum, penis, and prostate (Wilson et al., 1993). In the absence of DHT, female-type external genitalia develop, and the prostate remains rudimentary. Testicular testosterone production is dependent first on placental secretion of human chorionic gonadotropin (hCG) and increasingly on pituitary secretion of luteinizing hormone (LH). Another gonadotropin, follicle stimulating hormone (FSH), stimulates Sertoli cell proliferation in the testis and folliculogenesis in the ovary. Both gonadotropins are stimulated by hypothalamic gonadotropin releasing hormone (GnRH).

Estrogens do not seem to play an essential role in sexual differentiation, since normal development is possible in the absence of estrogen receptors (Smith et al., 1994; Couse & Korach, 1999) and the aromatase enzyme that is needed for conversion of androgens to estrogens (Morishima et al., 1995). However, excess estrogens can inhibit insulin-like hormone 3 activity and thereby contribute to cryptorchidism (Emmen et al., 2000; Nef et al., 2000). Imbalance in the androgen/estrogen ratio has been suggested to be a reason for testicular disruption during development (Sharpe, 2003).

Although the precise mechanisms for puberty initiation remain unclear, it is under central nervous system control and involves complex neuroendocrine interactions. In infancy, serum concentrations of gonadotropins and sex hormones are similar to those of children with normal puberty. However, in the months and years after birth, hypothalamic–pituitary–gonadal activity decreases; this period is known as the juvenile pause (Styne, 2003). In primates, when the time is right (probably due to size and internal clock), the KISS-1 gene activates production of the peptide hormone kisspeptin, which initiates the release of the puberty-inducing hormone GnRH. GnRH in turn stimulates the pituitary to release the gonadotropin hormones, triggering changes in the ovaries and testes (Shahab et al., 2005). Windows of susceptibility in reproductive system development are discussed in section 4.3.2.

3.6.4 Endocrine system

The primary purpose of the endocrine system is to maintain homeostasis — that is, to maintain a relatively constant internal environment in the face of a constantly changing external environment. The endocrine system consists of hormones and the glands and tissues that produce the hormones. A hormone is a chemical substance released by certain cells to effect the function of other distant cells (endocrine function). Many compounds act as endocrine hormones as well as having paracrine and autocrine functions. Paracrine and autocrine describe actions on nearby cells and on other cells that produce the substance, respectively. There is considerable overlap between substances classified as hormones and other chemical messengers such as neurotransmitters and cytokines. Many substances function in more than one of these categories. For example, epinephrine and norepinephrine function as both neurotransmitters and adrenal medullary hormones.

3.6.4.1 Hypothalamic–pituitary axis

The endocrine system can be broadly divided into the hormones of the hypothalamic–pituitary axis and the glands and target organs they regulate and other endocrine hormones and glands that are not part of this axis (Figure 6). The hypothalamus regulates the hormones of the anterior pituitary gland by secreting releasing hormones (GnRH, thyrotropin releasing hormone, corticotropin releasing hormone, somatocrinin/growth hormone releasing hormone) or inhibiting hormones (dopamine, somatostatin) into the portal circulation. These hormones act on specialized groups of cells in the anterior pituitary gland to stimulate or inhibit the secretion of other hormones. Figure 6 also illustrates the central concept of negative feedback, whereby a hormone regulates the secretion of another hormone, which in turn feeds back to inhibit the secretion of the first hormone. This maintains the levels of both hormones within a narrow range.

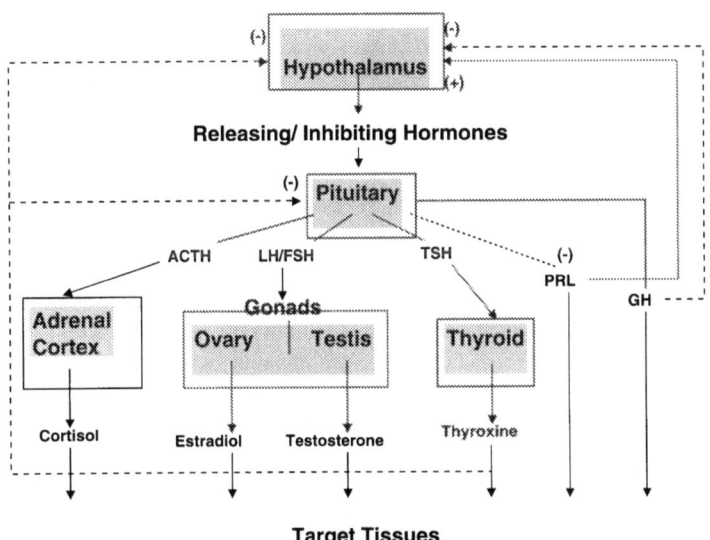

Fig. 6. Hormones of the hypothalamic–pituitary axis and the glands and target organs they regulate (ACTH = adrenocorticotropic hormone; LH = luteinizing hormone; FSH = follicle stimulating hormone; TSH = thyroid stimulating hormone; PRL = prolactin; GH = growth hormone).

The hypothalamus regulates the hormones of the posterior pituitary gland via direct neural connections. Thus, hypothalamic neuroendocrine magnicellular neurons terminate in the posterior pituitary, where they secrete oxytocin and vasopressin into the general circulation. Other endocrine organs that are not part of the hypothalamic–pituitary system include the islet cells of the pancreas, which secrete insulin, glucagon, and somatostatin; the parathyroid glands, which secrete parathyroid hormone; the parafollicular cells of the thyroid, which secrete calcitonin; the pineal gland, which secretes melatonin; and the gut, which produces several hormones, including gastrin, secretin, and cholecystokinin.

The anterior and posterior lobes of the pituitary gland have different embryonic origins, with the anterior pituitary being of oral ectodermal origin and the posterior pituitary of neural ectodermal origin. The anterior pituitary develops from an upgrowth of the roof of the primitive mouth, called Rathke's pouch. The posterior pituitary develops from a downward growth of the neural ectoderm of the floor of the prosencephalon or forebrain. As these two outgrowths converge, the stalk joining Rathke's pouch with the mouth regresses, while the stalk from the diencephalon remains to form part of the infundibulum or pituitary stalk. The other part of the infundibulum arises from the upgrowth of Rathke's pouch.

The pituitary gland begins to synthesize and secrete hormones during weeks 8–12 of gestation in humans (Porterfield & Hendry, 1998; Sadler, 2000; Marty et al., 2003). The target organs of the pituitary gland hormones are depicted in Figure 6. The hypothalamic–pituitary–thyroid and hypothalamic–pituitary–gonadal axes begin to function during fetal life around week 12; gestation, however, and complete maturation of some of these target organs (e.g. gonads, adrenals) do not occur until after birth. The anterior pituitary hormone prolactin begins to be secreted at 11 weeks' gestation in humans. The most well known function of prolactin is its indispensability for milk production by the mammary glands; however, prolactin also plays important roles in modulating immune function and in the development of the dopaminergic tuberoinfundibular neurons (Shyr et al., 1986; Ben-Jonathan et al., 1996).

3.6.4.2 Thyroid gland

The genetic pathways involved in thyroid development have been recently reviewed (Jahnke et al., 2004). Thyroid hormones are critical for normal central nervous system development (Porterfield & Hendry, 1998; Sher et al., 1998). Thyroid hormones regulate cellular proliferation within the developing central nervous system. They also regulate cytoskeletal and microtubular assembly and stability, which are important for cellular migration and neuronal outgrowth. They regulate the expression of genes that are critical for synaptic development, neuronal growth, and myelination. During the embryonic period and the early fetal period, the developing human is entirely dependent on maternal thyroid hormones. The fetal thyroid begins to function during week 12 of pregnancy, but the maternal thyroid gland contributes thyroid hormones throughout gestation. In both humans and rodents, full maturation of thyroid system function does not occur until four weeks after birth (Jahnke et al., 2004). Thus, the effects of congenital hypothyroidism are partially counteracted in utero by maternal thyroid hormones; after birth, however, it is critical to identify these infants so that thyroid hormone replacement can begin as quickly as possible. Thyroid hormones are also involved in development of the male reproductive system in humans and rodents, by promoting Sertoli cell differentiation (Jahnke et al., 2004).

3.6.4.3 Adrenal glands

Histologically, the human adrenals comprise an outer cortex, the site of steroid hormone synthesis, and an inner medulla, the site of catecholamine synthesis. The steroidogenic tissue arises from coelomic mesoderm in the genital ridge of the embryo. In both humans and mice, the fetal adrenal cortex contains a definitive or adult outer zone that surrounds a fetal zone. The apoptotic degeneration of the fetal zone occurs at puberty in male mice and after the first pregnancy in female mice. The definitive cortex is itself composed of four zones that synthesize different hormones. The outer zone glomerulosa synthesizes the mineralocorticoid aldosterone. Next comes the zona intermedia, which does not appear to synthesize hormones, followed by the zona fasciculata and zona reticularis, which synthesize glucocorticoids (primarily cortisol in humans). The catecholaminergic cells arise from the neural crest and migrate into the developing cortex, forming the medulla. The nuclear receptor/ transcription factor SF-1, which was discussed above as being critical for gonadal development, is also necessary for adrenal gland development (Bland et al., 2003).

The adrenal glands play an important role in pubertal development. Termed adrenarche, the maturation of a prominent zona reticularis, the innermost layer of the cortex, begins around age six to eight in girls, resulting in increased secretion of the adrenal androgens, dehydroepiandrosterone (DHEA) and DHEA sulfate (Beckman & Feuston, 2003). The rise in these hormones leads to the development of pubic and axillary hair. Recent evidence suggests that premature adrenarche may be associated with subsequent development of polycystic ovarian syndrome and the related syndrome X/metabolic syndrome, characterized by obesity, insulin resistance, dyslipidaemia, and high blood pressure (Ibanez et al., 2000).

3.6.4.4 Gonads

Gonadal development and the hormones of the reproductive system are discussed in section 3.6.3.

3.6.4.5 Somatotropin (growth hormone), calcium homeostasis, and bone development

During the first two months of embryonic life, there is extensive differentiation of progenitor cells, without rapid cell replication. Thereafter, in the fetal period, the highest growth rates of these cells are observed. Growth slows in late gestation and continues to decline in childhood. The high growth rate of the fetus compared with the child is mostly the result of cell replication; the proportion of cells that are dividing becomes progressively less as the fetus becomes older. Insulin-like growth factors (IGFs, also called somatomedins) are the primary factors that drive intrauterine growth. During gestation, growth hormone receptors are expressed at very low levels, and growth hormone is not the primary regulator of IGFs. Instead, fetus insulin, which in turn is regulated by fetus glucose levels, is the primary regulator of IGF-1 (Gluckman & Pinal, 2003). This pattern of regulation of IGF-1 continues until about six months after birth, by which time growth hormone receptor populations have increased and growth hormone regulation of IGF-1 takes over (Gluckman & Pinal, 2003). IGFs cause growth of the epiphyseal regions of the long bones by stimulating the proliferation of chondrocytes, the cartilage-producing cells.

3.6.4.6 Pancreas

The endocrine islet cells comprise only 1–2% of the pancreatic tissue. They synthesize the hormones insulin, glucagon, somatostatin, and pancreatic polypeptide. Insulin and glucagon maintain glucose homeostasis via their actions on lipid, carbohydrate, and protein metabolism. The pancreas originates from two patches of epithelium in the duodenum during the fifth week of gestation in humans. The endocrine pancreatic cells begin to differentiate very soon after the pancreas begins to bud (Murtaugh & Melton, 2003). These endocrine cells then delaminate from the epithelium and aggregate into islets. The transcription factors SOX17, PDX1, HLXB9, and PTF1a are known to be essential for normal pancreatic development based on knockout mouse models (Murtaugh & Melton, 2003). It is during the second half of gestation that the endocrine cells begin to differentiate into the specialized cell types containing a single hormone (Hellerstrom & Swenne, 1991). By term, the islets have the appearance of adult tissue, but there are still considerable changes in size and arrangement of the islets for four or more years in humans. Specific susceptible windows of development for the various endocrine components are discussed in section 4.3.3.

3.6.5 Cardiovascular system

The formation of the heart is one of the earliest events in development, as it is essential for the delivery of oxygen and nutrients to the rapidly developing cells of the embryo. The molecular decision to form cardiac cells is made at the time of gastrulation. The heart begins to beat at three weeks of embryonic age. Important elements of cardiac formation include formation of the heart forming fields as cells migrate out of the primitive streak; the segregation of cell lineage (myocardial and endocardial) within the fields; the elongation and segmentation of the tubular heart; the internal differentiation/septation of first the atria and later the ventricle; and development of the conducting system. The heart also descends as it is developing, starting cephalic to the somites and winding up at the mid-thoracic level. All this development takes place while the heart is performing a critical function for the rest of the developing embryo (O'Rahilly & Muller, 1992; Markwald et al., 1997). Molecular control factors for cardiac morphogenesis are being elucidated, including T-box transcription factors (Stennard & Harvey, 2005), homeobox transcription factors (Akazawa & Komuro, 2005), and growth factors and extracellular remodelling (Corda et al., 2000) (see section 4.3.4).

3.6.6 Immune system

The immune and haematopoietic systems arise from pleuri-potent stem cells (West, 2002; Holsapple et al., 2003). As gestational development proceeds, these give rise to haematopoietic stem cells that produce the array of haematopoietic and immune cell populations. In humans, many of the critical steps in formation of specific lineages within immune development occur during the first and second trimesters of pregnancy. Lymphocyte progenitors are present in the liver by weeks 7–8 of gestation (Migliaccio et al., 1986). Holsapple et al. (2003) discuss the evidence indicating that lineage-specific progenitors are at potential risk by 7–10 weeks post-conception. Around this same window, the thymus stroma forms and T cell progenitors migrate from the liver to the thymus. Also, in the first trimester, B cell progenitors appear in the blood, and the gastrointestinal tract–associated lymphoid tissues emerge. This might be considered an early window of susceptibility. West (2002) discusses lymphogenesis within the human bone marrow that emerges within this same window of susceptibility. In general, early B and T cell differentiation seem to occur in parallel (Holsapple et al., 2003). The thymic medulla and cortex areas begin to differentiate during the first trimester, and the areas are fully formed with maturational cell migration from the cortex to the medulla in the subsequent trimester (West, 2002).

Immune development is relatively delayed in rodents compared with humans; some rodent postnatal events occur prenatally in humans (Landreth, 2002; West, 2002). Human T cells can respond to several mitogenic and allogeneic stimulatory challenges prenatally, whereas significant responses in rodents usually appear after birth. However, despite the extent of prenatal human immune development, West (2002) identified several areas of continued immune development that occur during the early neonatal periods. The author pointed to the fact that, at birth, the human has a relatively low proportion of T cells, reduced myeloid and natural killer cell lineages in both numbers of cells and cytokine activation potential, and reduced development of plasma cells in the bone marrow. Increased susceptibility to some infectious agents may be linked to the relatively incomplete maturation and/or expansion of some immune cell lineages and the lack of a complete cytokine network (West, 2002). Further discussion of periods of susceptibility during immune system development can be found in section 4.3.5.

3.6.7 Respiratory system

Development of the human lung begins in the embryo and continues until the age of 18–20 years. Cellular differentiation and formation of the primary lung structures occur in stages during fetal development, but the majority of growth and maturation of the lung occurs postnatally through the processes of branching morphogenesis and alveolarization. The major antenatal and postnatal developmental milestones are summarized in Table 3.

Table 3. Normal development of the lungs in humans

Developmental stage	Process of lung development
Prenatal	• Airway branching to terminal bronchioles complete by 16 weeks
	• Functional smooth muscle by 8–10 weeks, to respiratory bronchioles by 26 weeks
	• Cartilage complete by 28 weeks
	• Blood vessels complete by 17 weeks
	• Lamellar bodies in Type II cells by 24 weeks
	• 30–50% of alveoli present by term
Postnatal	• Increase in airway size parallels somatic growth
	• Rapid increase in smooth muscle early
	• Alveolarization continues until at least 2 years
	• Maturation of microvasculature during the postnatal phase of alveolar development
	• Lung volume approximately doubles from birth to 18 months and again to 5 years
	• Lung growth continues until approximately 18 years in females and 20–23 years in males.

The lung originates in the embryo as an out-pouching of ventral foregut endoderm that grows into the surrounding mesenchyme tissue. The pseudoglandular period (weeks 5–17 of gestation) is a critical stage of cellular differentiation and is characterized by the formation of the bronchial tree and pulmonary vasculature. The development of the pre-acinar conducting airways is regulated by interactions between epithelium and mesenchyme tissue at the site of bronchial buds; by 16 weeks of gestation, the branching pattern of the bronchial tree is complete. During the canalicular phase (weeks 16–24 of gestation), the gaseous exchange regions evolve with adjacent capillary beds. Surfactant synthesis begins in the latter stages. Extracellular matrix components and acini form in the saccular phase, with alveolar formation beginning around 26 weeks' gestation and continuing postnatally until approximately 2 years of age. The precise age at which alveolarization ceases is not known because of the small number of normal lungs studied and the wide variability in the reported adult number of alveoli. Branching morphogenesis is characterized by enlargement of the airways and alveoli and continues well into adolescence. Up to 80% of alveoli develop postnatally in parallel with the growth of the lungs and with the increasing metabolic demands of the growing child.

Many of the studies on the effects of chemical exposures on the growth and development of the lungs have been performed in animals, especially rodents. However, the pattern of lung development differs between animals and humans. For example, alveolarization occurs exclusively postnatally in rats (Massaro et al., 1984; Massaro & Massaro, 1986) and almost completely prenatally in sheep (Davies et al., 1988). Early lung development in rabbits is similar to that in humans (Kovar et al., 2002), but alveolarization in rabbits continues until adult life. Because of these differences, extreme care must be taken when extrapolating the results from animal studies to human situations. The molecular development of the lung has been reviewed (Kumar et al., 2005; Bridges & Weaver, 2006; Pongracz & Stockley, 2006). Periods of susceptibility during respiratory system development are discussed further in section 4.3.6.

3.6.8 Kidney

Development of the metanephric kidney begins with an outgrowth of the ureteric bud from the distal region of the mesonephric (Wolffian) duct. The ureteric bud must grow into the mesenchyme of the nephrogenic cord. Upon contact, the mesenchyme epithelializes to form a nephron, and this process is repeated over and over as the ureteric bud branches. Ultimately, the branching of the ureteric bud results in the formation of the major and minor calyces (the large ducts that empty into the renal pelvis) and the system of collecting tubules. The two major calyces form from the first branching of the ureteric bud, around the end of the sixth week in humans. Secondary branches arise from these, which in turn give rise to tertiary branches. About 12 generations of branching occur by the end of the fifth month, which essentially completes the formation of the collecting duct system.

Although the general pattern of nephron formation is similar across mammals, there are marked species differences in the timing of development. The onset of nephron development starts at approximately the same stage of embryogenesis in all species that have been evaluated; because of differences in the length of the embryonic period, however, the day of gestation differs. In humans, metanephric kidney development starts around gestation day 35, whereas in the rat, it starts on gestation day 12, and in the mouse, gestation day 11. Induction and differentiation of nephrons occur continuously through the 38th week of gestation in humans and for 10–12 days postnatally in rats and mice. There are approximately 1.5 million nephrons per kidney in humans, and 1000–2000 in mice. Zoetis & Hurtt (2003b) published a review on comparative aspects of kidney development. The molecular development of the kidney and subsequent implications for altered renal development have been the subject of a recent review (Ruan et al., 2005).

The renin–angiotensin system is essential for normal renal development (Guron & Friberg, 2000). Expression of angiotensinogen in rats is higher in late gestation than in the adult, and the angiotensinogen is localized in the proximal tubules (Niimura et al., 1997). Renin is also expressed at a higher level during late gestation, and again the localization is different from the adult animal; instead of being expressed in the juxtaglomerular cells as in adults, renin is found in renal arteries in the fetus. The distribution and type of angiotensin II (AT_2) receptors are altered in the fetus, and the receptor subtypes show a characteristic spatiotemporal pattern, with AT_2 receptors showing dominance over the AT_1 receptor. This reverses after birth. The AT_2 receptors are primarily located in the undifferentiated mesochyme within the nephrogenic zone. Blockade of this system either pharmacologically or by using gene knockouts leads to extensive renal vascular abnormalities (Tufro-McReddie et al., 1994). Nephrogenesis is complete prior to birth in the human, although substantial growth and maturation of function still occur postnatally. The periods of susceptibility of the kidney during development can be found in section 4.3.7.

3.7 Summary and conclusions

The information presented in this chapter illustrates the complex role and interplay of molecular and physiological factors in the functional and structural development of the various organ systems. These factors ultimately influence the toxicokinetics and toxicodynamics of chemicals. The developing organs are particularly susceptible to toxic insult, given the increased rate of cell division and immaturity of functional systems. The age at which specific organs undergo their most rapid rate of development and the age at which development is completed have major implications for the susceptibility of growing animals. For example, toxicity that is dependent on rates of cell proliferation (DNA/RNA replication and protein synthesis) might affect different tissues to different degrees at various stages of development. Additionally, the fact that a number of factors determining absorption, distribution, metabolism, and excretion of chemicals change as a function of age signifies that the target tissue dose in children may differ from that in adults for a given exposure situation. Furthermore, the individual toxicokinetic processes and determinants may change in different ways within each developmental stage, and this information must be considered in toto to understand the net impact on the internal dose in children. In this regard, physiology-based models are likely to be useful tools. For developing physiology-based toxicokinetic models in neonates, however, liver blood flow rate data are lacking. Such information is critical to better understanding the metabolism and clearance of xenobiotics by the liver. Additionally, in neonates, data on cofactors involved in Phase II reactions (e.g. glucuronide, sulfate) are required.

Limited data are available on male–female differences in physiological data for the various age groups of children. Most of the current data were obtained in boys, with the exception of a few physiological parameters (e.g. cardiac output, breathing rate, fat volumes). Such sex-specific data should facilitate the construction of biologically based models for simulating uptake and deposition of inhaled gases and particulates in children. There is also a need for data on the expression, development, and maturation of various transporters that play a critical role in the cellular flux of chemicals in children of various age groups. Finally, the availability of data on age- and tissue-specific rates of cell proliferation and molecular events in organ development would be useful for constructing biologically based models for the conduct of child-specific risk assessments.

4. DEVELOPMENTAL STAGE–SPECIFIC SUSCEPTIBILITIES AND OUTCOMES IN CHILDREN

4.1 Introduction

In chapter 3, the structural and functional features that potentially convey special susceptibilities of children to environmental exposures were detailed for a number of key organ systems. In this chapter, we highlight the impacts of exposure to environmental agents on those organ systems as a function of life stage. The overview is not meant to be an exhaustive review of the literature; rather, it is intended to be illustrative of the potential outcomes. Each of the organ systems discussed here presents different periods of susceptibility during critical windows in its development. It is clear that the timing of exposure to chemicals or other insults is critical in determining the consequences to children's health. Because of the differing windows of susceptibility, the same dose of the same chemical during different periods of development can have very different consequences. Structural malformations are most likely to occur as a result of exposures to chemicals during the embryonic period, when organs are beginning to differentiate. Hence, historically, the focus of concern has been on environmental factors that result in adverse pregnancy outcomes such as fetal loss, intrauterine growth restriction (IUGR), or birth defects. However, even after the basic structure of an organ has been established, disruption of processes such as growth and cell migration can have lifelong consequences on the function of key organ systems. It is also important to bear in mind when assessing the susceptibilities of children that there are similarities and differences in the timing of these periods between humans and commonly used laboratory animal species. For example, as documented in chapter 3, some developmental events that occur prenatally in humans occur after birth in rodents.

Table 4 provides examples of the types of outcomes and critical life stages for organ systems that are influenced by environmental agents. The susceptibilities identified in Table 4 are covered in greater detail throughout this chapter. To a large extent, the review has focused on what is known about the effects of chemicals on human

Table 4. Examples of adverse effects of developmental stage–specific exposures on various organ systems[a]

A.

Period of susceptibility for exposure	Neurological	Reproductive	Renal	Endocrine
Preconception Preimplantation	Periconceptional use of folic acid supplements decreases rate of neural tube defects (Bailey et al., 2003)			
Embryonic age	Neural tube defects from retinoic acid, arsenic, and valproic acid (Adams, 1993; Bennett & Finnell, 1998)	Decreased fertility in female rats exposed to dioxin (TCDD) (Gray & Ostby, 1995)	Hydronephrosis with dioxin exposure during embryonic or fetal periods in rats (Couture-Haws et al., 1991; Birnbaum, 1995)	
Fetus	Decreased intelligence, increased behavioural problems with lead (Bellinger et al., 1994; Rice, 1996) Cerebral palsy, mental retardation with high-dose methylmercury (Harada, 1978); subtle neurobehavioural effects with low doses (Grandjean et al., 1997)	Exposure to several phthalates induces reduced AGD and malformations in male rats (Mylchreest et al., 1999; Gray et al., 2000) Delay in pubertal development from exposure to PBBs Vaginal adenocarcinoma in young women due to DES (Herbst et al., 1971)	ACE fetopathy with neonatal renal failure from maternal exposure to angiotensin inhibitors (Tabacova et al., 2003)	Maternal smoking causes decreased birth weight and increased risk for later diabetes (Montgomery & Ekbom, 2002) and osteoporosis (Cooper et al., 2002) Decreased T3/T4 levels in infant and juvenile rats (Brouwer et al., 1998) exposed to PCBs

Developmental State–Specific Susceptibilities and Outcomes

Table 4 (Contd)

Period of susceptibility for exposure	Neurological	Reproductive	Renal	Endocrine
Neonate			Hydronephrosis with dioxin exposure during neonatal and infantile periods in rats (Birnbaum, 1995)	
Infant	Exposure of juvenile mice to pesticides caused Parkinson-like declines in dopaminergic neurons in adulthood (Cory-Slechta et al., 2005)			Maternal grooming affects ability to respond to stress in adulthood in rats (Gilbert, 2005)
Child	Brain tumours and meningiomas after therapeutic high-dose ionizing radiation to the head (Ron et al., 1988b; Kleinschmidt & Lillehei, 1995)			Lead poisoning causes abnormal bone structure and poor growth (Osterloh, 1991)
Adolescent		Delayed puberty with ethanol consumption (Dees et al., 1998) Delayed puberty with atrazine exposure in rats (Laws et al., 2000; Ashby et al., 2002)		

Table 4 (Contd)

B.

Period of susceptibility for exposure	Cardiac	Immune	Respiratory	Cancer
Preconception				
Preimplantation				Exposure of male mice to X-rays or urethane causes cancer in their offspring (Anderson et al., 2000)
Embryonic age				
Fetus	Decreased heart rate variability in children exposed prenatally to methylmercury (Grandjean et al., 2004)	Decreased cell-mediated immunity in males following perinatal exposure of rats to methoxychlor (Chapin et al., 1997) and heptachlor (Smialowicz et al., 2001; Smialowicz, 2002)	Altered airway growth with increased collagen deposition in airway walls with exposure to maternal smoking (Sekhon et al., 2001)	Inorganic arsenic in drinking-water caused adrenal tumours in male offspring and ovarian and lung tumours in female offspring as adults (Waalkes et al., 2003)
	IUGR (e.g. due to poor maternal malnutrition) increases risk of coronary heart disease in adulthood (Lau & Rogers, 2005)	Lead exposure reduces Th1 immune capability, causing a shift towards increased Th2 responses in rats (Dietert et al., 2004; Dietert & Lee, 2005)	Altered control of breathing response postnatally with maternal smoking in utero (Ueda et al., 1999)	

Developmental State–Specific Susceptibilities and Outcomes

Table 4 (Contd)

Period of susceptibility for exposure	Cardiac	Immune	Respiratory	Cancer
Neonate				
Infant			Increased incidence of respiratory mortality following exposure to particulates in the air (Glinianaia et al., 2004)	
Child		Leukaemia in children due to radiation from atomic bomb (IARC, 2000)	Exacerbation of pre-existing asthma from exposure to particulates in the air (Parnia et al., 2002)	Ionizing radiation and leukaemia in childhood and adulthood (Chow et al., 1996; Ron et al., 1988a)
			Chronic ozone exposure decreases lung function (Kunzli et al., 1997)	Radioisotopes of iodine from Chernobyl disaster and thyroid carcinoma (Pacini et al., 1997)
Adolescent				Breast cancer in adulthood with high-dose ionizing radiation (Boice et al., 1996)

ACE, angiotensin converting enzyme; AGD, anogenital distance; DES, diethylstilbestrol; IUGR, intrauterine growth restriction; PBBs, polybrominated biphenyls; PCBs, polychlorinated biphenyls; T3, triiodothyronine; T4, thyroxine; TCDD, tetrachlorodibenzo-p-dioxin; Th1, T helper 1; Th2, T helper 2

[a] This table is not intended as a comprehensive review. Only selected examples are provided.

development; however, where there was good supporting evidence from animal models or where particularly illustrative information was obtained solely from animal models, such information was included in the chapter.

Exposures to chemicals during early life stages can result in adverse effects during the stage when exposure occurred, or the effects may not manifest themselves until later stages. Depending on the dose of the chemical and the susceptibility during that life stage to the mode of action of the chemical, effects can range in severity from functional deficits to growth restriction to malformations to mortality. Mortality, growth restriction, and birth defects will be discussed in the next section, and functional deficits in particular organ systems will be discussed in subsequent sections.

4.2 Mortality, growth restriction, and birth defects

4.2.1 Mortality

Because there is currently no sensitive and specific biomarker of conception in humans, the prevalence of preimplantation embryonic mortality is not accurately known; however, studies of preimplantation pregnancy losses after in vitro fertilization suggest that as many as 50% of conceptions are followed by death of the embryo prior to implantation (Mesrogli & Dieterle, 1993). It is often stated that exposures occurring between conception and implantation result in either death of the embryo or no effects. However, experiments in rats have shown that exposures to mutagens such as ethyl methanesulfonate, 5-azacytidine, and methyl nitrosourea during the preimplantation period can also cause malformations (Rutledge & Generoso, 1998). At higher doses, these agents cause death prior to or around the time of implantation (Rutledge & Generoso, 1998).

In contrast to preimplantation mortality, more exact estimates of the incidence of spontaneous abortions (miscarriages occurring prior to 20 weeks' gestation) have been possible with the development of sensitive assays for hCG, which begins to be secreted by the conceptus at implantation. These studies show that about one third of postimplantation pregnancies end in spontaneous abortion. Of these, about two thirds occur prior to the recognition of pregnancy (Wilcox et al., 1988). These studies used predominantly Caucasian, college-educated populations. Occupational exposure of the mother to a variety of agents during pregnancy has been associated with spontaneous abortion in epidemiological studies. For example, maternal exposure to organic solvents has been associated with spontaneous abortion in several studies (Pastides et al., 1988; Taskinen et al., 1989; Lindbohm et al., 1990; Lipscomb et al., 1991; Windham et al., 1991; Schenker et al., 1995). However, a meta-analysis of five of these studies resulted in a non-significant odds ratio (McMartin et al., 1998). Two recently published prospective pregnancy studies reported an increased risk of pregnancy loss associated with serum levels of dichlorodiphenyltrichloroethane (DDT) and its metabolite, dichlorodiphenyldichloroethene (DDE). Risk of having had a prior pregnancy loss (or loss occurring prior to the index pregnancy) was higher for women with higher serum DDE concentrations upon enrolment into a prospective pregnancy study and for women recruited preconceptionally who were prospectively followed through pregnancy (Longnecker et al., 2005; Venners et al., 2005). Longnecker et al. (2005) reported a significant increased risk of prior fetal loss associated with a 60 µg/l increase in serum DDE (odds ratio [OR] = 1.4; 95% confidence interval [CI] = 1.1–1.6). A 10 ng/g increase in serum DDT significantly increased the risk of early pregnancy loss as measured by hCG assays (Venners et al., 2005). In fact, a positive monotonic exposure–response association was observed between preconception serum total DDT and risk of early pregnancy loss. However, this pattern was not seen among women with later clinically recognized pregnancy losses, underscoring the importance of capturing early pregnancies confirmed by hCG assays.

Stillbirths (death of the fetus after 20 weeks' gestation) are much less common than spontaneous abortions, occurring in about 7 per 1000 pregnancies in the United States (NCHS, 1997). About 5 of 1000 liveborn babies die annually during the neonatal period, and about 3 per 1000 die annually during the post-neonatal period in the United States. Rates of neonatal and infant mortality vary widely between and within countries, with some countries reporting rates in excess of 100 per 1000 (Kramer, 2003). Maternal smoking during pregnancy increases the risks of pregnancy loss, stillbirth, and infant mortality (Platt et al., 2004).

The potential for exposure to pollutants to increase mortality in children has been recognized since the 1950s (Ministry of Public

Health, 1954). Several studies have investigated the impact of air pollution on neonatal (birth to 28 days) and infant (28 days to one year) mortality (Bobak & Leon, 1999a; Dejmek et al., 2000; Ha et al., 2003; Glinianaia et al., 2004). While exposure to particulate air pollution is not consistently associated with increased neonatal or infant mortality in general, it is associated with increased mortality from respiratory causes, such as pneumonia and sudden infant death syndrome (Glinianaia et al., 2004). There is also sufficient evidence for a causal relationship between exposure to ETS and sudden infant death syndrome (Anderson & Cook, 1997), with the risk of death from sudden infant death syndrome increased by up to 150% by exposure to both pre- and postnatal ETS (NHMRC, 1997). Increased respiratory mortality in children under five years of age associated with nitrogen dioxide levels originating from diesel exhaust emissions has been suggested, but little attention was paid to potential confounders (Saldiva et al., 1994).

Embryonic or fetal mortality can also lead to altered sex ratio at birth if one sex is more susceptible than the other to the exposure (Taylor et al., 2006). Sex ratios (ratio of male to female live births) in the offspring of angler populations (sports fishermen/women) have received some study given their higher potential for exposure stemming from consumption of contaminated sport fish (Faulk et al., 1999). A reduced sex ratio was reported among the offspring of Swedish anglers' wives who lived on the Baltic Sea when compared with the offspring of wives who lived near the less contaminated Swedish west coast (Rylander et al., 1995). Equivocal results exist in relation to parental serum polychlorinated biphenyl (PCB) concentrations among angler populations. A reduced sex ratio (fewer males) was observed among mothers in the highest PCB quintile compared with the lowest quintile, although no relation was observed for paternal exposure, suggesting a maternally mediated effect (Weisskopf et al., 2003). Conversely, a higher sex ratio or male excess was observed in the offspring of a sample of Michigan anglers and their spouses for paternal but not maternal PCB exposure (Karmaus et al., 2002). Paternal consumption of cooking oil contaminated with PCBs, polychlorinated dibenzofurans (PCDFs), and polychlorinated dibenzo-p-dioxins (PCDDs) was reported to be associated with a significantly lower odds of having a male infant in Taiwan, China (del Rio Gomez et al., 2002). After an accidental release of dioxin in Seveso, Italy, exposed fathers under the age of 19 sired significantly more girls than boys compared with those

Developmental State–Specific Susceptibilities and Outcomes

fathers who were unexposed (Mocarelli et al., 2000). No significant change in the sex ratio was observed in Fukuoka and Nagasaki, Japan, following accidental contamination of rice oil with dioxin-like compounds (Yoshimura et al., 2001). Using a causality algorithm, Jarrell (2002) concluded that dioxin, dibromochloropropane, and hexachlorobenzene reduce the number of male births.

The possibility that early-life exposures can lead to increased mortality rates in later childhood and during adulthood will be discussed in subsequent sections that deal with the influence of early-life exposures on the risk for developing diseases (e.g. diabetes and heart disease) later in life.

4.2.2 Growth restriction

Effects of prenatal chemical exposure on growth have most commonly been measured as changes in birth weight. Low birth weight is defined as less than 2500 g at birth; however, birth weight is a continuous variable, and many exposures that affect birth weight do not necessarily result in low birth weight. Therefore, recent studies have emphasized the concept of diminished birth size, which can be assessed via several end-points: weight, length, head and abdominal circumference. Preterm birth is defined as birth prior to 37 weeks' gestation. Because birth weight is highly dependent on gestational age, another measure, IUGR, also known as small-for-gestational-age, has been defined as weighing less than the 10th percentile of weight-for-gestational-age standards for a given population. Maternal smoking is clearly associated with about a twofold increase in low birth weight and IUGR in multiple studies (Bosley et al., 1981; Wang et al., 2002). Wang et al. (2002) showed that there is an interaction of maternal smoking with maternal polymorphisms in GST T1 and CYP1A1. Women who smoke during pregnancy and who have one or both of these polymorphisms are at an even greater risk of having a low-birth-weight baby than women who smoke and do not have these specific polymorphisms. Maternal exposure to ETS is associated with smaller decreases in birth weight than is maternal smoking. In a meta-analysis of 19 studies (Windham et al., 1999), it was estimated that exposure to ETS lowers birth weight by an average of 31 g. Maternal smoking is thought to be the single most important factor for determining birth weight in developed countries (DiFranza et al., 2004). Smoking may induce growth restriction via at least two mechanisms: 1) by lowering maternal uterine blood flow from the uterus to the placenta and 2) by raising maternal and fetal carboxyhaemoglobin levels (DiFranza et al., 2004).

Epidemiological studies have also linked exposure to various components of air pollution to growth restriction. An overview and analysis of these studies were provided by Srám et al. (2005). Exposure to particulate matter less than 10 μm in diameter (PM_{10}) or less than 2.5 μm in diameter ($PM_{2.5}$) during pregnancy was significantly associated with low birth rate at term and IUGR (Bobak & Leon, 1999a; Dejmek et al., 1999; Bobak et al., 2001; Jedrychowski et al., 2004). Other components of air pollution, including carbon monoxide (Ritz et al., 2000, 2002), sulfur dioxide (Bobak & Leon, 1999b), and PAHs (Perera et al., 1998; Dejmek et al., 2000) have also been associated with low birth weight or IUGR. At this time, it is not clear which, if any, of the components of air pollution cause the observed decreases in embryonic and/or fetal growth.

Reduced birth weight has also been associated with prenatal exposure to persistent organochlorine compounds (Rylander et al., 1995). In a cohort of girls exposed prenatally to PCBs and polybrominated biphenyls (PBBs), estimated prenatal PCB exposure, but not estimated prenatal PBB exposure, above 5 μg/l in serum was associated with reduced weight adjusted for height at 5–24 years of age. Mothers with PCB serum levels above the median value had daughters whose current adjusted weights were 5 kg lower than for daughters whose mothers had levels below the median. This study provides evidence that prenatal exposure to PCBs may affect child growth (Blanck et al., 2002).

4.2.3 Birth defects (structural malformations)

Development of the child during pregnancy is a complex biological process, as organs and tissues develop from the union of a an egg and a sperm that must differentiate in a perfectly organized and well timed sequence. During that process, there may be divergences from the normal development that result in a high rate of spontaneous abortions and stillbirths, as was discussed above.

An estimated eight million children — about 6% of total births worldwide — are born with major birth defects annually. Additional

Developmental State–Specific Susceptibilities and Outcomes

anomalies will be diagnosed in about 3% of the children up to the age of seven years. These anomalies will include mental retardation, neurological impairment, and a variety of morphological and functional defects in different organs. Although the prevalence of major malformations detected at birth is about 3% of live births, these malformations are responsible for about 20% of the infant mortality rate and the majority of paediatric hospitalizations. Birth defects therefore have a tremendous impact on society and are a major cause of infant mortality, particularly in developed countries (Lynberg & Khoury, 1990).

A birth defect, a synonym for the clinical term "congenital anomaly", is defined as an anatomical and/or functional defect resulting from disturbance of normal developmental processes. This definition includes a wide range of defects, from a visualized structural defect such as spina bifida to microscopic and metabolic defects such as phenylketonuria. Terms such as malformation, disruption, deformation, and sequence have been utilized to describe various manifestations (Jones, 1988).

Distinguishing between the above-mentioned categories is of clinical importance for the prognosis and risk evaluation of the pregnancy outcome and of the newborn. In view of the fact that most of the birth defects are considered to be "malformations" (Martinez-Frias et al., 2000), the more specific clinical terms "major" and "minor" malformations were established. Major congenital malformations represent a status of a newborn that requires significant medical or surgical care due to an abnormality in an essential anatomical structure; minor malformations are less threatening to health and need less medical intervention. Examples of major malformations include congenital heart disease, neural tube defects, and cleft lip/cleft palate. Nail hypoplasia, auricular deformities, and broad nasal bridge are examples of minor malformations. Umbilical and inguinal hernia are examples of anomalies that may be categorized in each of these groups, depending on the severity. Most surveillance programmes focus on major malformations; thus, limited data are available on the incidence of minor malformations.

4.2.3.1   Etiology

Research suggests that about 15–25% of all birth defects can be attributed to genetic background, 4% to maternal conditions, 3% to maternal infections, 1–2% to deformations, <1% to chemicals and other environmental influences, and 55–65% to unknown etiologies (Brent & Beckman, 1990). As embryonic development is an outcome of the combination of intrinsic hereditary factors and the surrounding environmental influence, the etiology of most birth defects is likely to be the consequence of both independent or synergistic environmental and genetic factors. Since the exposure to environmental factors (as opposed to genetic factors) can be altered or prevented, studies on the role of environmental factors is important in spite of the low direct attributable risk.

In humans and in experimental animal models, different environmental factors, including chemical agents, have been shown to affect every stage of embryonic and fetal development, and therefore a wide range of defects has been observed. For example, excess amounts of retinoic acid may affect several developmental processes via interaction with retinoic acid receptors; the outcomes resulting from excess amounts of retinoic acid in experimental animals have been shown to be highly developmental stage specific (Shenefelt, 1972; Matt et al., 2003). In humans, inadequate periconceptual folic acid intake was shown to be responsible for a large percentage of neural tube defects. Subsequent studies showed that a 70–80% reduction in these defects was possible with periconceptional folic acid supplementation (Bailey et al., 2003). Public health and food fortification efforts to ensure that all women of child-bearing age have adequate folic acid intake have been accompanied by reductions in neural tube and other birth defects (Botto et al., 2004). Recent work in mice suggests that the beneficial effects of folate in preventing birth defects may be mediated by increasing methylation of transposable elements within DNA (Gilbert, 2005). These studies have shown that supplementing the diet of pregnant mice with methyl donors like folate significantly increases DNA methylation in a dose-dependent manner.

Given that practically every chemical may have a harmful influence at some dosage and stage of embryonic development, depending on the species studied, understanding the mechanism of action and the ways of disturbing embryogenesis for each agent has tremendous importance. There are several reference materials that review the evidence for the embryotoxic teratogenic potential of drugs, chemicals, and infections. These include *Drugs in Pregnancy and Lactation* (Briggs et al., 2002), *Maternal–Fetal Toxicology* (Koren, 2001), *Shepard's Catalog of Teratogenic Agents* (Shepard, 2004), *Teratogenic Effects of Drugs: A Resource for Clinicians* (Friedman & Polifka, 2000), and the TERIS (Teratogen Information System) database. The TERIS database is available via the Internet (http://depts.washington.edu/~terisweb/teris/) as a subscription-based teratogen information service to assist physicians and healthcare professionals. REPROTOX (http://reprotox.org/) is another Internet-based information system that provides information on the effects of environmental hazards on human reproduction and development.

Examples of chemicals that cause birth defects in various organ systems are discussed in subsequent sections, along with periods of susceptibility of chemicals for these organ systems and for cancer.

4.2.3.2 *Functional developmental toxicity*

Observations in children whose mothers were exposed to methylmercury or PCBs (see section 4.3.1.2) have made it increasingly obvious that many manifestations of developmental defects occur in the absence of gross morphological changes. Early studies focused largely on alterations in the function of the central nervous system, prompting the use of the term behavioural teratology; later, the term developmental neurotoxicity was used to cover this research area (Rodier, 1994). However, other organ systems are also at risk as a result of developmental toxicity (USEPA, 1991; Holladay & Luster, 1994; Lau & Kavlock, 1994; IPCS, 2002). The critical periods for such effects extend well beyond the period of major organogenesis and include postnatal stages as well. In extrapolating findings between species, it is important to consider comparative rates of development, since what may be a prenatal event in humans could well be equivalent to postnatal periods in the animal species commonly used in toxicology assays. More recently, the concept of the intrauterine environment influencing the onset of adult diseases such as coronary heart disease, hypertension, and type 2 diabetes has come into prominence. A number of epidemiological studies have associated changes in birth weight (as a proxy for

IUGR) with elevated risk levels of these diseases (Lau & Rogers, 2005). The basis of the association is believed to be that alterations in nutrient availability (or other environmental stressors) lead to short-term adaptive measures in the fetus (involving altered homeostatic set-points) that later result in metabolic disorders when the stressor is relieved. The metabolic alterations, in turn, then gradually contribute to increased risk with ageing. It is important to note that functional developmental toxicity may be evident only after long latency periods and may be difficult to ascertain due to the functional reserve capacity of many organ systems.

4.3 Specific organ systems

4.3.1 Nervous system

Section 3.6.2 describes the normal development of the nervous system.

The developing nervous system is more susceptible than the adult brain to the disrupting effects of toxic chemicals. Levels of exposure that produce few, or no, obvious effects on the mature nervous system in adults may pose a serious risk to the developing nervous system (Faustman et al., 2000). The lengthy period of brain development and the extensive number of neural processes available for disruption during development contribute to the susceptibilities of the developing nervous system to toxicants (Rodier, 1994). The process by which normal central nervous system development unfolds requires the precise orchestration of neuronal proliferation, migration, differentiation, synaptogenesis, gliogenesis, myelination, and apoptosis (Rice & Barone, 2000). These developmental processes need to occur in specific brain regions at specific times. This complex array of processes can be disturbed by both genetic and environmental influences, which may lead to long-term losses in the structural and functional integrity of the nervous system (Rodier, 1995; Barone et al., 2000). To understand the action of neurotoxicants on the developing child, it is important to explore both normal and abnormal pathways of brain development. Section 3.6.2 describes the normal development of the nervous system. This section provides a brief overview of how exposure to neurotoxicants at early life stages can alter the biological foundations of behaviour.

Developmental State–Specific Susceptibilities and Outcomes

4.3.1.1 Periods of susceptibility and consequences of exposures

To understand the consequences of chemical exposures on the central nervous system and, ultimately, the implications of such exposures on childhood growth and development, it is important to consider the concept of critical or sensitive periods in development. Critical periods, in the context of neurotoxicology, are used to describe time points when the brain is highly susceptible to perturbation from exposure to chemicals. The complexity and vast number of processes that take place during central nervous system development provide multiple opportunities for differential effects of chemical exposures. When evaluating toxicological studies in animal models for their relevance to humans, it is also important to keep in mind differences in the timing of critical events in nervous system development between humans and common laboratory animal species. For example, in rodents, considerable brain development occurs during the neonatal period, whereas most of this development occurs during the fetal period in humans.

Neurogenesis of different brain regions continues to occur throughout gestation and postnatally. The period of susceptibilities to agents that affect proliferation and migration will thus vary, depending on the brain region. For example, initial proliferation in the cerebellum occurs during the fetal period in humans and in rats. A second period of proliferation begins during the fetal period in humans and continues well into childhood, whereas in rats it occurs entirely postnatally (Rice & Barone, 2000). Disorders in neuronal proliferation, migration, and maturation, resulting from both genetic and environmental causes, can lead to both lethal and non-lethal congenital anomalies. Barone et al. (2000) and Rice & Barone (2000) provided extensive reviews of early brain development in which the timing and sequence of processes such as proliferation, migration, synaptogenesis, and apoptosis, as well as the critical roles of signalling and trophic molecules, are discussed. Perturbation of these processes in central nervous system development can result in malformations. For example, microcephaly (small brain and skull with mental retardation) is caused by faulty neuronal proliferation, and agenesis of the corpus callosum (usually associated with seizures and mental retardation) is caused by defects in neurulation and neuronal migration. The number of fetal brain malformations that have been clinically identified is too extensive to list in full. In the case of neuronal migration disorders alone (i.e. failure of neurons to move from their site of birth to where they will function in mature neural circuits), there are over 25 recognized clinical syndromes (http://www.ninds.nih.gov). Defects in genes that control neuronal migration are thought to play a leading role in the onset of these disorders, but the mechanisms that control these genes are not yet delineated.

1) Neurobehavioural (functional) deficits

Exposure to environmental chemicals such as methylmercury, lead, or certain pesticides at levels below those that cause structural defects may produce cellular or molecular changes that are expressed as neurobehavioural (functional) deficits (Adams et al., 2000) or as increased susceptibility to neurodegenerative diseases much later in life (Cory-Slechta et al., 2005). Scientists and health professionals must grapple with the fact that not all early central nervous system damage stemming from neurotoxic insult can be visualized with the eye or under the microscope. Functional loss, whether taking the form of mental retardation or subtle behavioural deficits, is a reflection of abnormal development and impaired central nervous system functioning. Moreover, neurotoxic insults during development that result in no observable phenotype at birth or during childhood could manifest later in life as earlier onset of neurodegenerative diseases, such as Parkinson disease. Only a small number of neurotoxins have been adequately studied to address their specific neurobehavioural consequences after prenatal or perinatal exposure. The developmental consequences of some of these compounds are briefly discussed below.

While behaviour is frequently difficult to tie to specific brain regions, there are some important generalities that can be gleaned from the fields of cognitive neuroscience and developmental neurobiology. As summarized by Rice & Barone (2000), working memory and executive functions are controlled by the prefrontal region, some aspects of learning and memory are dependent on medial temporal lobe structures, and sleep/wake cycles, autonomic nervous system functions, and regulation of arousal are a function of the brain stem. Each of these neural areas has a course of maturation that can be qualitatively (stages) and quantitatively (timing) distinct from those of other structures within the brain. Behaviours that depend on different brain systems will therefore be differentially affected by chemical exposure, depending on when the exposure occurred during development. The timing of the exposure is therefore critical in establishing what type of functional loss is likely to occur. While early-developing neural systems may be the most vulnerable to chemical insult, recent evidence from paediatric functional magnetic resonance imaging studies suggests that the behavioural and physiological foundations of cognition continue to develop during childhood and adolescence (Casey et al., 2005). Chemical exposures that occur late in childhood or adolescence should not be dismissed as inconsequential.

The effects of prenatal chemical exposure can be expressed across several domains of behaviour and can include adverse effects on intelligence/cognition, social behaviour or temperament, sensory development (vision, hearing), and physical growth (Vreugdenhil et al., 2004). Behavioural changes can be difficult to detect and even more difficult to link to specific pre- or perinatal risk factors, such as exposure to a drug or chemical. Depending on the timing and nature of the neurotoxicity, behavioural deviations in the developing child can range from mild (e.g. learning disabilities) to severe (e.g. mental retardation). Common neurodevelopmental disabilities such as autism, mental retardation, attention deficit hyperactivity disorder, and dyslexia affect approximately 3–8% of the babies born in the United States each year (Weiss & Landrigan, 2000; Newschaffer et al., 2005). The basis of the neurological damage in most developmental disorders can be established in only about 25% of affected children. Given our expanding knowledge of global chemical exposures, it remains plausible that there is a potential relationship between early neurotoxicant exposure, subtle central nervous system damage, and the rising number of children with major and minor neurodevelopmental disabilities.

Exposure to retinoic acid, methylnitrosourea, and clomiphene during the early embryonic period, prior to the induction of the neural plate (before day 18 in the human), results in an increased incidence of neural tube defects and other malformations in experimental animal models (Bennett & Finnell, 1998). In addition, exposure of rodents to teratogens such as retinoic acid, arsenic, and valproic acid during the period of neurulation results in neural tube defects such as spina bifida and encephaloceles (Adams & Lammer, 1993; Bennett & Finnell, 1998). Of these, therapeutic use of valproic acid has been associated with elevated rates of spina bifida in humans. A number of structural defects of the brain, including exencephaly, result from the failure of the rostral neuropore to properly close during the fourth week of human embryonic development. Various teratogenic agents, such as ionizing radiation (X-ray) and hydroxyurea, both antimitotic agents capable of stopping cell division, can experimentally induce these conditions in animal models (Hicks, 1954). As the rhombomeres form and the neural tube closes later during the embryonic period, valproic acid and thalidomide target the hindbrain, brain stem, and cranial nerve motor nuclei (Rodier et al., 1996; Rodier, 2004). Indeed, it has been speculated that insult to the cranial nerve motor nuclei during rhombomere formation may play a role in the development of autism, a serious developmental disorder affecting thousands of children annually.

The majority of malformations of the spinal cord are the result of the failure of the caudal neuropore to properly close by the end of the fourth week of development. The defective closure of the caudal neuropore results in serious neural tube malformations known generally as spina bifida. There are many types of spina bifida, and the clinical presentation, including neurological deficits, can range from minor (e.g. spina bifida occulta) to severe (e.g. spina bifida with myeloschisis). Spina bifida cystica has been associated with exposure of the mother to large doses of retinoic acid, or vitamin A, via ingestion (Moore, 1988).

4.3.1.2   *Specific examples*

1)   Methylmercury

Catastrophic episodes of human methylmercury poisoning have occurred in both Japan and Iraq, providing much of the information that is known about the effects of exposure to high doses of methylmercuy on development in human infants. At present, environmental methylmercury contamination is widespread, and low-level exposure to this toxicant occurs primarily through the consumption of contaminated fish. The fetus is particularly sensitive to methylmercury exposure, and adverse neurobehavioural effects in infants have been associated with exposure levels that result in few, if any, signs of maternal clinical illness or toxicity. Early life stage exposure to this organometal produces a broad spectrum of neurobehavioural effects that are clearly dose dependent (NRC, 2000b;

Developmental State–Specific Susceptibilities and Outcomes

Davidson et al., 2004). High-level exposure to methylmercury during fetal development can result in cerebral palsy, seizures, blindness, deafness, and mental retardation.

After the work by Kjellstrom and colleagues on low-level methylmercury exposure and child development (Kjellstrom et al., 1986, 1989), two large-scale longitudinal studies were undertaken to investigate the consequences of in utero methylmercury exposure from a maternal diet high in fish. The Faroe Islands study in the northern Atlantic Ocean is an epidemiological study that enrolled approximately 1000 children at birth (Grandjean, 1992). In Faroese neonates, neurological optimality scores taken at two weeks of postnatal age showed that increased cord blood mercury concentrations were associated with decreased neurological function and that this effect corresponded to a gestational age of about three weeks (Steuerwald et al., 2000). Analysis of behavioural data from children at seven years of age revealed significant methylmercury-related impairments in language, attention, and memory (Grandjean et al., 1997). Methylmercury effects on the latency of brain stem auditory evoked potentials were found at both 7 and 14 years, suggesting that some neurotoxic effects from intrauterine methylmercury exposure may be irreversible (Murata et al., 1999, 2004). Decreased heart rate variability, an indicator of autonomic nervous system function, was also observed at 7 and 14 years (Grandjean et al., 2004). Overall, results from the Faroe Islands study suggest that, in this population, low-level prenatal exposure to methylmercury from maternal consumption of fish and pilot whale is an important neurological risk factor for impaired behavioural development in infants and children.

The second prospective study of in utero exposure to methylmercury was initiated in the Republic of Seychelles and enrolled about 800 mother–infant pairs (Myers et al., 1995). In contrast to the Faroe Islands study, the investigation in the Seychelles did not find evidence of methylmercury-related adverse effects on the neurobehavioural development of children through nine years of age (Myers et al., 2003). In some instances, prenatal mercury exposure was actually associated with precocious behaviour, and important developmental milestones were reached more quickly in the most highly exposed subjects.

The differences in the outcomes of the studies in the Faroes and the Seychelles have been the subject of much deliberation (NTP,

1998; NRC, 2000b). Both assessments concluded that the two studies were credible and provide valuable insight into the potential health effects of methylmercury. Differences in the study designs and in the characteristics of the study populations might explain the differences in findings between the Faroes and the Seychelles studies. Differences include the ways in which methylmercury exposure was measured (i.e. in umbilical cord blood versus maternal hair), the types of neurological and psychological tests administered, the age of testing (7 years versus 5.5 years of age), and the patterns of methylmercury exposure. The United States National Academy of Sciences (NRC, 2000b) noted that the Faroe Islands population was also exposed to relatively high levels of PCBs. However, on the basis of an analysis of the data, the Committee on the Toxicological Effects of Methylmercury (NRC, 2000b) concluded that the adverse effects found in the Faroe Islands study, including those seen in the Boston Naming Test, were not attributable to PCB exposure and that PCB exposure did not invalidate the use of the results from the Faroe Islands study as the basis of risk assessment for methylmercury.

2) Lead

Lead is perhaps the best studied toxicant that has been clearly linked to central nervous system injury and adverse neurobehavioural outcomes in exposed children. It has long been recognized that high-level exposure to lead can result in encephalopathy, coma, and death (for a review of lead poisoning, see Needleman, 2004). In the 1970s, Needleman and colleagues began to examine the neurobehavioural consequences of developmental exposure to lead in exposed children. This body of work established that chronic, low-dose exposure to lead is associated with a significant decrease in intelligence quotient (IQ), as measured by standardized psychometric instruments (Needleman et al., 1979). In a recent publication, the relationship between environmental lead exposure and intellectual deficits in children was confirmed in an international pooled analysis (Lanphear et al., 2005). Children exposed prenatally to lead also display impaired performance on specific cognitive tests, such as reaction time and vigilance (Rice, 1996). These experimental findings suggest that in utero exposure to lead results in slower basic information processing and deficits in attention. These functional losses may play a large role in the decreased global IQ scores observed in lead-exposed children.

Research has also demonstrated that as early as age two, lead-exposed children exhibit more problem behaviours than their unexposed peers (Sciarillo et al., 1992; Wasserman et al., 1998). In a prospective study, the behaviour of lead-exposed children at eight years of age was measured by teacher ratings in the classroom, and total problem behaviour scores were significantly related to tooth dentine lead levels (Bellinger et al., 1994). These data suggest that social and emotional difficulties may be correlates of early lead exposure. One of the most significant relationships to emerge from the lead literature is that between antisocial behaviour and developmental lead exposure. In a longitudinal study of boys, a modest relationship was found between bone lead levels and teacher ratings of behaviour such as aggression and delinquency at seven years of age (Needleman et al., 1996). At 11 years of age, parental reports suggested an increase in antisocial behaviour and health complaints in children with higher lead levels. Teacher ratings corroborated the parental reports, in that children with higher bone lead levels were found to have more health concerns, depression/anxiety, and behavioural problems in the classroom. In a prospective, longitudinal study conducted by Dietrich and colleagues, both prenatal and postnatal lead exposure were related to antisocial and delinquent acts in adolescents (Dietrich et al., 2001). It is generally accepted in the scientific and medical communities that the adverse neurobehavioural consequences associated with developmental lead exposure are not reversible and remain in place across the human lifespan (Bellinger, 2004).

3) PCBs

PCBs are prevalent environmental pollutants that pose potential health risks to both humans and wildlife. In episodes of human PCB poisoning in Japan (Yusho) and Taiwan, China (Yucheng), people became ill after ingesting rice oil that was highly contaminated with PCBs and PCDFs (Kuratsune et al., 1971; Hsu et al., 1985). Infants born to mothers who consumed PCB-contaminated rice oil during pregnancy were at increased risk for low birth weight, abnormal brown pigmentation of the skin, and clinical abnormalities of the gingiva, skin, nails, teeth, and lungs (Yamashita & Hayashi, 1985; Rogan et al., 1988). Neurobehavioural deficits such as delayed attainment of developmental milestones, lower scores on intelligence tests, and higher activity levels were also reported in both cohorts of children (Guo et al., 2004). In most contemporary exposure scenarios, human infants are exposed to low-level complex PCB mixtures through the placenta during prenatal development and via breast milk during postnatal development. Although the effects of these compounds on the central nervous system are not well described, there is mounting evidence of developmental neurotoxicity from studies in Taiwan, China, the United States, the Netherlands, Germany, and the Faroe Islands (Schantz et al., 2003).

Studies of newborns suggest that lower levels of PCB exposure can affect a number of newborn behaviours. Exposed infants are more likely to exhibit signs that are consistent with immaturity of the central nervous system (e.g. increased startle response, abnormal reflexes) (Rogan et al., 1986; Huisman et al., 1995). In a longitudinal investigation in the United States of infants born to mothers who consumed fish contaminated with low-level PCBs, investigators found early recognition memory deficits in exposed infants, poorer scores on a preschool IQ test, and reduced verbal IQ and reading comprehension at 11 years of age (Jacobson & Jacobson, 2002a,b). The authors also found that adverse effects of developmental PCB exposure were observed less frequently in breastfed infants, suggesting a protective influence of breastfeeding on the behavioural development of exposed infants. Further studies of this cohort at 11 years of age have found evidence of increased impulsivity as well as deficits in concentration and working memory in exposed children (Jacobson & Jacobson, 2003). Again, adverse effects were primarily seen in subjects who had not been breastfed. A study from the Netherlands found that prenatal PCB exposure was related to longer and more variable reaction times in childhood, suggesting persistent deficits in basic cognitive processes (Vreugdenhil et al., 2004). Although these studies and others provide significant evidence of a relation between low-level PCB exposure and intellectual impairment, some studies have not observed such effects, and the relationship between PCB exposure and deficits in childhood cognition remains controversial (Gladen & Rogan, 1991; Gray et al., 2005).

4) Ethanol

Prenatal exposure to ethanol is the leading preventable cause of mental retardation in the United States, if not the world. The consumption of beer, wine, or spirits during pregnancy can have a profound impact on childhood development (Burbacher & Grant, 2006). The effects of ethanol are dose dependent, and children born to alcoholic or ethanol-abusing mothers are at highest risk for poor developmental outcome (Stratton et al., 1996). The most serious clinical outcome for infants who have been exposed in utero to alcohol is the development of fetal alcohol syndrome (Jones & Smith, 1973). Infants with this condition have a common facial dysmorphology that includes shortened palebral fissures (eyelid openings), smooth philtrum (area between the nose and upper lip), thin upper lip, low nasal bridge, and minor ear anomalies (Abel, 1984). It is now understood that some alcohol-exposed infants do not express the facial features commonly associated with fetal alcohol syndrome but do exhibit significant neurobehavioural delays. Children with this less severe constellation of behavioural effects are commonly referred to as having fetal alcohol effects.

It is now recognized that maternal intake of one drink per day, on average, is sufficient to result in neurological disturbances in exposed infants (Streissguth, 1993). Prenatal exposure to ethanol is clearly associated with central nervous system injury, and a broad spectrum of behaviours can be affected, including intellectual functioning (particularly arithmetic), language, abstract problem solving, working memories, attention, and executive functioning (e.g. planning, flexibility) (Streissguth et al., 1994; Mattson et al., 2001; Jacobson & Jacobson, 2002a,b). Attention appears particularly susceptible to the effects of alcohol exposure, and a recent study found that standardized tests of attention and distractibility can discriminate between exposed and control subjects with 92% accuracy (Lee et al., 2004). In general, children with a history of intrauterine ethanol exposure tend to lack the ability to stay focused and attentive over time and have difficulty analysing problems and forming effective response strategies. New evidence from South Africa indicates that gestational ethanol exposure also results in the disruption of the infant visual system (Carter et al., 2005). As children born to drinking mothers mature, deficits in social behaviour become more pronounced and are often expressed in the form of classroom aggression, impaired social judgement, and anti-social/delinquent behaviour (Allebeck & Olsen, 1998; Famy et al., 1998). Prenatal alcohol exposure is also a risk factor for the development of drinking problems in young adulthood, underscoring the intergenerational nature of ethanol abuse during pregnancy and the lifelong consequences of gestational exposure (Baer et al., 2003). In addition, adolescents and adults with a history of prenatal ethanol exposure are more likely to experience adverse life outcomes such as dropping out of school, arrest or confinement in a jail or psychiatric setting, or the expression of repeated inappropriate sexual behaviours (Streissguth et al., 2004).

5) Pesticides

It has been hypothesized that neurotoxic insults during development that result in no observable phenotype at birth or during childhood could manifest later in life as earlier onset of neurodegenerative diseases, such as Parkinson disease. Recent studies in mice provide support for this hypothesis (Cory-Slechta et al., 2005). Mice were exposed as juveniles only (postnatal days 5–19), as adults only, or during both stages to the pesticides maneb and paraquat. Both pesticides damage the dopaminergic pathways involved in Parkinson disease, but the two agents have different modes of action. Mice exposed as juveniles and again as adults had dramatically greater declines in nigrostriatal dopaminergic neurons at seven months of age than did mice exposed during either period alone (Cory-Slechta et al., 2005).

6) Other environmental chemicals

It is important to take into account the fact that, besides the above examples, the number of environmental chemicals that might affect the neurological development of children is increasing. Recently, cognitive effects have been shown for ETS (Yolton et al., 2005), arsenic (Calderón et al., 2001; Wasserman et al., 2004), manganese (Wasserman et al., 2006), and some mixtures of arsenic and manganese (Wright et al., 2006).

4.3.2 Reproductive system

Section 3.6.3 describes the normal development of the reproductive system.

Developmental State–Specific Susceptibilities and Outcomes

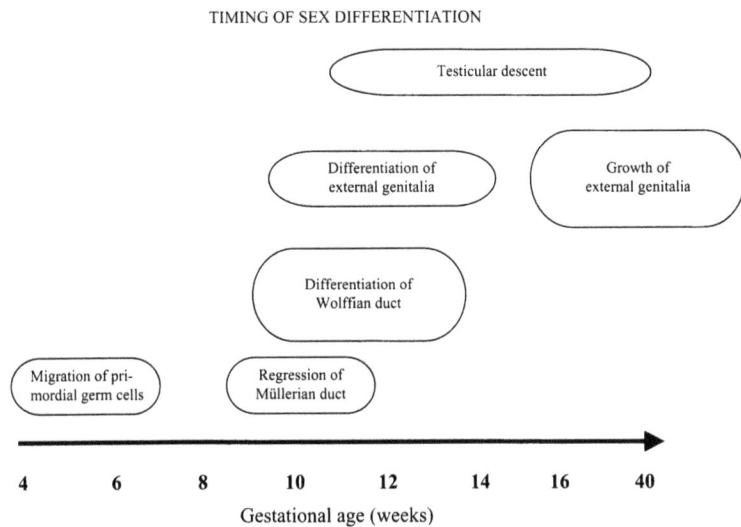

Fig. 7. Key events of sex differentiation and their timing in pregnancy.

4.3.2.1 Periods of susceptibility

Reproductive organs develop throughout gestation, as demonstrated in Figure 7. Many gene activities, such as those of SRY, SOX9, and AMH, are strictly time dependent, and disruption of those activities can occur only in a narrow time frame, whereas some other developmental phases take a long time. An example of the latter, testicular descent, starts with a transabdominal migration in mid-gestation and ends with an inguino-scrotal migration during late gestation. This long developmental period may partly explain why testicular maldescent cryptorchidism is so common (2–9% of newborn boys; Boisen et al., 2004). Male-type development is hormonally regulated, whereas female-type differentiation occurs in the absence of reproductive hormone action. Because the male phenotype is dependent on an induced, rather than default, pattern of gene expression, the male fetus tends to be susceptible to hormonal perturbations that modulate function of the androgen signalling pathways. Likewise, genotypic females will be masculinized by exposure to sufficient amounts of androgens. These effects do not need to be all or none, as the phenotype could be anywhere in the continuum between male and female (IPCS, 2002). Owing to accurate timing of gene activities, the same agent can cause very different effects at different times of development; for example, an antiandrogen exposure early in pregnancy could cause hypospadias, whereas later in pregnancy it would only cause cryptorchidism.

Puberty is a period of interrelated neuroendocrine processes that culminate in a physiologically mature reproductive system and, therefore, is another period of susceptibility to environmental influences. The form of pubertal alteration (maturational delay or acceleration) is a function of the nature of the insult (Colon et al., 2000; Den Hond & Schoeters, 2006). Effects on puberty can be the result of earlier life stage exposure or exposure concurrent with the maturational process. Comprehensive reviews of normal puberty and perturbations by exogenous influences in experimental animal models are available for the female (Goldman et al., 2000) and male (Stoker et al., 2000). Body composition changes across life stages, and the endocrine control of body composition by such factors as gonadal sex steroids, growth hormone, and IGF-1 also plays an important role in puberty (Veldhuis et al., 2005).

4.3.2.2   *Consequences of exposures*

Outcome after chemical exposure depends on the mechanism and type of action, the timing of exposure, and the dose of the chemical. Adverse effects can be manifest at birth (e.g. hypospadias and cryptorchidism in humans), in puberty (as delay or precocity), or in adulthood (e.g. infertility, alterations in accessory sex organs, disturbances in pregnancy maintenance, endometriosis, or premature reproductive senescence) (Pryor et al., 2000; Buck Louis et al., 2005). In the following, we discuss some specific chemicals that have been reported to affect one or several reproductive outcomes. Where possible, the discussion will focus on effects that are observed in humans. The list of chemicals that have been reported to have adverse effects on reproductive organs is much longer than presented here, and the selected examples serve only to illustrate the types of reproductive toxicants and their different effects. The general order in which they are presented is based on the life stage in which exposure is associated with the outcome, regardless of whether the outcome was observed concurrent with the exposure or in a subsequent life stage.

Developmental State–Specific Susceptibilities and Outcomes

1) Diethylstilbestrol (DES) and other estrogen agonists

In utero exposure of men to DES, a synthetic non-steroid estrogen, has been linked to increased incidence of meatal stenosis, epididymal cysts, testicular hypoplasia, cryptorchidism, microphallus, and sperm abnormalities (Henderson et al., 1976; Gill et al., 1977, 1979; Stillman, 1982). In females, adenosis, clear cell adenocarcinoma, and structural defects of the cervix, vagina, uterus, and fallopian tubes have been linked to in utero exposure to DES (Stillman, 1982).

2) Phthalates

Fetal exposure of male rats to some phthalate esters (e.g. diethylhexyl phthalate, dibutyl phthalate, and butyl benzyl phthalate) results in many changes in the male reproductive tract, such as decreased anogenital distance, hypospadias, cryptorchidism, disturbed development of prostate, epididymis, vas deferens, and seminal vesicles, retained nipples, and decreased sperm production (Mylchreest et al., 1998, 1999, 2000, 2002; Gray et al., 2000; Kavlock et al., 2002a,b,c,d,e; Lottrup et al., 2006; Skakkebaek et al., 2006; Weisbach et al., 2006). The critical window for all of these effects is the latter half of gestation (days 12–21), which is the time during which male sexual differentiation occurs (Mylchreest et al., 1999). The critical window has been further refined for undescended testes and the reduction of anogenital distance in males to gestational days 15–17 (Ema et al., 2000; Selevan et al., 2000).

In utero exposure of male rats to dibutyl phthalate on gestational days 13–21 permanently alters the testis and produces foci of testicular dysgenesis (immature seminiferous tubules with undifferentiated Sertoli cells, Sertoli cell–only tubules, Leydig cell hyperplasia, morphologically distorted tubules, and the presence of abnormal germ cells), which persist in the adult animal (Fisher et al., 2003). Subsequent research demonstrated a coordinated, dose-dependent reduction in expression of key genes and proteins involved in cholesterol transport and steroidogenesis and a corresponding reduction in testosterone in the fetal testes (Lehmann et al., 2004). In humans, similar dysgenetic changes in the histology of the testis have been found in patients with testicular cancer, subfertility, or cryptorchidism (Sohval, 1954, 1956; Berthelsen & Skakkebaek,

1983; Hoei-Hansen et al., 2003; Skakkebaek et al., 2003). Furthermore, men with rare genetic abnormalities that cause testicular dysgenesis (e.g. 45X/46XY and androgen insensitivity) also have high risk of testicular cancer, often combined with cryptorchidism and hypospadias (Savage & Lowe, 1990). It has been proposed that all these human disorders (testicular germ cell cancer, cryptorchidism, hypospadias, and low sperm counts) have common origins in fetal life, and thus they all represent different symptoms of the same underlying entity called testicular dysgenesis syndrome (Aarskog, 1970; Scully, 1981; Sharpe & Skakkebaek, 1993; Skakkebaek et al., 2001, 2006; Sharpe, 2003; Asklund et al., 2004). Since the testicular and other changes in dibutyl phthalate–exposed rats have also been reported in human testicular dysgenesis syndrome, it has been proposed that in utero exposure of the rat to dibutyl phthalate is a possible model for studying human testicular dysgenesis syndrome (Fisher et al., 2003).

Perinatal exposure of rats to butyl benzyl phthalate causes reduced anogenital distance, reduced testis weight, permanent nipples, hypospadias, cryptorchidism, and testicular malformations (Gray et al., 2000). Also, reduced daily sperm production has been linked to gestational and lactational exposure to butyl benzyl phthalate in rats (Sharpe et al., 1995).

3) Polybrominated biphenyls (PBBs)

In humans, exposure to high levels of PBBs in utero and via breastfeeding has been linked to an earlier age at menarche. Perinatal exposure to PBBs has been associated with earlier menarche (pubic hair stage) in breastfed girls (Blanck et al., 2000).

4) Antineoplastic agents

Many antineoplastic agents are well known to cause amenorrhoea and premature ovarian failure in women and oligospermia or azoospermia in men (Howell & Shalet, 1998). The likelihood of ovarian failure after chemotherapy treatment increases with increasing age and is thought to be due to lower ovarian reserves in older women (Howell & Shalet, 1998). There are few data on the effects of in utero exposure to antineoplastic drugs on reproductive function in adulthood. However, evidence from animal studies suggests that the fetal ovary may be more sensitive to these agents than the

Developmental State–Specific Susceptibilities and Outcomes

prepubertal or adult ovary. Fetal exposure to busulfan causes reduced numbers of oogonia and primordial follicles in rats (Merchant, 1975; Hirshfield, 1994), and high-dose exposure causes preterm ovarian exhaustion (Shirota et al., 2003). Also in humans, high-dose busulfan regimens cause ovarian failure in young women (Cicognani et al., 2003). Complete destruction by the alkylating agent cyclophosphamide of primordial and primary follicles is achieved at lower doses in prepubertal mice than in adult mice (Shiromizu et al., 1984; Plowchalk & Mattison, 1991). In young men, the use of multiple chemotherapy regimens is associated with a risk of permanent sterility, and the cumulative dose of cyclophosphamide has been shown to be an important determinant of recovery to normospermic levels after azoospermia (Meistrich et al., 1992).

5) Lead

Rats chronically exposed to lead (starting in utero) show delay in sexual maturity (Ronis et al., 1998). In a study concerning girls from the United States, higher blood lead levels were associated with delayed attainment of pubic hair and menarche (Wu et al., 2003). Compared with concentrations of 1 µg/dl, lead concentrations of 3 µg/dl were associated with decreased height ($P < 0.001$), after adjustment for age, race, and other factors, but not with body mass index or weight. Blood lead concentrations of 3 µg/dl were associated with significant delays in breast and pubic hair development in African American and Mexican American girls. The delays were most marked among African American girls; in this group, the delays in reaching Tanner stages 2, 3, 4, and 5 associated with a lead concentration of 3 µg/dl as compared with 1 µg/dl were 3.8, 5.3, 5.8, and 2.1 months, respectively, for breast development and 4.0, 5.5, 6.0, and 2.2 months, respectively, for pubic hair development; the associated delay in age at menarche was 3.6 months. In Caucasian girls, there were non-significant delays in all pubertal measures in association with a lead concentration of 3 µg/dl (Selevan et al., 2003).

6) Polycyclic aromatic hydrocarbons (PAHs) and smoking

Women who smoke have decreased fecundity and earlier menopause than non-smokers (Jick & Porter, 1977; Baird & Wilcox, 1985). Women whose mothers smoked while they were in utero also have reduced fecundity compared with women whose mothers did not smoke (Weinberg et al., 1989). Treatment of mice with PAHs, which are present in tobacco smoke, has long been known to cause dose-dependent destruction of oocytes (Mattison & Thorgeirsson, 1979). More recently, it has been appreciated that lower doses of PAHs, which cause limited oocyte depletion in adult mice, cause much greater oocyte depletion in the offspring when given to pregnant mice (Matikainen et al., 2002). Exposure to PAHs induces the expression of the gene BAX in oocytes, which is followed by apoptosis. This results in fewer oocytes at birth and premature ovarian failure. The same cascade can also be induced in human ovarian explants (Matikainen et al., 2001, 2002). In men whose mothers smoked tobacco while they were pregnant, reduced semen quality, smaller testis size, and reduced fecundability odds ratios have been observed (Jensen et al., 1998, 2005).

7) Atrazine

Peripubertal exposure to atrazine causes delayed vaginal opening in rats (Laws et al., 2000; Ashby et al., 2002), indicating delayed puberty. Studies examining the effect of both prenatal and lactational exposure to atrazine on pubertal indicators in rats have shown that in utero exposure can cause delays in the development of the mammary gland, whereas delayed vaginal opening seems to be mediated via lactational exposure (Rayner et al., 2004). Atrazine has been shown to alter serum LH and prolactin levels in female rats by changing hypothalamic control of these hormones (Cooper et al., 2000).

8) Alcohol

Consumption of alcohol during early adolescence has been linked to delays in the onset of female puberty. The response appears to be related to alcohol's effect on the function of IGF-1, which is synthesized in the liver and which is active in the brain to coordinate overall physical growth. Long-term consumption of alcohol inhibits the production of IGF-1, and short-term consumption of alcohol may alter IGF-1 function within the brain (Dees et al., 1998).

Developmental State–Specific Susceptibilities and Outcomes

4.3.3 Endocrine system

Section 3.6.4 describes the normal development of the endocrine system.

The diverse glands, hormones, and other chemical messengers that make up the endocrine system exert effects on virtually every organ system and cell within the body. Endocrine systems regulate metabolic, nutritional, reproductive, and behavioural processes, as well as growth, responses to stress, and the function of the digestive, cardiovascular, renal, and immune systems. Disruption of endocrine function can have severe health consequences in adults, and exposures that interfere with the development of the endocrine system during early life stages can have even more far-ranging consequences (Barr et al., 2000; Damstra et al., 2002). Like the other systems discussed in this chapter, the development of the endocrine system involves intricately orchestrated processes of cell proliferation, migration, and death, which, if disrupted, can lead to permanent consequences. In addition, programming of endocrine set-points is a unique aspect of endocrine system development, which is also susceptible to disruption. This section will discuss periods of susceptibility and consequences of exposures for non-reproductive components of the endocrine system. The endocrine regulation of reproduction and consequences of its disruption are discussed in chapter 3 and in section 4.3.2, respectively.

4.3.3.1 Periods of susceptibility

The endocrine glands have early windows of susceptibility during the embryonic period, when the glands first begin to develop. The later period of differentiation of the glands, which occurs mostly during the fetal period, constitutes another set of susceptible periods for the endocrine system. While homeostasis via feedback loops is central to the functioning of all endocrine systems, the set-points or narrow ranges within which the levels of hormones are regulated must first be programmed. The term programming generally describes a process whereby a stimulus or insult, when applied at a critical or sensitive period of development, results in a long-term or permanent effect on the structure or function of the organism. Importantly, it is during fetal/neonatal development that programming of the endocrine system occurs. Exposures to toxicants during this critical period of programming can result in permanent abnormalities in endocrine function.

In human embryos, weeks 4–8 of gestation, when the pancreatic buds first appear and then begin to proliferate, represent an early window of susceptibility for the pancreas (Sadler, 2000). Weeks 10–14 during the fetal period, when differentiation is occurring and alpha, beta, and delta cells of the endocrine pancreas appear, constitute another period of susceptibility during the development of the pancreas (Sadler, 2000) (Figure 8). The formation of distinct islets of endocrine cells occurs during the later fetal period, but the islets continue to grow and rearrange until about four years of age (Hellerstrom & Swenne, 1991). Similar stages of pancreatic development occur in mice during equivalent developmental periods, and much has been learned in recent years about the genes that control pancreatic development from knockout mice that have disruption of these genes (Figure 8).

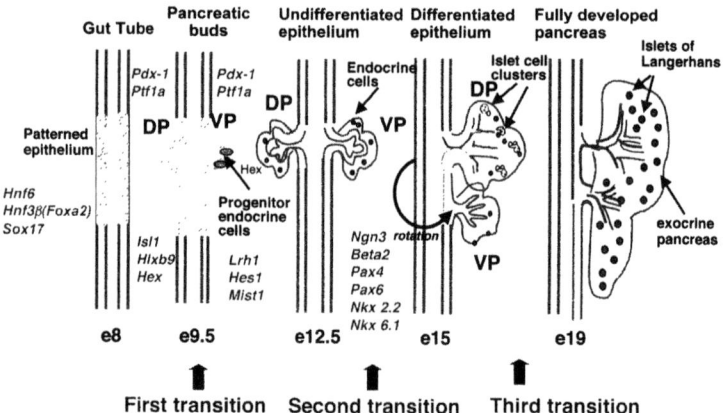

Fig. 8. Genes that control pancreatic development in mice. DP = dorsal pancreas; VP = ventral pancreas; e = embryonic day. [Figure reproduced from Habener et al. (2005) with permission from the Society for Endocrinology, Bristol, U.K.]

Evidence from epidemiological studies demonstrates that exposures during early life stages can impact susceptibility to diabetes and obesity later in life (Lau & Rogers, 2005). In particular, numerous studies have linked poor maternal nutrition with later risk for these adverse health outcomes. The Dutch Hunger Winter was a short defined period of famine; therefore, it has been possible both to assess the role of early nutrition in future susceptibility to disease and to identify critical time windows (G.P. Ravelli et al., 1976; A.C. Ravelli et al., 1998). It was shown that poor maternal nutrition, especially during the last trimester of pregnancy, was associated with poor glucose tolerance and insulin resistance in the offspring. In terms of obesity, individuals who were exposed to the famine during the first half of pregnancy were more obese at age 19. In contrast, those who were exposed to the famine during the last trimester of pregnancy and in early postnatal life had reduced obesity (Ravelli et al., 1976). This suggests that the critical time windows for increased risks of obesity and type 2 diabetes differ.

Studies of twins have been used to address the importance of the intrauterine environment in determining future susceptibility to type 2 diabetes and insulin resistance. The advantage of carrying out studies in monozygotic twins is that they are genetically identical and are not influenced by gestational age or sex. One such study was carried out on twin pairs in Denmark (Poulsen et al., 1997). Midwife-recorded birth weights were traced for middle-aged twin pairs (identified from the Danish Twin Register) who were discordant for type 2 diabetes. Birth weights were significantly lower in both diabetic monozygotic and diabetic dizygotic twins who had diabetic mothers compared with their non-diabetic co-twins (Poulsen et al., 1997). It was therefore concluded that a non-genetic (environmental) intrauterine factor (such as intrauterine malnutrition) played an important role in the development of type 2 diabetes much later in life. A second study in Italian twins has reported similar findings. In this study, both monozygotic and dizygotic twins with hyperinsulinaemia and/or hyperglycaemia during an oral glucose tolerance test were found to have significantly lower birth weights than their co-twins with normal glucose tolerance and normoinsulinaemia. They also had higher levels of triglycerides, total cholesterol, insulin, and C-peptide (Bo et al., 2000). In humans, migration of endodermal cells from the pharynx to the site of the future thyroid during weeks 5–6 of gestation constitutes an early period of susceptibility to disruption by chemicals, and the subsequent period of thyroid differentiation during weeks 8–9 of gestation constitutes a second window of susceptibility (Sadler, 2000). Fetal thyroid hormone synthesis begins by weeks 10–12 (Sadler, 2000) and is potentially susceptible to agents that affect thyroid hormone synthesis or metabolism.

In an attempt to understand the molecular basis of the relationship between early growth restriction and development of subsequent disease and to investigate the specific nutrients that may be involved, a number of animal models have been developed. Maternal protein restriction, maternal caloric restriction, maternal high fat feeding, and maternal anaemia have all been shown to result in features of the metabolic syndrome in the offspring (reviewed in Ozanne, 2001). The phenotypic outcomes of these different insults have been remarkably similar, suggesting that these act through a common pathway. Elevation of glucocorticoid levels in the fetus has been suggested as a key element of this common pathway (Philips et al., 1998; Lau & Rogers, 2005).

Thyroid hormones are essential for normal central nervous system development. They play roles in neuronal and glial proliferation and migration, in neuronal outgrowth and myelination, and in the development of the dopaminergic and cholinergic neuronal systems. The developing central nervous system is sensitive to disruption of thyroid homeostasis throughout the embryonic and fetal periods and continuing through early postnatal life, as demonstrated by studies of infants whose mothers were hypothyroid during pregnancy or who themselves have congenital hypothyroidism. Maternal hypothyroidism, which causes inadequate levels of thyroid hormone to the embryo/fetus prior to the onset of fetal thyroid hormone secretion, causes lowered IQ, poor word discrimination, decreased reading comprehension, and learning deficits (Haddow et al., 1999). Congenital hypothyroidism, if untreated, causes late disappearance of infantile reflexes, delayed acquisition of acquired reflexes, speech and learning disorders, spasticity or hypotonia, and tremors (Porterfield & Hendry, 1998). Even when treated from an early age, children born with congenital hypothyroidism display increased learning and behavioural disorders, as well as impaired memory, spatial perception, and fine motor coordination (Porterfield & Hendry, 1998). Even more severe effects are observed when both mother and fetus are hypothyroid, once common in parts of the world that lacked adequate iodine in the diet, causing endemic cretinism. These children have deaf-mutism, spasticity, gait disturbances, complete or partial inability to stand, and profound mental retardation (Porterfield & Hendry, 1998).

Developmental State–Specific Susceptibilities and Outcomes

1) Periods of susceptibility during pituitary gland development

   An early period of susceptibility for the pituitary gland occurs during weeks 4–9 of gestation in humans, when Rathke's pouch from the embryonic oral cavity grows up to form the anterior pituitary and the infundibulum, while a downgrowth from the floor of the diencephalon forms the posterior pituitary. Weeks 8–13 of gestation, when the differentiation of the five cell types that form the anterior pituitary occurs, constitute another period of susceptibility. Corticotropes, which secrete adrenocorticotropic hormone, appear at 8 weeks; thyrotropes, which secrete thyroid stimulating hormone, somatotropes, which secrete growth hormone, and lactotropes, which secrete prolactin, all appear at 11 weeks of gestation. Gonadotropes, which secrete LH and FSH, appear at 12–13 weeks of gestation (Sadler, 2000).

2) Periods of susceptibility during adrenal development

   In humans, the adrenal cortex is sensitive to disruption by environmental chemicals during gestational weeks 5–8, when mesoderm from the urogenital ridge proliferates to form the embryonic adrenal cortex, which develops both a fetal zone that regresses during the neonatal period and a definitive zone (Sadler, 2000; Hammer et al., 2005). A second period of susceptibility occurs during week 12 of gestation, when the adrenal medulla begins to differentiate, a process that is completed 12–18 months after birth (Sadler, 2000). The definitive zones of the adrenal cortex do not begin to differentiate until 7–8 months after birth in humans, constituting another critical window for the cortex; however, the adrenal cortex does not fully reach its adult form until puberty (Figure 9) (Sadler, 2000). While many of the same genes appear to regulate adrenal development in mice and other laboratory animal species and in humans, the pattern of adrenal development differs between mice and humans (as shown in Figure 9). Mice are born with less developed adrenal glands compared with humans. The mouse X-zone (analogous to the human fetal zone) appears 10–14 days after birth. In male mice, the X-zone degenerates at puberty, whereas in females, it regresses during the first pregnancy (Hammer et al., 2005).

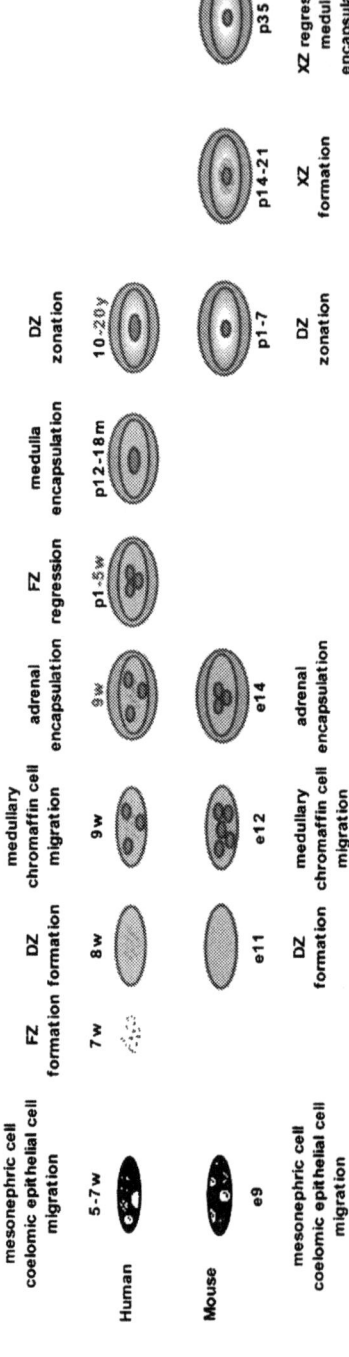

Fig. 9. Comparison of adrenal gland development in humans and mice. Abbreviations: w, weeks; m, months; y, years; e, embryonic; p, postnatal; FZ, fetal zone; DZ, definitive zone; XZ, X zone (from Hammer et al., 2005)

Cortisol production by the fetal adrenal gland is critical for maturation of the lungs, glycogen production in the liver, and synthesis of enzymes in the brain, pancreas, and gut (Sadler, 2000). Fetal stress has been associated with increased size of the fetal adrenal cortex (Barr et al., 2000) and with increased glucocorticoid hormone levels, leading to permanent reprogramming of the hypothalamic–pituitary–adrenal axis (Lau & Rogers, 2005). Since the adrenal cortex continues to develop until puberty, one might expect that the susceptibility to exposures would extend into the neonatal and childhood periods. In the rat, maternal grooming behaviour towards her pups during the neonatal period profoundly affects the pups' ability to deal with stress later in life. Pups whose mothers groomed and licked them intensively as neonates retained methylation of a portion of the promoter region of the glucocorticoid receptor gene that binds the Egr-1 transcription factor (Gilbert, 2005). As adults, these pups had more glucocorticoid receptors in the hippocampal region of the brain and were better able to respond to stress (Gilbert, 2005).

3) Consequences of alterations in growth hormone and glucocorticoid signalling

Congenital failure of growth hormone/somatotropin synthesis and secretion causes dwarfism, whereas oversecretion causes gigantism. Less severe perturbations of growth hormone and of the hypothalamic–pituitary–adrenal axis during development have been linked to the development of osteoporosis later in life. The long bones have their most rapid period of growth during the second trimester of pregnancy. The main adaptive response to a lack of nutrients and oxygen during this period of growth is to slow the rate of cell division. This results in permanent reduction in peak skeletal proportions attained later in life. Thus, several studies have shown that body weight in infancy is positively associated with adult bone mass (Cooper et al., 1997). Low rate of childhood growth has been associated with increased risk of hip fracture later in life (Cooper et al., 2002; Javaid & Cooper, 2002). Experiments in rats, mice, sheep, and pigs have also demonstrated that protein or caloric restriction of the mother during pregnancy and lactation is associated with smaller offspring that have lower bone mineral content and bone area in adulthood (Cooper et al., 2002; Javaid & Cooper, 2002). The effects of birth weight and weight in infancy on the pathogenesis of osteoporosis appear to be mediated by effects on growth hormone and cortisol in these individuals, who have lower basal levels of growth hormone and elevated cortisol, as well as increased rates of bone loss, in late adult life (Fall et al., 1998; Dennison et al., 1999). Offspring of female rats maintained on low-protein diets have reduced bone marrow alkaline phosphatase activity and reduced responsiveness to growth hormone, IGF-1, and vitamin D (Cooper et al., 2002).

Vitamin D deficiency during childhood leads to the disease rickets, a disorder of mineralization of the bone matrix that involves both the epiphysis (growth plate) and newly formed bone. Children with rickets commonly develop a bowed deformity of the legs, as well as deformities of the back, skull, and sternum. Evidence of a gene–environment interaction has been observed for the vitamin D receptor. The relationship between lumbar spine bone mineral density and vitamin D receptor genotype varies according to birth weight. Among individuals in the lowest third of birth weight distribution, spine bone mineral density is higher in individuals with vitamin D receptor genotype "BB". In contrast, individuals with this genotype in the highest third of birth weight distribution have reduced spine bone mineral density (Keen et al., 1997).

4) Consequences of disruption of hypothalamic regulation of pituitary prolactin secretion

Maternal prolactin via the milk is required for normal development of the tuberoinfundibular neuronal system of the hypothalamus during the neonatal period in rats (Shyr et al., 1986). Blocking the suckling-induced rise in maternal prolactin levels causes abnormal tuberoinfundibular function, with decreased inhibition by dopamine of prolactin secretion in the offspring later in life. The resulting chronically elevated prolactin levels cause prostatitis in the male offspring (Tangbanluekal & Robinette, 1993).

4.3.3.2 Consequences of exposures

The consequences of chemical disruption of the development of the endocrine system or of endocrine function during early life have only begun to be explored (Damstra et al., 2002; Dietert et al., 2002). Importantly, exposures during gestation or childhood may not manifest immediately. In some cases, the latency period between exposure and effect may be years. Some examples of environmental chemicals and other environmental factors that are known to affect the human endocrine, metabolic, and cardiovascular systems with developmental consequences are discussed in this section.

A number of environmental chemicals alter thyroid homeostasis. In animal models, many polyhalogenated aromatic hydrocarbons, such as dioxins and PCBs, suppress levels of thyroxine (T4) and triiodothyronine (T3) by upregulating metabolic enzymes, leading to increased glucuronidation and excretion of these hormones (Brouwer et al., 1998). In rats, PCB exposure during gestation has been shown to increase enzymatic activity of type II thyroxine 5'-deiodinase in fetal brain (Brouwer et al., 1998). This is likely a compensatory response to decreased circulating levels of T4, as this enzyme converts T4 to T3, the more active form. Hydroxylated metabolites of PCBs also inhibit binding of T4 to the serum binding protein transthyretin, resulting in increased availability of free T4 for metabolism (Brouwer et al., 1998; Cheek et al., 1999). Transthyretin binding of PCB metabolites has been shown in animal studies to result in increased transport of these compounds from the maternal to the fetal compartment and to the fetal brain (Brouwer et al., 1998). There is concern that alterations in thyroid hormone signalling by these compounds during fetal and neonatal life could disrupt central nervous system development. There have been several long-term epidemiological studies of the neurobehavioural effects of in utero exposure to PCBs. Some of these studies have found significant associations between PCB exposure and cognitive and behavioural deficits, while others have not (NRC, 1999; Winneke et al., 2002; Jacobson & Jacobson, 2003). Thus far, there have been few studies that have directly linked neurobehavioural effects of exposure to polyhalogenated hydrocarbons to disruption of thyroid hormone signalling. One example is a study that showed that low-frequency hearing loss caused by developmental exposure of rats to PCBs could be partially reversed by replacement of T4 (Goldey & Crofton, 1998).

Perchlorates, which inhibit iodine uptake by the thyroid gland, reducing T4 and T3 synthesis, constitute another class of environmental chemicals that affect thyroid function. In the past, high doses of these compounds were used to treat hyperthyroidism. In recent years, there has been concern that contamination of drinking-water supplies with perchlorates from industrial sites could suppress fetal thyroid hormone synthesis, disrupting central nervous system development. Several ecologic studies have addressed this issue, with some finding increased rates of congenital hypothyroidism in communities with detectable perchlorate levels in the drinking-water (Brechner et al., 2000) and others observing no such difference (Lamm & Doemland, 1999; Kelsh et al., 2003). Clarification of this issue awaits the results of additional studies.

Several environmental exposures have been associated with poor growth and increased risk of diabetes, osteoporosis, and hypertension later in life. Lead poisoning in children causes poor growth and abnormal bone structure. The mechanism is thought to be interference by lead with the metabolism of 25-hydroxycholecalciferol to the active form of vitamin D, 1,25-dihydroxycholecalciferol (Osterloh, 1991). Maternal smoking and poor nutrition during pregnancy are associated with reduced neonatal bone mineral content, presumably via effects on fetal nutrient supply and subsequent bone accretion (Cooper et al., 2002). There is also direct evidence that poor maternal nutrition (Ravelli et al., 1998) and maternal smoking (Montgomery & Ekbom, 2002) cause both a reduction in birth weight and subsequent loss of glucose tolerance. Adult humans exposed to dioxins have increased risk of diabetes, hyperinsulinaemia, and abnormal glucose tolerance (Henriksen et al., 1997; Michalek et al., 1999). In contrast, exposure to dioxins causes hypoinsulinaemia and hypoglycaemia in adult rats and rabbits (Gorski & Rozman, 1987; Ebner et al., 1988). Unfortunately, the effects of exposure to dioxins during early life stages on glucose homeostasis and the risk of developing diabetes have not been studied in humans or animals. Low-birth-weight individuals also have increased risk of developing hypertension later in life. It has been suggested that reduced growth of the kidneys during gestation, leading to a decreased number of nephrons, may be a causal factor (Brenner et al., 1988). The reduction of the filtration area leads to systemic hypertension via sodium retention and subsequent increased extracellular fluid volume. These cause increased cardiac output, total peripheral resistance, and, thus, increased arterial blood pressure. This leads to increased glomerular capillary pressure and glomerular sclerosis, exacerbating the reduced surface area. From this, it can be seen that individuals who suffer poor conditions in utero could be more susceptible to hypertension, as they already have a reduced number of nephrons.

The herbicide atrazine suppresses pituitary prolactin secretion in adult rats and suppresses suckling-induced increases in prolactin secretion in lactating rats by stimulating hypothalamic dopamine secretion (Stoker et al., 1999; Cooper et al., 2000). By altering prolactin secretion in the mother, atrazine exposure during lactation causes elevated prolactin levels in the male offspring at puberty (Stoker et al., 1999). Subsequently, these males develop persistent inflammatory changes in the lateral prostate (Stoker et al., 1999).

4.3.4 Cardiovascular system

Section 3.6.5 describes the normal development of the cardiovascular system.

The cardiovascular system is, out of necessity, the first of the organ systems to develop. The heart itself forms from a primordium from mainly splanchnic mesoderm (Kaufman & Navaratnam, 1981) and begins as a tubular structure that becomes a four-chambered structure after looping and septation. The development of a primary vascular plexus begins by the differentiation of precursor cells into endothelial cells that, after proliferation, cluster and form long extending endothelial processes. This primitive plexus outgrows into a complex network by the process of angiogenesis (Carmeliet, 2000). These processes require a variety of growth factors, genes, and transcription factors, including vascular endothelial growth factor, transforming growth factor-beta (TGF-β), ephrins, and integrins (Risau, 1998). However, these do not exclusively control the process; both haemodynamic and metabolic factors can also alter the development of the cardiovascular system. Hypoxia acts via the redistribution of cardiac output to cause "brain sparing" (Cohn et al., 1974). This results from an increase in peripheral sympathetic outflow as well as catecholamine release. The process of generating arteries is by no means completed by the formation of the endothelial tube. Cells from the mesenchyme differentiate into vascular smooth muscle cells, and this process is controlled by a different set of growth factors (Hellstrom et al., 1999). The thickness of the vascular smooth muscle cells is linked with cardiovascular disease and may continue to change in early postnatal life.

4.3.4.1   Periods of susceptibility

The most susceptible period of prenatal development of the heart occurs between weeks 2 and 8 in humans. Congenital cardiac anomalies occur in about 5 in 1000 to 1 in 8000 live births, and one third of these are severe (Kirby, 1997). The proportion of cardiac anomalies that are primarily of environmental origin is unknown. The most frequent types of defects are intraventricular septal defects, coarctation of the aorta, transposition of the great vessels, and tetralogies. Because of the significant changes in blood distribution at birth (closing of the foramen ovale and ductus arteriosus, which shunts blood to the lungs of the newborn), changes in cardiac development resulting from prenatal exposures do not manifest until the neonatal period. During this transition to neonatal life, there is also a progression of functional changes, which include decreasing pulmonary vascular resistance, increasing pulmonary blood flow, increasing volume of the left atrium, and increasing systemic vascular resistance (O'Rahilly & Muller, 1992).

4.3.4.2   Consequences of exposures

In experimental animal models, developmental cardiac anomalies have been associated with a broad spectrum of agents and altered metabolic conditions. For example, cardiomegaly is induced by thyroid hormone, carbon monoxide, and monocrotaline; cardiac glycosides and catecholamines produce arrhythmogenic effects; and agents that affect the plasma osmolality, such as mirex, trypan blue, and 2-methoxymethanol, induce characteristic changes in the fetal electrocardiogram (Lau & Kavlock, 1994). There is evidence from mechanistically oriented experimental studies that malformations and other effects in the fetus induced by antihypertensive, antiarrhythmic, and sympathomimetic drugs are secondary to haemodynamic alterations causing fetal hypoxia rather than direct effects on the heart (Danielsson & Webster, 1997). However, as the chronotropic (rate) and inotropic (contractile force) responses of the heart are regulated by the autonomic nervous system and as adrenergic innervation in particular has been implicated in controlling growth and development of the cardiac muscle, direct or indirect changes in adrenergic tone during critical periods can produce long-lasting effects in the cellular development of the myometrium. In experimental animal models, several factors that alter adrenergic tone have been known to influence the prenatal maturation of the heart, including hormones (thyroid and glucocorticoid), therapeutic drugs (opiates and antihypertensives), and environmental compounds (e.g. mercury). This period of susceptibility also extends into the neonatal period in experimental animals (Lau & Kavlock, 1994). For instance, Meyer et al. (2004) studied the immediate and long-term effects of exposure of neonatal rats to the organophosphate pesticide chlorpyrifos on gestation days 9–12 and 17–20 or postnatal days 1–4 and 11–14. Cardiac responses were measured by pharmacological challenge of adenylyl cyclase activity with forskolin, isoproteronol, and glucagons. Effects were most prominent in adulthood, with exposure of the three earlier stages the most effective. Interestingly, the effects on cell signalling pathways did not appear to be related to the inhibition of acetylcholinesterase, the pesticidal mode of action of chlorpyrifos (Song et al., 1997).

There are suggestions that environmental contaminants can affect cardiac development in humans. The effects of ambient air pollution (carbon monoxide, nitrogen dioxide, ozone, and PM_{10}) on the risk of cardiac malformations were evaluated using the California Birth Defect Monitoring Program in Southern California, USA, between 1987 and 1993 (Ritz et al., 2002). The odds ratio for a ventricular septal defect increased with increasing concentration of carbon monoxide during the second month of pregnancy. For the fourth quartile of exposure, the odds ratio was 2.95 (95% CI 1.44–6.05). Ritz et al. (2002) also observed increased risks for aortic artery and valve defects during the second month of pregnancy.

4.3.5 Immune system

Section 3.6.6 describes the normal development of the immune system.

The development of the immune system as it relates to comparative developmental toxicology has been considered in several publications over the last decade (Barnett, 1996; Dietert et al., 2000; Holladay & Smialowicz, 2000; Chapin, 2002; Holladay & Blaylock, 2002; Holsapple, 2002; Holsapple et al., 2003; Luster et al., 2003; Luebke et al., 2004). Immune development is a dynamic process involving cellular proliferation, migration, recognition, selection, apoptosis, clonal expansion, dissemination to peripheral sites, and, finally, cell cooperation and function. Because many of the changes require exquisitely timed differentiation events occurring in more than one site, there is ample opportunity for environmental interventions that can alter, delay, or abrogate specific elements of immune development. Environmentally induced events altering immune development can be directed at immune cells. However, immunotoxic changes can also arise if the physiological microenvironment necessary to promote immune cell maturation is modified through environmental exposure. An example of the latter would be perinatal changes in immune function linked to the thyroid–immune axis (Rooney et al., 2003). Obviously, such indirect changes could include the endocrine, neurological, hepatic, or lymphoid organ supporting tissues. Operationally, one may need to consider only the relative developmental stage of toxicant exposure and the potential for serious outcomes later in life. Mechanistically, however, it is useful to understand the potential for both direct immune cell insult and indirect developmental alterations in supportive non-immune tissues, such as thymic stroma, bone marrow, and reticuloendothelial cell components that contribute to immune cell development. Ironically, potentially subtle or transitory changes in these non-lymphoid cells, if occurring at a critical time of immune development, might produce severe and prolonged immunotoxicity. From a risk assessment perspective, it is helpful if those windows of greatest immune system susceptibility can be identified.

4.3.5.1   Periods of susceptibility

If one examines immune development, there are specific functionally distinct windows during which the immune system might be expected to have different susceptibilities based on critical biological events. By defining functionally distinct immune developmental windows, it is possible to make direct comparisons of differential immunotoxic susceptibilities using exposure assessment.

The immune "windows", along with developmental windows for the respiratory system, were identified at a workshop sponsored by the USEPA and the March of Dimes (see Dietert et al., 2000; Holladay & Smialowicz, 2000; Landreth, 2002). They include 1) initiation of haematopoiesis, 2) migration and expansion of stem cell populations, 3) colonization events, including bone marrow colonization, pre–T cell seeding to the thymus, T cell education, T cell repertoire establishment, then seeding of the periphery by mature T cells, 4) acquisition of immunocompetence, and, finally, 5) the capacity to develop immunological memory. While the exact placement of these five "immunological boxes" on a gestational/perinatal timeline would differ between rodents and humans, the sequence of immune developmental events is similar (Figure 10). This approach of carving up development into distinct segments, or boxes, for direct sensitivity testing would seem to offer advantages that are not restricted solely to the immune system. Recently, additional developmental immune windows have been described that emphasize heightened perinatal susceptibilities (Dietert & Piepenbrink, 2005).

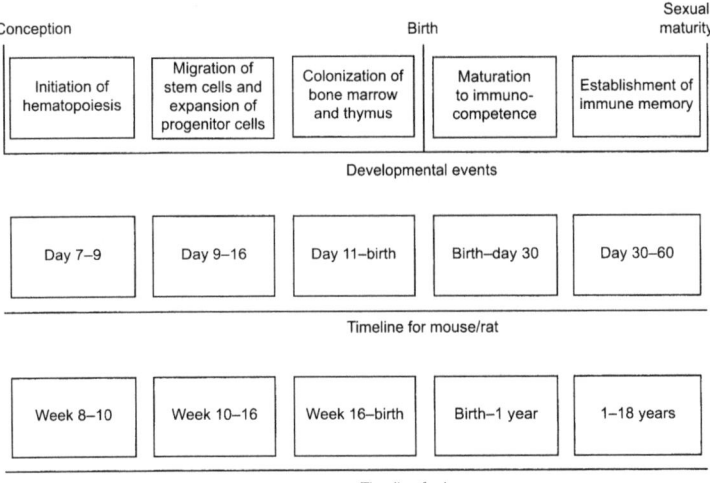

Fig. 10. Timeline for mouse/rat and human for developmental events indicating functionally distinct immune developmental windows (from Dietert et al., 2000).

Exposure to a low level of an immunotoxicant during these different immune developmental windows might be expected to produce different outcomes. This is based on such factors as the specific target cells present at the time of exposure, the cellular interactions in progress during exposure, the dependency on cell proliferation or migration, and the extent to which immunotoxic damage might be contained or possibly reversed after environmental insult. As is discussed below, the limited data available to date suggest that the developmental timing of exposure is critical in determining the nature and extent of environmentally induced immune alteration.

One of the tenets of early immune development that has emerged in recent years is the apparent differential timeline for the development of certain immune capacities. In particular, several investigators have proposed that T helper 2 (Th2)–driven capacity is the earliest to form during ontogeny, whereas T helper 1 (Th1)–dependent functions emerge in later development (Peden, 2000; Bellanti et al., 2003). The implication of this differential timeline is that Th2-associated capacity is a likely default function, with useful immune balance being achieved when Th1 capacity can develop fully. If environmental exposures delay, impair, or reduce the efficiency of timely Th1 development, then the neonate and potential subsequent life stages might face a skewed immune capacity towards Th2-driven functions. This could result in an increased risk of allergy and atopy as well as certain types of autoimmunity at the expense of protective antiviral and antitumour Th1-driven responses (Bellanti et al., 2003). Therefore, chemical exposures that interfere with optimum Th1 maturation could leave the individual at increased risk for diseases requiring effective Th1-driven immune function. Additionally, some allergic and autoimmune conditions exacerbated by overzealous Th2 function could become prevalent in segments of the population experiencing chemically induced Th1 depression. Neonatal production capacity for interleukin 12 may be a factor in juvenile Th1/Th2 balance among responses (Prescott et al., 2003). The status of the maternal system appears to be an important risk factor for allergic disease, at least within some subpopulations. Maternal stress has been identified as a contributing factor to altered T cell differentiation and potential risk of postnatal allergic disease (Von Hertzen, 2002). This suggests that fetal and perinatal environmental exposures may not need to target the immune system directly to disrupt subsequent T cell–associated immune capabilities. Several studies on endocrine disrupting gestational exposures support this likelihood (Walker et al., 1999; Karpuzoglu-Sahin et al., 2001; Dietert et al., 2003). Furthermore, some early environmental exposures during specific windows of gestation appear to result in unexpected physiological responses when the juvenile or adult offspring encounters postnatal stressors (Karpuzoglu-Sahin et al., 2001; Lee et al., 2002).

An additional component of the T helper balance issue is a postnatal concern known as the "hygiene hypothesis". This states, in its purest form, that exposure of the neonatal immune system to certain infectious agents and/or their immunostimulatory components (such as lipopolysaccharide of Gram-negative bacteria) is an important component of immune maturation and may be necessary for appropriate Th1 development (Strachan, 1989, 1999; Cremonini & Gasbarrini, 2003). However, other researchers dispute the "hygiene hypothesis" in favour of a tenet that it is the development of robust anti-inflammatory responses early in life that helps protect against or minimize allergic disorders (Yazdanbakhsh et al., 2002).

4.3.5.2 *Consequences of exposures*

Numerous toxicants have been reported to alter the immune response capabilities and health outcomes following early exposure. The majority of these appear to alter thymus-associated T cell development and/or T cell–dependent functions. However, changes are not restricted to T cell function, and some, like the pesticide chlordane, target other immune cell lineages (Theus et al., 1992; Blyler et al., 1994). Even in the case of the heavy metal lead, most notably known as a T cell toxin, early fetal exposure seems directed more against macrophages than against T cells (Bunn et al., 2001a; Lee et al., 2001). Therefore, for some chemicals, it may be useful to specify the primary immune target of toxic exposure in the context of developmental life stages.

As might be expected, the outcomes of early life stage–induced immunotoxicity take several forms. T cell–dependent functions are frequently impaired, and these alterations may be more persistent than with similar adult toxicant exposure (Dietert et al., 2003; Luebke et al., 2004). The heightened sensitivity of T cell–dependent function to early-life immunotoxicant exposure may be linked to the dramatic reversal of T helper balance and changes in dendritic cell maturation that occur before and after birth (reviewed in Dietert & Piepenbrink, 2005). This can lead to increased susceptibility to both infectious diseases and cancer. Additionally, asthma, atopy, and some forms of autoimmunity may be at an increased risk based on specific cell-mediated immune changes. Sex differences have been seen following certain exposures (Blyler et al., 1994; Chapin et al., 1997; Bunn et al., 2000, 2001b,c). Little is known at present about the impact of early toxicant exposure on the onset and rate of immune senescence.

While the database for developmental immunotoxicants is relatively modest, several chemicals have received considerable research attention. For example, Luebke et al. (2004), in a report to the USEPA, reviewed the comparative age-related sensitivities of the human and rodent immune systems for four developmental immunotoxicants: DES, lead, diazepam, and tributyltin. These authors concluded that DES, a strong estrogenic compound, produced similar immune alterations at similar doses following exposure of adult rodents and embryos or neonates. However, the immune changes persisted following early exposure, whereas adults appeared to be able to recover post-exposure.

With the heavy metal lead, the evidence suggests that rodent fetuses are sensitive to lower doses of lead than are required to produce adult immune alterations. Immunotoxicity is persistent following early exposure, and, depending upon the timing (the critical window) of exposure, different combinations of juvenile and adult immune changes will result. Immune sensitivities appear to be comparable to those reported for the neurological system (Canfield et al., 2003; Dietert et al., 2003). Rodent data suggest that early exposures to lead (producing blood lead levels of <8 µg/dl at or near birth) are associated with subsequent immunotoxicity (Snyder et al., 2000; Bunn et al., 2001b; Dietert et al., 2003; Luebke et al., 2004). Furthermore, in rats, lead exposure from mid-gestation appears to reduce Th1 capabilities, skewing immune responses towards Th2 (Heo et al., 1997; Miller et al., 1998; Bunn et al., 2001c; Dietert & Lee, 2004; Dietert et al., 2004). This would be expected to increase the risk of allergy and asthma while decreasing certain antiviral and antitumour responses. Additionally, changes in autoimmune responses have been reported (Bunn et al., 2000). There is an immune developmental period in which the capacity of low-level lead exposure to modulate T cell response in the offspring appears to be the greatest. This period of increased sensitivity (compared with adult-induced immunotoxicity) corresponds to the developmental period during which stem cells migrate, progenitor cell populations expand, and the bone marrow and thymus are colonized (Dietert et al., 2000; Landreth, 2002).

Developmental State–Specific Susceptibilities and Outcomes

In a study on diazepam, a drug in the benzodiazepine family, Luebke et al. (2004) concluded that late gestational and early neonatal exposure of rodents produced severe immunosuppression at lower doses than were required for similar effects in adults. Furthermore, the cellular and humoral immunosuppression following fetal and neonatal exposures was persistent, whereas the adult-induced immunosuppression appeared to be short-lived. With the organotin wood preservative compounds found in some paints (tributyltin oxide and tributyltin chloride), the results appeared to be similar (Luebke et al., 2004). The tributyltin compounds appear to target the thymus, producing thymic atrophy and widespread immunosuppression in rodents with exposure at sufficient doses. However, the doses required for adult-induced suppression appear to be significantly greater than those found to produce immunosuppression after perinatal exposure (Smialowicz et al., 1989).

2,3,7,8-Tetrachlorodibenzo-p-dioxin (TCDD) is another important developmental immunotoxicant that has been extensively examined in animal models (Vos & Moore, 1974; Faith & Moore, 1977). TCDD can target very early precursor T cells in the bone marrow (Fine et al., 1989), cause profound atrophy of the thymus (Gehrs et al., 1997; Gehrs & Smialowicz, 1999), inhibit thymocyte maturation (when given during gestation) (Holladay et al., 1991; Blaylock et al., 1992), persistently depress T cell–dependent immune responses, including delayed-type hypersensitivity (Gehrs & Smialowicz, 1999), and increase susceptibility to infectious diseases and tumour cells (Holladay & Smialowicz, 2000). It appears not only that early life stages are more sensitive to lower doses than are adults (at least in rodents), but that early exposure produces more persistent immunosuppression (Holladay et al., 1991; Gehrs & Smialowicz, 1999; Holladay & Smialowicz, 2000). Smialowicz (2002) discussed the capacity of TCDD to suppress the delayed-type hypersensitivity response following perinatal (Gehrs & Smialowicz, 1997, 1999; Gehrs et al., 1997) compared with adult (Fan et al., 1996) exposure. He concluded that placental plus lactation exposure were the most sensitive exposure windows for delayed-type hypersensitivity depression in the rat and that the differential age-related sensitivity for TCDD exposure is greater than two orders of magnitude for this delayed-type hypersensitivity suppression.

Two organochlorine pesticides have also been evaluated in animal models using early life stage exposures. Methoxychlor (Chapin et al., 1997) and heptachlor (Smialowicz et al., 2001) were evaluated for immunotoxicity after perinatal plus juvenile exposure of rats. In the case of methoxychlor, T cell–dependent antibody responses were depressed persistently in males but not females (Chapin et al., 1997). For heptachlor, early exposure of Sprague-Dawley rats, using doses relevant to human exposure, produced persistent impairment of antibody responses in males but not females. No adult-exposure immunotoxicity was observed at the doses examined, suggesting that there is an increased susceptibility of the prenatal and/or early postnatal life stages to this pesticide (Smialowicz et al., 2001; Smialowicz, 2002).

Two recent studies have reported on the immune effects of exposure to PCBs and DDE in humans (Dewailly et al., 2000; Dallaire et al., 2004). In both of these studies, Inuit infants were recruited and followed during the first year of life for the occurrence of infections of various kinds. This population has high exposure to PCBs and other organochlorines because of their high consumption of carnivorous fish and marine mammals. Various PCBs and DDE were measured in cord blood and/or maternal plasma at delivery (Dewailly et al., 2000; Dallaire et al., 2004) and in the infants' blood at follow-up (Dallaire et al., 2004). In both studies, the risk of otitis media during the first year of life increased with increasing prenatal exposure to PCBs and DDE (Dewailly et al., 2000; Dallaire et al., 2004), although most of the associations did not reach statistical significance. In the latter study, the risk of all infections combined was significantly increased with increasing prenatal PCB level (Dallaire et al., 2004).

In summary, early life stage exposure to environmental hazards can produce significant and persistent immunotoxicity. For some chemicals, adult-induced immunotoxicity has not been observed, or the effect is transitory. Consequences following early exposure can include increased susceptibility to infectious disease and cancer, increased risk for asthma and atopy, and an increase in some forms of autoimmune disease. For some chemicals, sex differences have been noted, and the developing immune system may have greater than an order of magnitude difference in dose sensitivity compared with the adult immune system. Additionally, evidence suggests that the expected outcome of exposure can differ depending upon the

Developmental State–Specific Susceptibilities and Outcomes

window of immune development when exposure occurs. Hence, the developmental status of the immune system during environmental insult is a key factor in determining the likely health risk.

4.3.6 Respiratory system

Section 3.6.7 describes the normal development of the respiratory system.

Many of the studies on the effects of chemical exposures on the growth and development of the lungs have been performed in experimental animals; however, patterns of lung development differ between animals and humans. Because of these differences, extreme care must be taken when extrapolating the results from animal studies to human situations.

4.3.6.1 Periods of susceptibility

The respiratory system has a number of critical windows of exposure and periods of susceptibility (Pinkerton & Joad, 2000). Lung development occurs through six stages: embryonic, pseudoglandular, canalicular, saccular, alveolar, and vascular maturation. The first four of these stages are complete during fetal development, and about 85% of alveoli are present in the human at birth, as shown in Figure 11 (Zoetis & Hurtt, 2003a). As lung development is a continuous process from embryo to adolescence, it is logical to surmise that children may be more susceptible to the effects of respiratory toxicants than adults, whose lung growth is complete. Alveoli number and lung surface area begin to level off between two and four years of age, whereas lung expansion continues up to eight years of age. Immature (neonatal) differentiating cells of the respiratory tract are more sensitive to injury following exposure to respiratory toxicants than mature cells, and at dose levels that cause no effects in adult cells (Plopper et al., 1994). Lung injury in the early postnatal period impairs cellular differentiating capacity and proliferation, producing abnormal postnatal lung growth and development in rabbits (Smiley-Jewell et al., 1998). Exposure of neonatal primates to oxidative insult (via ozone exposure) has been shown to impair the development of pulmonary gas exchange units and bronchioli (Tyler et al., 1988). Experimental studies in rats clearly defined the critical window of exposure to ETS as both the pre- and

EHC 237: Principles for Evaluating Health Risks in Children

postnatal periods (Joad et al., 1995, 1999). Clinical parallels are seen in studies of human infants born to smoking mothers, demonstrating reduced lung function in those exposed to ETS in utero and postnatally (Tager et al., 1983; Hanrahan et al., 1992).

Many studies try to distinguish between environmental exposures that induce disease in previously normal hosts and those that trigger exacerbations of pre-existing disease. From the above discussion, we contend that this is an artificial distinction and is more likely to result from the developmental phase of the host when the exposure took place rather than an intrinsic property of the exposure agent. More research has concentrated on relating environmental exposures to triggering exacerbations of respiratory disease, as this is technically easier. Studies designed to understand the role of environmental exposures in the induction of disease are more difficult, and longitudinal assessment of exposures and disease outcomes is required. Birth cohort studies are particularly powerful in this respect, but they are expensive and require a long-term commitment.

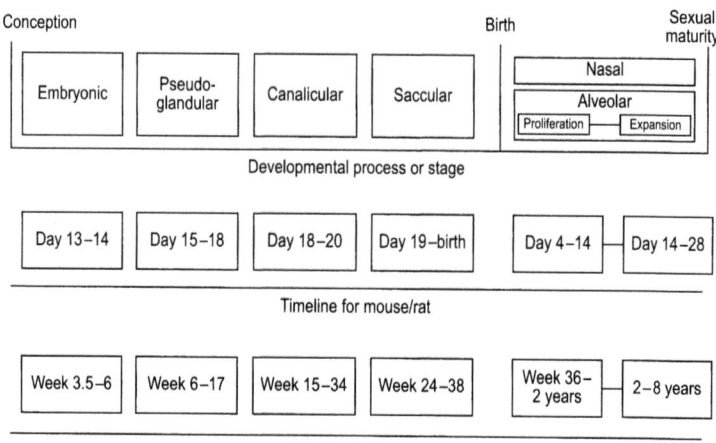

Fig. 11. Parallel timelines for development of the lung in mouse/rat and human (from Dietert et al., 2000).

4.3.6.2 Consequences of exposures

Air pollution, both outdoor and indoor, has been identified as a potential risk factor for both the initiation/induction and the exacerbation of respiratory diseases, especially asthma. Pollutants or irritants that may influence immune system development and the induction or exacerbation of respiratory diseases include:

- combustion-related products formed by the burning of organic fuels, including nitrogen dioxide, particulate matter, and diesel exhaust particulates;
- bioaerosols, including moulds, allergens, and bacterial products (e.g. lipopolysaccharide);
- air toxics, including formaldehyde and other volatile organic compounds (VOCs); and
- pesticides, PCBs, and heavy metals.

1) Indoor air

Indoor air is potentially the most important source of pollution affecting child respiratory health, given that children spend up to 90% of their time indoors and the large range of pulmonary irritants found in the home (Woodcock & Custovic, 1998). The burning of solid fuels (coal and wood) is a major source of indoor air pollution. Worldwide, approximately 50% of all households and 90% of rural households utilize solid fuels for heating or cooking (Smith & Mehta, 2003; WHO, 2004b). Infants and young children, in particular, have little control over their exposure to pollutants in the home environment and are vulnerable to the impact of adult activities (particularly ETS). Exposure to pollutants in the home environment in developed countries has increased with improved insulation and reduced ventilation and the use of chemical detergents and building or furnishing constituents that contain noxious pulmonary irritants. Common indoor air pollutants include nitrogen dioxide, formaldehyde and other VOCs, and ETS.

Studies examining the effect of indoor nitrogen dioxide on the respiratory health of children, although inconsistent, identify nitrogen dioxide as a potential hazard. The principal source of nitrogen dioxide in westernized homes is gas cooking and heating appliances, although combustion of unprocessed fuels such as wood and coal and tobacco smoke contribute to nitrogen dioxide exposure globally. The extensive use of gas appliances in homes suggests that large populations of children are at risk of exposure (IEH, 1995). Nitrogen dioxide levels have been associated with increased risk of cough and wheezy bronchitis in children (Dodge, 1982; Pershagen et al.,

1995), and rises in ambient nitrogen dioxide levels of 30 $\mu g/m^3$ are reported to increase the risk of respiratory illness in children by 20% (Hasselblad et al., 1992). Asthmatic children may be particularly susceptible to the effect of nitrogen dioxide, experiencing airflow limitation and increased use of inhalant therapy (Jarvis et al., 1998; Ng et al., 2001). Studies have linked indoor nitrogen dioxide levels to increased asthma risk and increased bronchial hyper-responsiveness in preschool children (Volkmer et al., 1995; Salome et al., 1996).

VOCs are components of household detergents, adhesives, and furnishings. Ambient levels of VOCs, including formaldehyde, have been linked to reported asthma in children (Krzyzanowski et al., 1990; Ware et al., 1993; Garrett et al., 1999; Rumchev et al., 2000, 2002). The weight of evidence currently available linking VOCs to ill-health in adults suggests that ambient levels found in homes are unlikely to cause adverse effects, but research focusing on the impact of VOCs on the respiratory health of children is sparse. Formaldehyde has been associated with increased prevalence of atopy (Garrett et al., 1999) and higher levels of specific immunoglobulin E (Wantke et al., 1996) in children. Formaldehyde, at levels typically encountered in homes in developed countries, is associated with airway inflammation in both healthy children (Franklin et al., 2000) and adults (Wieslander et al., 1997). Exposing animals to formaldehyde (200 $\mu g/m^3$) enhances sensitization to inhaled allergens (Riedel et al., 1996), an observation that supports the role of formaldehyde as a cofactor for postnatal Th2 boosting. A study by Lehmann et al. (2002) found that maternal exposure to VOCs was associated with increased Th2 cytokines (IL-4) and decreased Th1 cytokines (IFN-γ) in the cord blood of neonates.

ETS, which contains not only combustion-related pollutants but also a large number of air toxics and carcinogens, including particulate matter, nitrogen oxides, aldehydes, and oxygen free radicals that act as pulmonary irritants or ciliotoxins, is another important contributor to indoor air pollution. The effects of passive smoking begin in utero, where constituents of tobacco smoke, such as PAHs, nicotine, and carbon monoxide, cross the placenta and are concentrated in the fetal circulation (Perera et al., 1999). Fetal enzymatic pathways are immature and do not effectively detoxify and clear tobacco smoke, leading to an accumulation of toxic metabolites at a period of intense cellular differentiation and growth (Ruhle et al., 1995).

The potentially mutagenic effects of tobacco smoke may impair normal cellular division and differentiation in the respiratory tree, leading to reduced lung function and increased bronchial hyper-responsiveness (Collins et al., 1985; Young et al., 1991; Cook et al., 1998). Animal studies demonstrate histological changes, including hyperplasia of bronchial muscles and prematurity of lung tissues in the fetal lung secondary to the effects of in utero exposure to tobacco smoke (Neslon et al., 1999). The decreased lung function and increased bronchial hyper-responsiveness observed in infants born to mothers who smoked in pregnancy may predispose infants to wheezing and lower respiratory tract illnesses (Tager et al., 1983, 1995; Hanrahan et al., 1992).

Prenatal and postnatal exposures to ETS are independently related to an increased risk of incident asthma (Strachan & Cook, 1998a; Cook & Strachan, 1999; Infante-Rivard et al., 1999). Parental smoking of more than 10 cigarettes per day increases the risk of asthma among children 2.5 times (Martinez et al., 1992) and may increase their risk of atopic sensitization in a dose–response pattern (Ronchetti et al., 1990; Braback et al., 1995). Major meta-analyses show that lower respiratory tract illness is up to 60% higher among children exposed to ETS during the first 18 months of life (NHMRC, 1997), and risks of chronic and recurrent otitis media are significantly increased (Strachan & Cook, 1998b).

Bioaerosols that have also been implicated in the development of asthma and other allergies include inhaled allergens (house dust mites and other insects, moulds, pets, pollens) and bacterial (lipopolysaccharide) and fungal (glucans) products. Sensitization to one or more common inhalant allergens is consistently associated with childhood asthma, especially in developed countries (Sporik & Platts-Mills, 2001). However, the relationship between exposure to inhaled allergens in early life and the development of asthma or wheeze in childhood is controversial (Burr et al., 1993; Sporik et al., 1995; Lau et al., 2000). Indeed, it seems that early exposure to some allergens may be protective of later development of asthma (Hesselmar et al., 1999) (see also discussion of the "hygiene hypothesis" in section 4.3.5). For example, some studies have found that exposure to lipopolysaccharides in early life protects against the development of allergy in children who have regular contact with farm animals compared with those without contact (von Mutius, 2002). Children raised in farming environments with livestock are exposed to very high levels of lipopolysaccharides (Gereda et al., 2000a). The mechanism for the protective effect of exposure to farm animals is thought to be via induction of Th1 immune responses (Gereda et al., 2000b). Interestingly, increased exposure to lipopolysaccharides in non-farming domestic environments has been associated with an increased risk of recurrent wheeze during the first year of life in children with a family history of allergy (Park et al., 2001); however, the levels of exposure are substantially less than those experienced by farmers' children. A recent study of rural Iowa children seems to contradict the "hygiene hypothesis" that early-life exposure to farm animals is protective against allergic diseases. Merchant and co-workers (2005) found that exposure to farm animals early in life was not protective against asthma. Those children living on farms that raised swine actually had significantly higher rates of diagnosed asthma and/or asthma symptoms compared with those not living on farms or those living on farms that did not raise swine (Merchant et al., 2005). These authors suggested that previous studies that considered only doctor-diagnosed asthma may have underestimated the true prevalence of asthma among farm children (Merchant et al., 2005).

Another source of exposure to pollutants in the indoor environment is via the combustion of biomass (such as dung, charcoal, wood, or crop residues) or coal. WHO estimates that, worldwide, approximately 50% of all households and 90% of rural households use such fuels for cooking or heating. Biomass fuel emissions include respirable particulates, carbon monoxide, nitrogen oxides, benzene, formaldehyde, 1,3-butadiene, and PAH compounds, such as benzo[*a*]pyrene. Women and young children are most heavily exposed to indoor air pollution from biomass combustion. Children under five years of age have been estimated to have a strong elevated risk of acute lower respiratory tract infections, particularly in developing countries. One example of such a study in India provided an elevated risk of 2.3-fold (WHO, 2004b).

2) Ambient air

There is a consistent body of evidence that exposure to ambient air pollution is associated with increased respiratory symptoms of cough, bronchitis, respiratory infection, and upper respiratory tract illness in children (Dockery et al., 1989; Raizenne et al., 1996;

Schwela, 2000). Although the effects of pollutants appear small, they occur at levels within the national ambient air quality standards of most countries and have the potential to affect large populations of children. Most studies attribute respiratory symptoms to particulate matter, although the close correlation of particulate matter levels with nitrogen dioxide and sulfur dioxide levels makes the contribution of individual pollutants difficult to determine. In Switzerland, moderate levels (below the national ambient air quality standards) of PM_{10}, sulfur dioxide, and nitrogen dioxide were associated with increased reporting of chronic cough and bronchitis (Braun-Fahrlander et al., 1997). This relationship was stronger among those children with a family history of asthma. An estimated relative risk for reported cough of 1.16 for every 20 $\mu g/m^3$ rise in PM_{10} was reported in Swiss preschool children (Braun-Fahrlander et al., 1992). Similar results were seen in a review of three cross-sectional surveys of children in the former German Democratic Republic between 1990 and 1998, with odds ratios for cough and bronchitis of 1.20 per 10 $\mu g/m^3$ increase in PM_{10} (Heinrich, 2003). The decline in pollution levels over this period was associated with an age-adjusted decrease in respiratory symptoms of bronchitis by 16%, cough by 1.2%, otitis media by 4%, and upper respiratory tract illness by 8%. This suggests that the respiratory symptoms caused by air pollution are potentially reversible (Heinrich, 2003). Pollutant exposure has also been linked to increased reporting of upper respiratory tract infection (Jaakkola et al., 1991; Heinrich, 2003). Ozone may cause a small increase in reported respiratory symptoms of cough and bronchitis at peak levels greater than 160 $\mu g/m^3$ (Braun-Fahrlander et al., 1997). Diesel exhaust emissions have been associated with increased reporting of cough and nonspecific respiratory symptoms in children (Nakatsuka et al., 1991; Nitta et al., 1993; Wjst et al., 1993; Oosterlee et al., 1996; Hirsch et al., 1999). Children living in close proximity to major freeways with high truck density experience increased cough, wheeze, and rhinitis (Van Vliet et al., 1997), and children less than two years of age may be the most vulnerable (Gehring et al., 2002).

Most of the literature to date on air pollution and asthma has concentrated on acute exacerbations resulting from environmental exposures. The role of environmental irritants in the induction of asthma is much less well understood. Various air pollutants can enhance allergic sensitization in animal models (Gilmour, 1995) and are thought to play an important adjuvant role in the development of asthma. Several studies have demonstrated that prenatal exposure to air pollutants has an effect on cytokine profiles in cord blood (Lehmann et al., 2002; Perera et al., 2003) and on the inflammatory effects in human airways (Parnia et al., 2002). Further research is required to elucidate the mechanisms by which environmental irritants modulate the development of asthma and atopy.

Oxidant gases such as nitrogen dioxide and ozone have also been studied with regards to their role in the development of asthma. Both of these gases have been associated with asthma exacerbations (Parnia et al., 2002), have increased airway responsiveness to inhaled allergens in asthmatic subjects (Jenkins et al., 1999), and can produce inflammatory changes in the airways (Davies & Devalia, 1993; Devalia et al., 1999). Asthmatic children exposed to exhaust emissions experience more symptoms and reduction in peak flow measurements and increased hospital admissions for asthma exacerbations (Wyler et al., 2000).

Acute exposure to ozone, nitrogen dioxide, sulfur dioxide, and particulate matter is known to cause transient reversible decreases in lung function (Vedal et al., 1998; Pekkanen et al., 1999). It is plausible that cumulative exposure to pollution throughout childhood could adversely affect airway maturation and therefore lung function. Reduced lung function in children and adolescents associated with chronic exposure to ozone (Kunzli et al., 1997) and particulate matter (Raizenne et al., 1996) has been shown, although studies are not consistent (Dockery et al., 1989; Roemer et al., 1999) and are limited by assumptions that measured ambient levels reflect personal exposure. Particulate matter, nitrogen dioxide, sulfur dioxide, and ozone (individually and synergistically) have been implicated in reductions in lung function capacity in children and adolescents. Expiratory flows, calculated from maximal forced expiratory manoeuvres (proxy measurements of large and small airway growth), appear primarily affected. For example, lung function, as measured by forced expiratory flow and volume, were reduced significantly in preadolescent children exposed to high levels of acid vapour and $PM_{2.5}$ in California, USA (Gauderman et al., 2002). Studies in Austria found a 2% reduction in forced vital capacity and FEV_1 (forced expiratory volume in 1 s) for every 20 µg/m^3 rise in ozone levels in seven-year-olds exposed to relatively low levels of ambient ozone (Horak et al., 2002) and large decrements in FEV_1

Developmental State–Specific Susceptibilities and Outcomes

(−84 ml per year) and FEF_{25-75} (forced expiratory flow between 25% and 75% of exhaled vital capacity; −329 ml per year) for every 10 µg/m^3 increase in PM_{10} in children exposed to particulate levels below the national ambient air quality standards in the United States. Increments in FEF growth rates in children have been observed upon relocation to residences with lower ambient pollution levels (Avol et al., 2001), again suggesting that the detrimental effect of pollution is potentially reversible. Reduced lung function among children living close to freeways has been described (Brunekreef et al., 1997). Personal exposure studies are required to confirm these findings and their clinical implications to determine whether lung function deficits persist into adulthood.

4.3.7 Kidney

Section 3.6.8 describes the normal development of the kidney.

4.3.7.1 Periods of susceptibility

As evident from the developmental sequence of ureteric bud outgrowth, induction, proliferation, and sculpting, the critical period for susceptibility of the developing kidney to toxicants is prolonged. Lau & Kavlock (1994) provided a representative list of renal teratogens and related critical periods for renal teratogenesis. In general, exposures during the time of early kidney development tend to cause the most severe structural and functional alterations, perhaps because they alter the earliest interactions and therefore have the most profound consequences on kidney development. Direct-acting cytotoxicants (e.g. chlorambucil) are very effective at disturbing development during periods of rapid cell proliferation, which occurs during induction of the anlagen. Alteration of differentiation of the ureteric epithelium or inhibition of breakdown of the ureteric membrane (e.g. by dioxin) can result in hydronephrosis. In the fetus, excessive disturbance of normal physiology due to pharmacological agents working on immature feedback can alter amniotic fluid production, with secondary consequences to the lungs. Guignard & Gouyon (1988) reviewed the effects of a variety of vasoactive or diuretic drugs, angiotensin converting enzyme inhibitors, and adrenergic agents and noted that several drugs used to treat sick, and often premature, infants also posed a risk of compromising renal function due to poorly developed feedback loops.

Alteration in trophic signals that regulate cell proliferation and differentiation during the rodent postnatal period (e.g. by methylmercury) can result in altered organ growth. Finally, direct effects on cell proliferation during histogenesis (e.g. by gentamicin) can also alter renal development. Because nephrogenesis continues postnatally in the rat, toxic insult during the neonatal period may still produce permanent developmental effects. For example, treatment with difluoromethylornithine (Gray & Kavlock, 1991) or gentamicin (Gilbert et al., 1987) reduces growth and differentiation of the kidney when given to newborn rats.

4.3.7.2 Consequences of exposures

A species comparison of the effects of angiotensin converting enzyme inhibition (Tabacova et al., 2003) is important to understanding why the human fetus suffers adverse consequences from exposure whereas rodent fetuses do not. The greater susceptibility of the human fetus to pharmacological agents such as enalapril and other angiotensin converting enzyme inhibitors is a function of the relative maturity of the kidney and the renin–angiotensin system, which are the specific targets during intrauterine development. In humans, these systems begin developing at the end of the first trimester, with continuing susceptibility throughout pregnancy. The timing is quite different in most animal species tested: these target systems develop close to birth and after the exposure period in standard developmental toxicity protocols has ended. At these later stages, these systems are relatively more mature and less susceptible to the pharmacological effects. For this reason, animal studies that follow standard protocols and evaluate developmental toxicity only for exposures during embryogenesis miss developmental effects arising secondary to disruption of target systems that develop after the period of major organogenesis. Thus, differences in the timing of development of the critical target organ systems, the renal system and renin–angiotensin system, explain the absence of definitive structural abnormalities in test animals.

It is important to note that there does not appear to be a good concordance between those agents that induce renal toxicity in the adult versus those that induce developmental renal toxicity. This is the result of the different cellular processes involved in organ development versus organ function. It is also interesting to note that the developing kidney is not always more sensitive to a toxicant than the adult kidney. Thus, while treatment with the proximal tubular toxicant gentamicin has been used to study reduced glomerular function in the neonatal rat, the age class is remarkably resistant to other proximal tubular toxicants (mercury(II) chloride, sodium fluoride, and dichlorovinylcysteine). The former result is probably due to the immature status of the brush border in the neonatal rat, whereas the latter is probably reflective of immaturity in biochemical differentiation, as the agent requires activation by β-lyase.

4.4 Cancer

Cancer is uncommon during the first two decades of life, but is nonetheless a substantial concern. In the United States, cancer is diagnosed in approximately 12 400 children and adolescents annually and is the most common cause of death from any kind of disease between 1 and 19 years of age. In the United States and other developed countries, lymphoid neoplasms (leukaemia, lymphoma) and cancers of the central nervous system are the most common paediatric malignancies. Other kinds of childhood tumours include embryonal tumours of the retina, sympathetic nervous system, kidney, and liver; tumours of bone and soft connective tissues; and certain gonadal neoplasms. Different kinds of cancer (e.g. carcinomas of liver or thyroid) may predominate in children in parts of the world where specific environmental risk factors are more prevalent.

Exposures to cancer-causing agents preconceptionally, during intrauterine life, or in early childhood may result in the development of cancer during later childhood or during subsequent adult life (Figure 12). Cancers that arise many years after carcinogenic exposures early in life may originate from different cell types and occur in different organs from the cancers that characteristically occur in infants and children.

There is direct evidence that children are more susceptible than adults to at least some kinds of carcinogens, including certain chemicals and various forms of radiation. Data from controlled experimental studies in animals also support the concept that susceptibility to some chemical carcinogens and to various forms of ionizing radiation is greatest during the early stages of life, both before and after birth (Tomatis & Mohr, 1973; Napalkov et al., 1989; Birnbaum & Fenton, 2003). There is also evidence of increased or even unique early-life susceptibility to cancers that result from infection with certain oncogenic viruses, including Epstein-Barr virus and hepatitis B virus. Anderson et al. (2000) reviewed epidemiological and experimental animal studies that investigated the relative susceptibility to carcinogens at different life stages. Windows of enhanced susceptibility were observed for many agents and organ systems during the embryonic, fetal, and neonatal periods (Anderson et al., 2000).

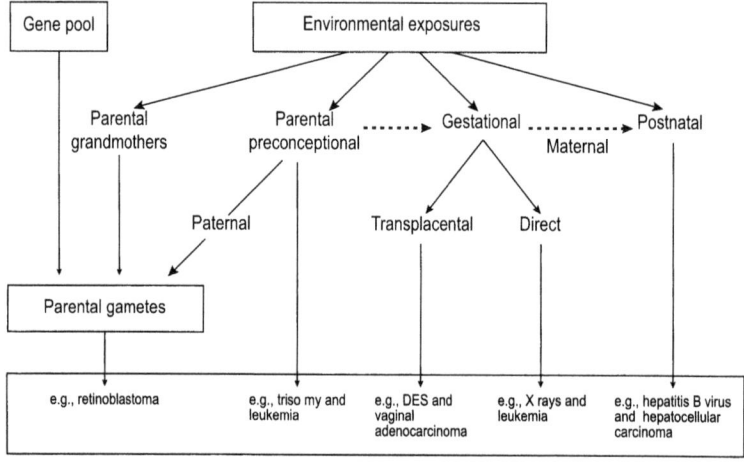

Fig. 12. Impact of timing of developmental exposure on the type of cancer developed (from Anderson et al., 2000)

4.4.1 Childhood cancers that may have environmental causes

4.4.1.1 Lymphoid tissues

Leukaemia was the first cancer to be linked with exposure to radiation from the atomic bombings at Hiroshima and Nagasaki, Japan. Excess relative risk for leukaemia was higher than for any other neoplasm in bomb survivors and for people exposed as children. Radiation-related leukaemia started to occur two to three years after the bombing, reached its peak within six to eight years, and has declined steadily since then. For people exposed as adults, the excess risk was lower than that of people exposed as children, but the excess risk appears to have persisted throughout the follow-up period (IARC, 2000). Small increases in childhood leukaemia may also have occurred in some populations that were exposed to radioactive fallout from nuclear weapons tests, but different studies of this possible association have not produced consistent findings (Chow et al., 1996).

Prenatal diagnostic X-irradiation has also been linked to increased risk of leukaemia in offspring, as has therapeutic, high-dose, ionizing radiation in childhood for other cancers and for various non-neoplastic conditions (Ron et al., 1988a; Chow et al., 1996).

Chemical exposures that are related to childhood leukaemia include high-dose therapies for cancer and other serious diseases. Cancer chemotherapeutic regimens that included topoisomerase II inhibitors have caused acute myeloid leukaemia in children with acute lymphoblastic leukaemia who were treated with these regimens (Pui, 1991). Cancer chemotherapeutic regimens that included alkylating agents for treatment of various childhood cancers increased the risk of developing leukaemia as a second malignancy (Tucker et al., 1987). Use of the antibiotic chloramphenicol has also been associated with subsequent development of acute leukaemia in children (Shu et al., 1987; Chow et al., 1996).

Infection with Epstein-Barr virus in early childhood is common worldwide; in combination with malarial infection, however, it causes a characteristic non-Hodgkin lymphoma in equatorial African children. African Burkitt lymphoma (small non-cleaved B cell lymphoma, Burkitt type) accounts for 30–70% of childhood cancers in equatorial Africa, with about 5–10 cases per year per 100 000 children below the age of 16 years and a peak incidence between 5 and 10 years of age. The disease is an extranodal lymphoma, involving the kidneys, ovaries, adrenals, and characteristically the jaws and the orbit. It is overwhelmingly associated with Epstein-Barr virus infection and holoendemic malaria: the neoplasm occurs most frequently in a geographic belt across Africa that has high rainfall and abundant mosquitoes. It is thought that malarial infection stimulates the B cell system and facilitates the emergence and proliferation of Epstein-Barr virus–infected and potentially neoplastic B lymphocytes (IARC, 1997). African Burkitt lymphoma is an example of a locally common paediatric malignancy that is caused entirely by infectious processes, without a discernible etiologic contribution by chemical agents, ionizing radiation, or major predisposing genetic factors.

4.4.1.2 Liver

Hepatitis B viral infection is spread by transfusion of blood from infected individuals and from mothers to children during the perinatal period. Hepatitis B virus can cause a chronic active infection that leads to hepatocellular carcinoma (Blumberg, 1997). Risk of hepatocellular carcinoma is greatly increased by the combination of hepatitis B viral infection and dietary exposure to naturally occurring aflatoxins, which can heavily contaminate certain staple food crops, including maize and peanuts (IARC, 2002; Turner et al., 2002). In regions of the world where prevalence of chronic hepatitis B viral infection is high and aflatoxin contamination of foodstuffs is also common, hepatocellular carcinoma often develops during childhood. Liver cancer is sufficiently common in children 6–14 years of age in Taiwan, China, that this age group has been used to evaluate the efficacy of hepatitis B vaccination for prevention of infection in offspring of infected mothers and to confirm that successful vaccination reduces the incidence of hepatocellular carcinoma (Chang et al., 2000). Aflatoxin has been detected in cord blood and breast milk in areas of Africa and Asia that have high rates of food contamination with this fungal toxin. In Thailand, 17 of 35 samples of cord sera contained aflatoxin at concentrations of 0.064–13.6 nmol/ml, whereas only 2 of 35 samples of maternal sera contained aflatoxin (Denning et al., 1990). Aflatoxin was detected in 37% of Sudanese, 28% of Kenyan, and 32% of Ghanaian breast milk samples (Maxwell et al., 1989). In Gambia, the amount of aflatoxin excreted in the breast milk is estimated to be 0.09–0.43% of the dietary intake (Zarba et al., 1992). Further, infants in Gambia receive not only in utero exposure but also continuing postnatal exposure to aflatoxin, as the aflatoxin B1 level in the sera of children does not differ markedly from that of adults (Wild et al., 1990). To what extent embryonic, fetal, and neonatal exposures compared with later exposures to aflatoxin contribute to the development of liver cancer in children is not known.

4.4.1.3 Thyroid

The Chernobyl nuclear reactor accident in April 1986 caused an epidemic of thyroid carcinomas in children. Vast quantities of

Developmental State–Specific Susceptibilities and Outcomes

radionuclides, including ^{131}I, other short-lived isotopes of iodine, and ^{137}Cs, were released, mainly during a period of 10 days following the accident, and contaminated large areas of the Ukraine, Belarus, and the Russian Federation. A significant increase in the incidence of thyroid cancer, generally of the papillary type, has occurred as a result in children in these three countries since 1990. Most of the tumours have been observed among individuals who were very young at the time of the accident (IARC, 2001). In Belarus, over half of the tumours occurred in people who were less than six years old at the time of the accident. In a series of 472 children with thyroid cancer diagnosed up to 1995 in Belarus, only 2% had been conceived after the accident; 9% had been exposed in utero, and 88% were under 15 years of age at the time of diagnosis (Pacini et al., 1997). What is unique about thyroid cancers resulting from the Chernobyl accident is the very early age at which the cancers have begun to be diagnosed. The unique susceptibility of the thyroid gland to external ionizing radiation during childhood is one of the most striking examples in human experience of special sensitivity to a carcinogen other than an infectious agent occurring exclusively during pre-adult life.

4.4.1.4 Brain and nervous system

Brain tumours have occurred in children who had received therapeutic doses of ionizing radiation to the head, especially for the treatment of tinea capitis (Ron et al., 1988b) or lymphoid neoplasms (Brustle et al., 1992). Iatrogenic tumours are, however, a very small fraction of all paediatric brain tumours. Except for certain genetic factors, causes of the most common brain tumours of childhood, including primitive neuroectodermal tumours and astrocytomas, remain unknown (Rice, 2004).

4.4.1.5 Other organ sites

Survivors of the Hiroshima and Nagasaki atomic bombings who were exposed to ionizing radiation in utero have experienced a significantly increased risk of solid tumours in childhood. Individuals exposed after birth have experienced no such increased risk. It has been suggested that this difference may result from the tumour precursor cells being susceptible to neoplastic transformation only during the prenatal period (Wakeford & Little, 2003). Both radiotherapy and chemotherapy for cancer are associated with increased risk of second cancers at various sites in children. Increased risk of bone sarcoma has been documented in children with various initial tumours who were treated with radiation or with cancer chemotherapeutic regimens containing alkylating agents (Tucker et al., 1987).

4.4.2 Adult cancers related to childhood exposures

Exposures to carcinogens during childhood have caused tumours that appear chiefly in adulthood. Examples include tumours of the brain, cranial nerves, and meninges after therapeutic irradiation of the head; thyroid carcinoma after therapeutic and environmental exposures to ionizing radiation; leukaemia and solid tumours in adult survivors of the Hiroshima and Nagasaki atomic bombs who were exposed in childhood; and skin cancer after intense childhood exposures to solar radiation. In addition, treatment of pregnant women with synthetic non-steroidal estrogens (e.g. DES) has caused tumours of the female reproductive tract in the adolescent and young adult offspring of these pregnancies.

4.4.2.1 Brain and nervous system

Therapeutic ionizing radiation to the head during childhood has been shown to cause tumours of the meninges and of the brain and cranial nerves in later life. For meningiomas, a clear dose–effect relationship has been recognized, with higher radiation dose leading to increased risk. Meningiomas typically occur in middle-aged and elderly individuals, but they also occur in children and in the very old. Meningiomas that result from radiation exposures during childhood can arise in late adult life, after latencies of 30 years or more, and can have extraordinarily long latencies; a case with a 63-year latency period has been reported (Kleinschmidt & Lillehei, 1995). As with chemical carcinogenesis in experimental animals, tumour latency is inversely proportional to intensity of exposure: average latencies of 35, 26, and 19–24 years of age have been reported for meningiomas induced by low-, moderate-, and high-dose radiation, respectively (Harrison et al., 1991; Kleinschmidt & Lillehei, 1995). Irradiation to treat tinea capitis at a retrospectively estimated mean X-ray dose per patient of 1.5 Gy was associated with a significantly increased relative risk of 8.4 for neurogenic tumours of the head and neck, including meningiomas (Ron et al., 1988a). This is a relatively low therapeutic dose, compared with what is used for antitumour therapy.

4.4.2.2 Thyroid

Between 1920 and 1960, radiotherapy was widely used to treat a variety of non-neoplastic conditions, including tinea capitis, tonsillar hypertrophy, and "thymic enlargement", which was not then recognized as the normal state of the thymus in childhood. Significantly increased risks of thyroid carcinomas later in life have resulted from these relatively low-dose therapeutic radiation exposures in childhood. Excess relative risks per gray averaged 32 for thyroid carcinomas following X-ray treatments for tinea capitis. Individuals exposed as very young children, less than 5 years old, had an excess relative risk more than twice that of children exposed between 5 and 15 years of age. In contrast, external exposures to ionizing radiation during adult life have not been linked convincingly to thyroid cancer (Ron, 1996). High-dose radiation exposures of paediatric cancer patients have also resulted in thyroid carcinomas as second cancers, with a positive linear dose–response above doses as low as 0.1 Gy.

Thyroid carcinomas are also increased in survivors of the atomic bombs at Hiroshima and Nagasaki who were children at the time of the bombings in 1945 and in inhabitants of the Marshall Islands who were accidentally exposed as children to fallout from one of the above-ground United States nuclear weapons tests in 1954 (Ron, 1996). These thyroid cancers, like the thyroid cancers in individuals exposed to radiotherapy as children, have occurred mostly in adults. Among survivors of the atomic bombings, the most pronounced risk for thyroid cancer occurred in individuals with an external radiation dose to the thyroid greater than 1 Sv before the age of 10 years, and the highest risk was seen 15–29 years after exposure (IARC, 2001). Radiation from the Chernobyl accident and from atomic bomb detonations differs fundamentally from what is used in therapeutic radiology, in that the exposures from Chernobyl and from atomic detonations included both external gamma radiation and internal irradiation from radionuclides of iodine that were selectively deposited in the thyroid.

4.4.2.3   Female breast

Ionizing radiation is a known environmental cause of female breast cancer. Breast cancer risk is significantly elevated in female survivors of the atomic bombings at Hiroshima and Nagasaki, but varies significantly depending on age at the time of radiation exposure. Relative risk at estimated exposure levels of 1 Sv was approximately 3–4 for women exposed before 10 years of age or between 10 and 20 years of age, but decreased to approximately 2 in women irradiated between 20 and 40 years of age and decreased even further in women exposed after 40 years of age (Boice et al., 1996).

4.4.2.4   Female reproductive tract

DES was extensively prescribed in developed countries from the late 1940s through the 1970s to women with high-risk pregnancies to prevent miscarriage and other complications of pregnancy. In 1971, Herbst et al. reported that prenatal DES exposure was associated with a rare form of female reproductive tract cancer, clear cell adenocarcinoma of the vagina, in daughters of women who had taken the drug during pregnancy (Herbst et al., 1971). Vaginal clear cell adenocarcinoma occurs in only 0.1% of women who were exposed to DES in utero, but this represents a 40-fold excess risk in comparison with the non-exposed general population. As of 1985, 519 cases of clear-cell carcinoma of the vagina and cervix had been recorded by the Registry for Research on Hormonal Transplacental Carcinogenesis at the University of Chicago (USA). Of these, 311 cases had a definite history of exposure to DES in utero, and 91% of these 311 cases were diagnosed between 15 and 27 years of age (Melnick et al., 1987). Cases were diagnosed up to 34 years of age (later extended to 48 years of age), at which time more than 700 cases had been recorded by the registry (Herbst, 1999). In contrast, men who were exposed to DES in utero do not have a clearly increased risk of any cancer, although a statistically non-significant threefold increased risk of testicular cancer has been reported (Strohsnitter et al., 2001).

4.4.2.5   Integument

Solar radiation and sunburn in childhood are significant risk factors for malignant melanoma of the skin. Numerous studies have assessed the carcinogenic effect of sunburn at different ages and concluded that childhood exposures were the most significant. A study in the United Kingdom assessed sunburn at different ages and found that the strongest association between elevated cancer risk and sunburn occurred at 8–12 years of age (Elwood et al., 1990). Duration of residence in Australia and the associated exposure to intense solar radiation are strongly associated with risk of developing malignant melanoma; and numerous studies indicate that childhood is an especially vulnerable life stage (IARC, 1992). For example, the Western Australia Melanoma Study showed a strong inverse correlation between age on arrival in Australia as an immigrant and risk of developing melanoma, indicating that individuals arriving there as early as 10 years of age were less likely to develop this cancer than native-born Australians of European descent or immigrants arriving at ages younger than 10 years, and that childhood exposure to the intense solar radiation of Australia was therefore a primary contributor to risk of melanoma (Holman & Armstrong, 1984).

4.4.2.6 *Other organ sites*

The Radiation Effects Research Foundation's Life Span Study of atomic bomb survivors has reported that for all solid tumours combined, there is clear evidence of a radiation dose–response relationship. Both excess relative risk and excess absolute risk are larger for individuals exposed as children than for those exposed as adults, and solid tumour risk continues to increase in later years (Kodama et al., 2003). Survivors of the atomic bombs also have increased risk of all kinds of solid tumours, including those of adult life, although the degree of susceptibility varies with age at the time of the bombings and is generally highest early in life.

4.4.3 *Chemical exposures of special concern*

Exposures to chemicals or chemical mixtures that are known to be carcinogenic to adults, especially DNA-reactive drugs, have also caused cancers in children. This occurs principally under the intense and prolonged exposure conditions that are associated with anti-tumour chemotherapy and certain other medical treatments (Chow et al., 1996).

Chemicals with DNA-damaging modes of action are likely to cause cancers in children if the children themselves, or their mothers during pregnancy, suffer sufficiently intense or prolonged exposures. It is prudent to regard any exposure to such substances as potentially carcinogenic. Whether children are likely to be more or less susceptible than adults to such chemicals is likely to depend on how a given chemical is absorbed, distributed in the body, and metabolized in younger versus older individuals, at the exposure levels encountered by children and pregnant women (Neri et al., 2006).

Tobacco smoke contains many DNA-damaging chemicals, including PAHs and 4-aminobiphenyl, and is categorized as a Class I carcinogen by the International Agency for Research on Cancer. These compounds are transplacentally transferred to the fetus. The genotoxicity of tobacco smoke to the fetal liver has been tested in an animal study. Sister chromatid exchange in the liver cells of fetal mice was analysed at the 16th day of gestation after short-term exposure (twice, on the 15th and 16th days of gestation), long-term exposure (starting four weeks before mating and stopping on the 16th day of gestation), and pre-pregnancy exposure (four weeks before mating). The number of sister chromatid exchanges was significantly increased in all exposure groups, and long-term exposure caused a significantly higher increase than did short-term exposure (Karube et al., 1989).

PAHs are metabolically activated to diol epoxides by Phase I drug metabolizing enzymes (e.g. cytochrome P450 and monooxygenase) and form DNA adducts by binding to genomic DNA. The formation of DNA adducts is an initiation step in mutagenesis and carcinogenesis as well as a useful marker of exposure to mutagens. The metabolism of carcinogens by fetal tissues and their extracts has been extensively studied in experimental animals (Anderson et al., 1989), and 10 of 28 human placentas examined had DNA adducts containing diol epoxide metabolites of the PAH benzo[*a*]pyrene (Manchester et al., 1988). Enzyme-linked immunosorbancy assays identified PAH–DNA adducts ($0.63–2.51/10^7$ nucleotides) in the livers of 4 of 15 spontaneously aborted human fetuses (gestational age 17–23 weeks) in the United States (Hatch et al., 1990). Administration of the PAH 3-methylcholanthrene to pregnant mice caused hepatic tumours in the offspring (Anderson et al., 1985).

Alkylating agents such as nitroso compounds are potent mutagens that bind to a nucleotide on genomic DNA without metabolic activation by monooxygenase. Some of these compounds are transplacentally transferred and cause mutagenesis and carcinogenesis. Administration of *N*-nitrosodimethylamine to pregnant mice induces DNA fragmentation in the livers of fetuses (Bolognesi et al., 1988). In addition, the treatment of pregnant rats with a single dose of ethyl methanesulfonate, ethyl-*N*-nitrosourea, *N*-nitrosodiethylamine, or methyl-*N*-nitrosourea causes alkylation and fragmentation of DNA (Robbiano et al., 1989). *N*-Nitroso compounds have been shown to exert transplacental carcinogenic effects (Anderson et al., 1989). For example, pregnant C3H mice were injected with *N*-nitrosodimethylamine (NDMA; 7.4 mg/kg of body weight) or *N*-nitrosoethylurea (41 mg/kg of body weight) on day 16 or 19 of gestation. Administration of NDMA on either gestational day 16 or 19 significantly increased the number of female offspring with hepatocellular carcinoma, and the incidence of hepatocellular carcinoma in male progeny was significantly elevated by administration of NDMA on gestational day 19. In addition, exposure to *N*-nitrosoethylurea on day 19 of gestation significantly increased the incidence of hepatocellular carcinoma among female offspring. These results indicate that sensitivity to *N*-nitroso compounds is dependent on gestational age.

Inorganic arsenic was long considered to be carcinogenic to adult humans but not to rodents, but it has recently been shown to be a multitissue transplacental carcinogen in mice. Sodium arsenite (As^{III}) given ad libitum in drinking-water to pregnant mice caused a significant dose-dependent increased incidence and multiplicity of hepatocellular adenomas and carcinomas and increased incidence of adrenal cortical adenomas in male offspring and dose-dependent increases in ovarian and lung tumours in females (Waalkes et al., 2003). Inorganic arsenic in various forms (including arsenic trioxide, As^{III}) has been previously tested extensively for carcinogenicity in adult rodents, with negative or equivocal results. At least in mice, inorganic arsenic is a much more potent carcinogen to the fetus than to adults.

Inorganic arsenic (arsenate plus arsenite) in drinking-water has recently been evaluated by IARC (2004) as being carcinogenic to humans, increasing risk of tumours of urinary bladder, lung, kidney, and skin. Inorganic arsenic is an important human carcinogen in parts of the world where very high levels of arsenic-contaminated drinking-water occur. The modes of carcinogenic action of inorganic arsenic in rodents and in humans are not yet fully understood, but the possibility exists that inorganic arsenic in drinking-water poses a special concern for pregnant women and their unborn infants. The toxic effects of arsenic in pregnant women and in young children may possibly include increased risk of carcinogenesis.

Vinyl chloride, a known occupational carcinogen, has been studied at different life stages in animals. Rats treated with vinyl chloride beginning during the neonatal period for one year had much higher rates of liver haemangiosarcomas than did rats treated for the same duration of time starting at age 11 weeks (Maltoni et al., 1981). Males treated from the neonatal period had a 16.7-fold higher incidence of the tumours than did males treated as adults. Females treated from the neonatal period had an even higher increased incidence; however, the ratio was not calculable because no cancers occurred in the females treated as adults only (Maltoni et al., 1981).

4.5 Summary and conclusions

In this chapter, we have attempted to highlight the importance of the timing of exposure to chemicals or other insults in determining the consequences to children's health. As illustrated in Table 4, the special susceptibilities of children relative to adults is clearly manifest looking across the various life stages, organ systems, and exposure scenarios. The fact that these susceptibilities exist, combined with the fact that the impacts are felt throughout the affected individuals' lifetime, raises the importance of understanding the contributions of environmental chemicals so that preventative measures can be taken to relieve the burden of disease. Several key points emanate from the analysis of the current state of the science:

- The windows of susceptibility of children are broad and extend from the preconception period through to the end of the adolescent period.

- Given the special nature of development, it is sometimes difficult to make predictions about which exposures might pose the greatest risks to children. However, those agents that influence key signal transduction pathways, modify cell proliferation or cell differentiation rates, activate apoptotic pathways, or react with DNA seem to present the most concern.

Developmental State–Specific Susceptibilities and Outcomes

- There are both qualitative and quantitative aspects to the potential heightened sensitivity of children. Thus, the target organ effects observed following exposure during early life stages are not necessarily the same as those seen following exposure during adult life. Whether or not there are similar target organs, exposures that are relatively without effect in adults can prove damaging during early development.

- For the early post-fertilization life stages, the true extent of susceptibility is difficult to gauge due to methodological difficulties in diagnosing early pregnancies, but several studies have shown this to be a period of high pregnancy loss, and the role of environmental factors cannot be ruled out.

- The manifestations of the effects are often delayed in appearance from the life stage where the critical exposure occurred, thus making determination of cause-and-effect relationships problematic. The greatest challenge is to detect effects related to functional alterations of organ systems. This is due to a combination of lack of easily applicable methods and the reserve capacity of organ systems that can modulate deficits in function. As epidemiological studies that have tracked children longitudinally are rather sparse, there is a tendency to rely on animal models to understand the potential extent of the problem.

- The comparative rate of development has to be understood when extrapolating the effects of exposures observed in laboratory animal models to humans. Major differences can occur in the interspecies extrapolation of both toxicokinetic and toxicodynamic information, depending on the comparative rates of organ maturation. This must be done on a organ system by organ system basis, as the relative rates of development vary among organ systems and across species.

- Unlike the general situation in adults, transient changes in physiology or endocrinology at critical periods of development can result in permanent changes in organ function.

- Even for adverse outcomes that have been clearly linked to exposures during specific life stages, there is a very limited understanding of the mechanisms by which the exposures cause the outcomes. For example, additional studies are needed on the mechanisms by which IUGR causes subsequent diabetes, cardiovascular disease, obesity, and hypertension and to understand the role of alterations in fetal thyroid function on subsequent neurobehavioural outcomes.

- There is clearly the potential for gene–environment–chemical interactions that can either ameliorate or enhance the risk of an adverse health outcome, depending on the nature of the influences and the life stage involved. Non-chemical environmental factors, such as socioeconomic status, are also capable of interacting with these chemical exposures.

- There is a pressing need to develop and validate sensitive, specific, and cost-effective biomarkers of exposure, susceptibility, and effect that can be applied to human studies so that the gaps in our understanding of the role of environmental stressors on children's health can be closed.

5. EXPOSURE ASSESSMENT OF CHILDREN

5.1 Introduction

Children's environmental health risks result from exposure of the parents before conception and of the child during the prenatal period and through childhood and adolescence. In this context, a child can be defined by a series of life stages from conception through adolescence, where each life stage has distinct anatomical, physiological, behavioural, and/or functional characteristics that contribute to potential differences in exposure, resulting in overall differences in susceptibility.

Children, like adults, may be exposed to chemicals through the air they breathe, the water they drink, the foods they eat, and the surfaces and materials they contact. Children also have unique routes of exposure, including transplacental exposure for the developing fetus and ingestion of breast milk for infants. Because of their unique physiology and behaviour, children's exposures may be higher than those of adults; as a result, children may have greater health risks than adults in the same environments.

In this chapter, we review general principles of exposure assessments and discuss methods for conducting exposure assessments, including biomonitoring of internal dose and other biomarkers. The unique characteristics of children that result in differential exposures for children at different ages or life stages are then discussed. Finally, we describe those situations that are likely to result in high exposures to children throughout the world because of their location, culture, socioeconomic status, or unique activities.

5.2 General principles of exposure assessments

Exposure is defined as the contact (at visible external boundaries) of an individual with a pollutant for specific durations of time (IPCS, 2004a). For exposure to occur, an individual must be present and must come in contact with a contaminated medium. Exposure usually results in absorbed dose when chemicals enter the body. Exposure is described in terms of the intensity, frequency, and duration of contact (USEPA, 1992a). The intensity of contact is typically expressed in terms of the concentration of contaminant per unit mass or volume in the medium to which humans are exposed. Exposure is expressed as mass per unit time. Absorbed dose may be expressed as total dose or mass per unit volume (e.g. µg/kg of body weight per day).

Exposure is one element in the environmental health framework depicted in Figure 13 that links contaminant sources to health effects. Exposure assessment evaluates the processes for identifying potentially exposed populations, identifying potential pathways of exposure, and quantifying the magnitude, frequency, duration, and time pattern of contact with a contaminant.

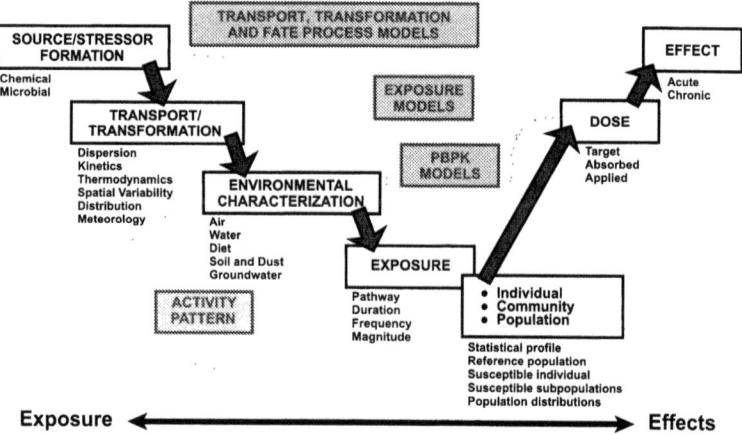

Fig. 13. Scientific elements for estimating exposure and source: Environmental health framework. PBPK = physiologically based pharmacokinetic.

The processes that are important for exposure assessment are shown in the boxes on the left-hand side of Figure 13. Starting in the upper left-hand corner, chemical or microbial contaminants are released from a source. Ambient sources are those that release contaminants into the outdoor environment and include automobiles, power plants, manufacturing facilities, waste sites, and agricultural spraying. Other sources release contaminants directly into indoor environments where people live, work, and play. These include consumer products, building materials, pesticide products, combustion sources for heating and cooking, and ETS.

Many contaminants can be transformed in the environment through a number of processes, including chemical reactions and biological degradation. Contaminants from ambient sources or their transformation products are transported through the environment to locations where people spend time and will be found in environmental media at these locations, including air, water, food, dust, and soil. Contaminants from indoor sources also distribute themselves among these media in the location where they are used. Exposure occurs when an individual actually comes in contact with a contaminated environmental medium and the contaminant is transferred to the individual. The amount of exposure depends upon the concentration of contaminant in the medium as well as the activity pattern of the individual, which defines the frequency, duration, and intensity of the contact. Exposure becomes absorbed dose when the contaminant moves across an absorption barrier; it becomes target tissue dose when the contaminant or metabolite interacts at the target site, which ultimately leads to an adverse health outcome.

The text under each pink box in Figure 13 shows the information that is needed to characterize the process represented in the box. This information is usually developed through laboratory and field measurement studies. The orange boxes show the types of models that are used to link the processes and to estimate exposure, absorbed dose, or target tissue dose.

Many chemicals, such as lead, dioxins, PCBs, and organochlorine pesticides, are persistent in the environment. Thus, exposures will continue to occur over time as long as there is contact with the contaminated medium. Longitudinal exposure can also occur for non-persistent chemicals, since sources for most chemicals provide recurring releases into the environment. Understanding both the frequency and the timing of exposures is very important for the developing fetus and young child. For many contaminants, there are discrete developmental windows during which exposure may lead to adverse health outcomes. For other pollutants, exposure accumulated over time is the important exposure metric.

Children's exposure to environmental contaminants is a complex process that can occur as a result of release of pollutants from many sources that can reach the child through a number of different routes and pathways (Cohen Hubal et al., 2000b). Aggregate exposure assessments evaluate exposure from all sources, routes, and pathways for a single contaminant. For example, a pesticide exposure may result from an agricultural application to foods as well as applications in homes, schools, day-care centres, and recreational areas to control pests. For children of agricultural workers, exposure can occur if the child stays with the parent in the field or if the parent transports pesticides into the home via his or her skin or clothing. For older children, direct occupational exposure to pesticides is an additional route. Several conceptual approaches have been developed for assessing children's aggregate exposure to chemicals (Armstrong et al., 2000; Reiss et al., 2003) as part of the USEPA's Voluntary Children's Chemical Evaluation Program. These approaches provide guidance for identifying and evaluating multiple sources and pathways for exposure.

Cumulative risk assessments evaluate the health risk for aggregate exposures accumulated over time and for multiple contaminants or stressors. In some contexts (e.g. USEPA pesticide risk assessments), cumulative refers specifically to combined exposures to chemicals that share a common mechanism of toxicity (see http://www.epa.gov/oppsrrd1/cumulative/). Populations may be defined by their location relative to sources, their activities and customs, and their susceptibility to exposures. In this context, populations can include different ethnic groups, different communities, or different age groups. Cumulative risk is a very important concept in understanding environmental health risks to children in different settings, particularly in underdeveloped countries where children may be facing multiple stressors.

Route of exposure is defined as the portal of entry to the body. Pathway is defined as the course that the contaminant takes from its source to the exposure medium, and then to the portal of entry. For a given source, exposure media and exposure routes can define the pathways. Depending upon the life stage of the child, exposure media can include amniotic fluid, breast milk, air, water, soil/dust/sediments, food, and objects/surfaces. Exposure routes include transplacental transfer, inhalation, ingestion, dermal absorption, and indirect (non-dietary) ingestion.

Exposure media will also change with life stage. For example, the fetus will be exposed via amniotic fluid, the infant to breast milk, the teething child to many objects (both intended and unintended) for mouthing, the school-age child to contaminants in the classroom, and the adolescent to vocational or recreational hazards.

Exposure factors are those factors related to human behaviour and characteristics that determine an individual's exposure to a contaminant. In a simple case, a child's exposure to ozone by the inhalation route is determined by factors that include the duration of time spent in different indoor and outdoor locations during the day and the child's breathing rates during the period of exposure. Differences in exposure factors, including location, activity, and behaviour, are primarily due to differences in age, sex, culture, geographical location, or socioeconomic status. Relative to body weight, children eat more food, drink more water, and breathe more air than adults. They also eat different foods. An extreme example is the almost total reliance of infants on breast milk for nutrition. Children are often in different environments than adults; even when in the same environment, however, they interact differently, to give more direct contact. A more complete discussion of the characteristics of children that affect exposure is given in section 5.4.

5.3 Methods for conducting exposure assessments

5.3.1 Direct methods

Direct assessments measure the contact of the person with the chemical in the exposure media over an identifiable period of time. Direct assessments are made through field monitoring studies of children in their everyday environments. In such studies, data are collected on pollutant concentrations in a variety of exposure media (e.g. air, drinking-water, food, house dust, surface residues), activities, and exposure factors so that exposure can be measured or estimated for each child in the study. When measurements are made on multiple people, the interpersonal variability in exposures can be evaluated. When the group of individuals for measurement is selected using probability sampling methods, then exposure distributions for the population can be estimated. Information on the highest exposures and the factors associated with these exposures is important for understanding and mitigating risks. Intrapersonal variability can be estimated by conducting repeated measurements on the same person over time. This information can be used to estimate intermittent or chronic exposures for individuals.

For assessing exposure, it is important to collect all of the data on exposure media concentrations, activities, and exposure factors that are required to quantify exposure (Cohen Hubal et al., 2000a; USEPA, 2001). As an example, Table 5 shows the data requirements for estimating exposure by several routes. For inhalation and dietary exposure, personal samples can be used to estimate exposure. For inhalation exposure, the concentration of contaminant in personal air samples is combined with breathing rate. For dietary ingestion, the concentration of contaminant in duplicate-diet samples is combined with the amount of food eaten. Methods for assessing exposure by indirect ingestion as a result of mouthing or eating soil or dust are less straightforward.

Table 5. Summary of the algorithms and data collection requirements by exposure route[a]

Parameter – measurement	How collected	Units
Inhalation exposure ($E_{ime/ma}$)		
$E_{ime/ma} = C_{ame} \times T_{me/ma} \times IR_{ma}$		
C_{ame} – Air concentration (C) in microenvironment (ame)	Measured with active sorbent collection	$\mu g/m^3$
$T_{me/ma}$ – Time (T) spent in each microenvironment/ macroactivity (me/ma)	Time–activity diary, questionnaire	h/day
IR_{ma} – Inhalation rate (IR) during each macroactivity (ma)	Estimated from size, age, and activity data collected with diaries and questionnaires using reference values	m^3/h
Dietary ingestion exposure (E_F)		
$E_f = \Sigma C_f W_f$		
C_f – Concentration (C) in the food (f) item	Measurement in individual food items or composite duplicate-diet samples	$\mu g/kg$
W_f – Weight (W) of food (f) item consumed	Measured in duplicate-diet sample	kg/day

Table 5 (Contd)

Parameter – measurement	How collected	Units
Indirect ingestion (dietary and non-dietary) exposure (E_{ingmi})		
$E_{ingmi} = C_{surfx} \times TE_x \times SA_x \times EF$		
C_{surfx} – Concentration (C) surface (surf) loading (total or transferable) on object x (x)	Measure by a wipe or press method	$\mu g/cm^2$
TE_x – Transfer efficiency (TE)[b] of object x (x)	Empirically determined from laboratory experiments	unitless
SA_x – Surface area contacted by object x (x)	Visual observation or videotape	cm^2/event
EF – Exposure frequency (EF), or frequency of mouthing events	Visual observation or videotape	events/day
Dermal exposure – macroactivity approach ($E_{dme/ma}$)		
$E_{dme/ma} = C_{surf} \times TC_{me/ma} \times AD_{me/ma}$		
C_{surf} – Concentration (C) surface loading (surf) (total or transferable) in each microenvironment	Measured by wipe, press, or roller methods	$\mu g/cm^2$
$TC_{me/ma}$ – Transfer coefficient (TC) for a specific microenvironment/ macroactivity (me/ma)[b]	Empirically determined for each microenvironment/ macroactivity from laboratory experiments or field studies	cm^2/h
$AD_{me/ma}$ – Activity duration (AD) in a specific microenvironment/ macroactivity (me/ma)	Time–activity diary, questionnaire	h/day

[a] From USEPA (2001).
[b] This parameter must be calculated using the same surface loading measurement method as used to measure C_{surf} factors that estimate the contact rate and the transfer rate. For dermal exposure, information on surface residues is combined with factors that estimate contact rate and transfer rates to the skin.

Here information on contaminant concentration in the environmental media (surface residue, dust, soil) is combined with factors that estimate the contact rate and the transfer rate. For dermal exposure, information on surface residues is combined with factors that estimate contact rate and transfer rates to the skin.

5.3.2 Biomarkers of exposure

Biomarkers do not measure exposure directly, but are an indicator of absorbed dose. A biomarker of exposure is defined as a xenobiotic substance or its metabolite(s) or the product of an interaction between a xenobiotic agent and some target molecules(s) or cell(s) that is measured within a compartment of an organism and can be related to exposure. Urine, blood, nail, saliva, hair, and faeces are common media collected for biomarker measurements. Maternal biomarkers of exposure can also be measured in amniotic fluid and breast milk. These matrices can also provide a measure of exposure for children, both prenatally and postnatally. Biomarkers in first teeth have also been used to assess early childhood exposure, whereas biomarkers in meconium and cord blood have been used to assess in utero exposures. Biomarkers of genetic damage (e.g. DNA adducts) have been extensively used to assess exposure to genotoxic agents (Neri et al., 2006).

When appropriately validated and understood, biomarkers present unique advantages as tools for exposure assessment (Gundert-Remy et al., 2003). Biomarkers provide indices of absorbed dose that account for all routes and integrate over a variety of sources of exposure (IPCS, 1993, 2001a). Certain biomarkers can be used to represent past exposure (e.g. lead in bone), recent exposure (e.g. arsenic in urine), and even future target tissue doses (e.g. pesticides in adipose tissue). Once absorbed dose is determined using biomarkers, the line has been crossed between external exposure and the dose metrics that reflect the pharmacokinetics and toxicokinetics of an agent (see section 5.3.3).

Currently, there are only a few cases where biomarkers can be used for quantitative exposure assessment. Biomarkers can be used to indicate that a person has been exposed and that the chemical has been absorbed into the body. They can often be used to rank exposure among individuals. Biomarkers alone cannot provide information on the source, route, or duration of exposure. Even with these limitations, biomarkers, when appropriately validated, can effectively be used to evaluate trends in these exposures (CDC, 2005) and determine the effect of exposure mitigation strategies as well as predict target tissue dose.

5.3.3 Modelling

Models use mathematical expressions to quantify the processes leading to exposure and dose. Models that predict dispersion, fate, transport, and transfer of chemicals are based on physical and chemical principles. Models that describe activities of individuals as they interact with the environment are based on statistical data from observational measurement studies. In Figure 13, the processes that must be accounted for from source to dose are described; the text above the orange boxes shows the types of models that can be used to quantify these processes. These models can be applied to predict exposure and dose for an individual; however, they are most effectively applied at the population level (IPCS, 2005).

Deterministic models use a single value for input variables and provide a point estimate of exposure or dose. Probabilistic models take into account the fact that most input variables will have a distribution of values. These models use probability distributions to develop a range of plausible exposures for the population of concern. Understanding exposure distributions will allow understanding of the range of exposures as well as prediction of risk for the entire population. It will also allow prediction of risk for the most highly exposed individuals. Sophisticated models can be used to develop distributions for different pathways and populations. They can also be used to develop information on interindividual variability and uncertainty in the estimated distributions and to predict the variables that are most important for both exposure and dose.

Exposure models use available information on concentrations of chemicals in exposure media along with information about when, where, and how individuals might contact the exposure media to estimate exposure. For population assessments, distributional data on exposure factors and environmental concentrations are used to estimate exposure distributions for a population. Examples of various exposure models are summarized in Table 6.

Physiologically based pharmacokinetic (PBPK) models are used to estimate the dose of toxic metabolites reaching target tissues. Model outputs provide internal dose estimates for specific life stages and differences between sexes, species, dose routes, and exposure patterns. These models provide a tool for understanding the physiological and biochemical characteristics of children that influence metabolism and disposition of chemicals at different stages of development. PBPK models can aid in evaluating the impact of parameters such as tissue growth rates and biochemical parameters such as enzyme induction on dose and health outcome. PBPK models can also be used as a tool for estimating exposure and dose for the developing embryo, fetus, or newborn (Corley et al., 2003).

Table 6. Examples of models for estimating exposure

Model	Type	Application	Reference
Integrated Exposure Uptake Biokinetic (IEUBK) model	Aggregate; stochastic with probabilistic output; sensitivity analysis	Estimates long-term lead exposure for children (6 months to 7 years old) across multiple pathways, routes, and environmental media, estimates blood lead concentrations	USEPA (2005e)
Stochastic Human Exposure and Dose Simulation (SHEDS) model	Aggregate; mechanistic modelling framework with statistical components and probabilistic capabilities; sensitivity analyses, uncertainty estimations, and inferences of source or pathway contributions	Estimates exposure and absorbed dose of several pollutant types across multiple pathways and routes of exposure and various environmental media; daily exposure through annual absorbed dose is simulated for any aged individual considering time series of exposure (up to 1-min resolution)	Zartarian et al. (2000); Burke et al. (2001)
LifeLine	Aggregate and cumulative; stochastic	Simulates daily pesticide exposures for periods from birth up to 85 years of pesticide applicators, residents of homes where pesticides are used, and the general population (dietary and tap water consumption)	LifeLine Group (2005)

Table 6 (Contd)

Model	Type	Application	Reference
RISK and Indoor Air Quality and Inhalation Exposure (IAQX)	Indoor air mass balance with multiple sources and sinks	Risk from inhalation exposure to VOCs, solvents, airborne particulate matter from indoor and outdoor sources	Guo (2002)
Dietary Exposure Potential Model (DEPM)	Model and database system for deterministic dietary exposure	Exposure from pesticides in diet; combines food consumption and residue data	USEPA (2003a)
Hazardous Air Pollutant Exposure Model (HAPEM)	Semistochastic, sequential simulation, producing aggregate exposure distributions	Used by USEPA to evaluate national exposures to hazardous air pollutants (part of Trim.Expo model)	Palma et al. (1996)
Air Pollutants Exposure (APEX) model	Stochastic time series simulation model producing probabilistic exposure distributions	Used by USEPA to evaluate national ambient air quality standards (also part of Trim.Expo model)	USEPA (2005b)

PBPK models can also be used for toxicokinetic assessments. Such assessments provide more precise estimates of internal dose, which, in turn, can be used to replace interspecies defaults for more precise risk assessments. Probabilistic assessments account for the range of interindividual variability and can be used to estimate the central tendency and upper bound of internal dose. Toxicokinetic assessments can also provide an understanding of the mechanism of toxicity by providing various estimates of internal dose that can be correlated with health effects (Ginsberg et al., 2004c).

5.4 Unique characteristics of children that affect exposure

Children's exposure to and dose from environmental contaminants are expected to be different from and, in many cases, much higher than those of adults. Both physiological and behavioural characteristics influence children's exposure to environmental contaminants.

Physiological characteristics influence exposure by affecting a child's rate of contact with exposure media or by altering the exposure–uptake relationship (as described in chapter 3). The developing fetus is the most unique case and is primarily exposed to chemicals through cord blood and amniotic fluid. For infants and young children, the primary source of food is often breast milk. Children have a much larger surface area relative to body weight than do adults. In addition to providing more area for dermal absorption, the larger relative surface area of children means that body heat loss will be more rapid, requiring a higher rate of metabolism. Children also need extra metabolic energy to fuel growth and development. The higher basal metabolic rate and energy requirements in children mean that both oxygen and food requirements are greater per kilogram of body weight. The higher breathing rate and food consumption rate required to meet these physiological needs can result in higher exposures to environmental contaminants in air and food relative to adults.

The distinct life stages for children, the major routes of exposure, as well as maternal exposures all affect total exposure levels as a child ages. During the prenatal stage, exposures to chemical and biological contaminants occur through the placenta, and the mother is the primary pathway for exposure. For the developing fetus, all maternal exposures are relevant, including occupational exposures, drug and alcohol consumption, and smoking. During infancy and young childhood, children may be exposed to chemicals in breast milk as well as through direct contact with all environmental media. Indirect ingestion may occur when children handle and eat foods that have come in contact with the floor or other contaminated surfaces. Young children's mouthing activities (hand-to-mouth and object-to-mouth) will result in indirect ingestion if the hands or objects are contaminated. For older children and adolescents, the mother is no longer a pathway for the child's exposure. In many countries, older children may enter the work force, and occupational exposures may become important.

Children's behaviour and the way in which they interact with their environment may have a profound effect on the magnitude of exposures to contaminants and differences in exposure at different ages. In other words, a child's exposure is greatly affected by where the child is, what the child is doing, and what the child ingests. Children crawl, roll, and climb over contaminated surfaces, resulting in higher dermal contact than would be experienced by adults in the same environment. They eat different foods, which may result in higher dietary ingestion (Cohen Hubal et al., 2000b). The USEPA's Risk Assessment Forum has proposed "Guidance on Selecting Age Groups for Monitoring and Assessing Childhood Exposures to Environmental Contaminants" (USEPA, 2006a). The development of these groupings takes into account behaviour as a function of developmental age and the impact it will have on exposure. Figure 14 gives the age groups in the document and illustrates how selected behaviours change within these age groups.

Not only are children's activities different from adults', but children (especially young children) can demonstrate very wide ranges in those activities that may affect exposure. Thus, children's exposures will be higher and more variable, with very high exposure at the upper tail of the distribution, as demonstrated by children's pica behaviours. It is important to understand that stages of biological development and susceptibility do not necessarily parallel the developmental stages that are important for exposure. Table 7 attempts to show the overlap between these stages. Information in the table extends the concept of exposures important for children to preconception (parental exposures) and embryo/fetal development. Methods that can be used for exposure assessment for different stages are also given.

Although developmental age is a critical element in determining children's activity patterns, other factors, such as geography, climate, culture, socioeconomic status, sex, season of the year, and areas (i.e. urban versus rural), can also have an important impact on activities and exposure. Thus, there is a need for caution when data about activity patterns generated in one region are used to estimate exposures in another region.

As an example, a comparison of activities, lifestyles, habitats, and diets in tropical areas and regions in the Arctic illustrates the differences that might exist in geographical regions. Likewise, different cultures have different diets and lifestyles that would be expected to impact exposures. Some folk medicines that contain chemical contaminants are commonly used. A good example is the use of azarcon, a lead-based product, for the treatment of gastrointestinal symptoms in Mexico (Yáñez et al., 1994). Traditional cosmetics

EHC 237: Principles for Evaluating Health Risks in Children

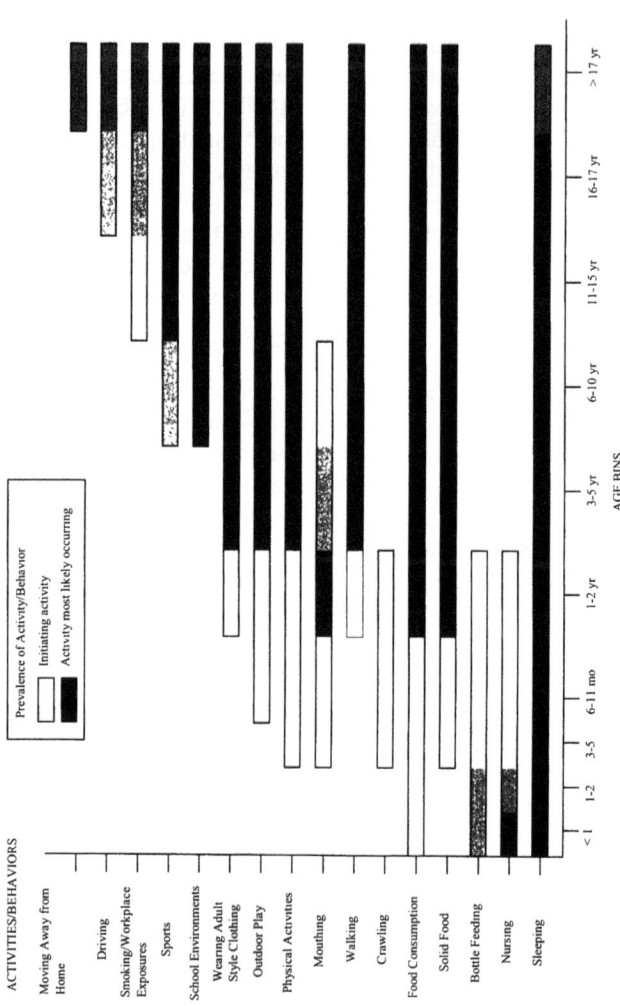

Fig. 14. Children's activities that impact exposure as a function of developmental age (from USEPA, 2003b)

Table 7. Considerations for exposure assessment at different developmental stages

Developmental stages	Exposure stages[a]	Exposure methods
Preconception	Reproductive-age adult	Material or paternal exposure measured or modelled using adult methods
Preimplantation embryo	Conception to birth	Maternal is the primary exposure route — maternal exposure measured or modelled using adult methods; fetal exposure modelled from maternal exposure or biomarker measurements (cord blood, amniotic fluid, meconium)
Postimplantation embryo – implantation to 8th week of pregnancy		
Fetus – 8th week of pregnancy to birth		
Perinatal stage – 29th week of pregnancy to 7 days after birth	Birth to 3 months	Child's exposure measured or modelled; biomarker measurements may be affected by differential uptake and metabolism depending upon age and birth condition
Neonate – birth to 28 days		
Infant – 28 days to 1 year		
	3 to 6 months	
	6 to 12 months	
Young child – 1 to 4 years	12 to 18 months	Exposure measured or modelled, differential exposure due to differing behaviours and contact with different environmental media
	18 to 24 months	
	24 to 30 months	
	30 to 36 months	
	3 to 5 years	
Toddler – 2 to 3 years	24 to 30 months	
	30 to 36 months	
Older child – 5 to 12 years	5 to 10 years	
	10 to 15 years	
Adolescent – usually 12 to 18 years	15 to 17 years	

[a] From USEPA (2006a).

used in some cultures can be sources of metals such as lead (al-Hazzaa & Krahn, 1995) and mercury (Sin & Tsang, 2003). Other exposures to potentially harmful chemicals can occur through several sources, including the use of lindane-based shampoos for the treatment of head lice and scabiasis (ATSDR, 1999) and contact with plastic toys and pacifiers that contain phthalates (Shea & American Academy of Pediatrics Committee on Environmental Health, 2003).

Gender has been identified as a factor influencing activity level and type of activity. Even for young children (ages 3–5 years), gender differences are observed in the types of games played, the frequency of play, and the activity level, with boys engaging in more active play. These patterns have also been observed for the activities of older children (Cohen Hubal et al., 2000b). In many cultures, there are important gender differences in activity patterns. Boys are more likely to attend school, while girls are more likely to work (Marcoux, 1994; UNICEF, 2005b). In other regions, it has been observed that females, especially young women, spend more time in contact with water. Thus, women would be at higher risk from exposure to contaminants via water.

5.5 Exposure as it relates to children around the world

5.5.1 Sources/geographical location

Proximity to sources, either natural or anthropogenic, is an important determinant for exposure to environmental contaminants. When considering ambient sources, contaminant concentrations in air, water, soil, and biota may be highest in areas that are closest to sources. Children who live in the most contaminated areas throughout the world may have high exposures and health risks simply because they live in these areas. For example, in mining areas, children can be exposed to metals as a result of contact with contaminated air, soil, and dust. Similarly, in agricultural areas, children could have high exposures to the pesticides that are applied to crops in the area. In the Antarctic area, children in countries such as Chile and New Zealand are at a higher risk of exposure to ultraviolet radiation due to a thinning ozone layer (McGee et al., 2002). High levels of arsenic or fluoride in drinking-water would be expected in areas receiving water from polluted aquifers. Finally, exposure to radon can occur in areas with a high natural concentration of radium in the soil (Vaupotic, 2002).

Figures 15–18 show areas of the world where pollutant levels are high and could impact the exposure and health of adults and children in the area.

5.5.2 Pathways of exposure

An exposure pathway is the course that a contaminant takes from its source to the individual. When contaminants are released from a source into the environment, they move through multiple environmental media to humans by many pathways. Air, water, soil, house dust, and food are important environmental media for human exposure. For children, several other media, such as breast milk, amniotic fluid, and cord blood, are also important. The remainder of this section discusses important pathways for children's exposure.

5.5.2.1 Ambient air exposure pathway

Contaminants in ambient air result in inhalation exposure either when the child is outdoors and breathes contaminated air or when contaminants in the air are transported indoors where the child spends time. Adverse health effects (acute and chronic) associated with inhalation of air contaminants are a common concern for people living in polluted cities, near hazardous waste sites, or close to point sources like smelters (Figure 15). Air emissions from past or current production processes, as well as volatilization of organic compounds, airborne particulates, and acid gases, may expose residents to contaminants at levels of health concern (ATSDR, 1994). In urban areas, mobile sources contribute substantially to organic, inorganic, and particulate air pollution. Fires, open burning, and wind-blown dust can also be major sources of ambient air pollution.

A relationship between ambient air pollution and daily mortality and morbidity rates has been reported for many cities throughout the world (Schwela, 2000; Stieb et al., 2002; Glinianaia et al., 2004; Gordon et al., 2004). The relevant contaminants include sulfur dioxide, suspended particulate matter, nitrogen dioxide, carbon monoxide, ozone, and lead (Schwela, 2000). Ambient air pollution has been declared an important health problem for developing countries. A considerable burden of disease has been reported for cities such as New Delhi, India (Pande et al., 2002); Santiago, Chile (Ostro et al.,

EHC 237: Principles for Evaluating Health Risks in Children

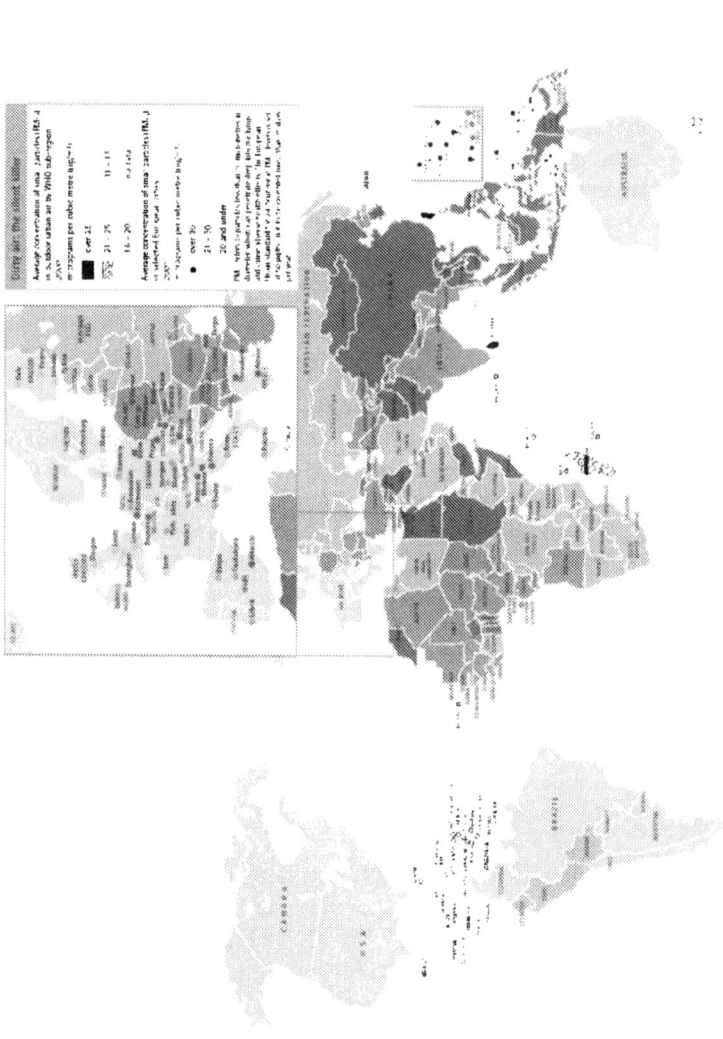

Fig. 15. Outdoor air pollution: Average concentration of small particles (PM$_{10}$) in outdoor urban air by WHO subregion (from WHO, 2004c).

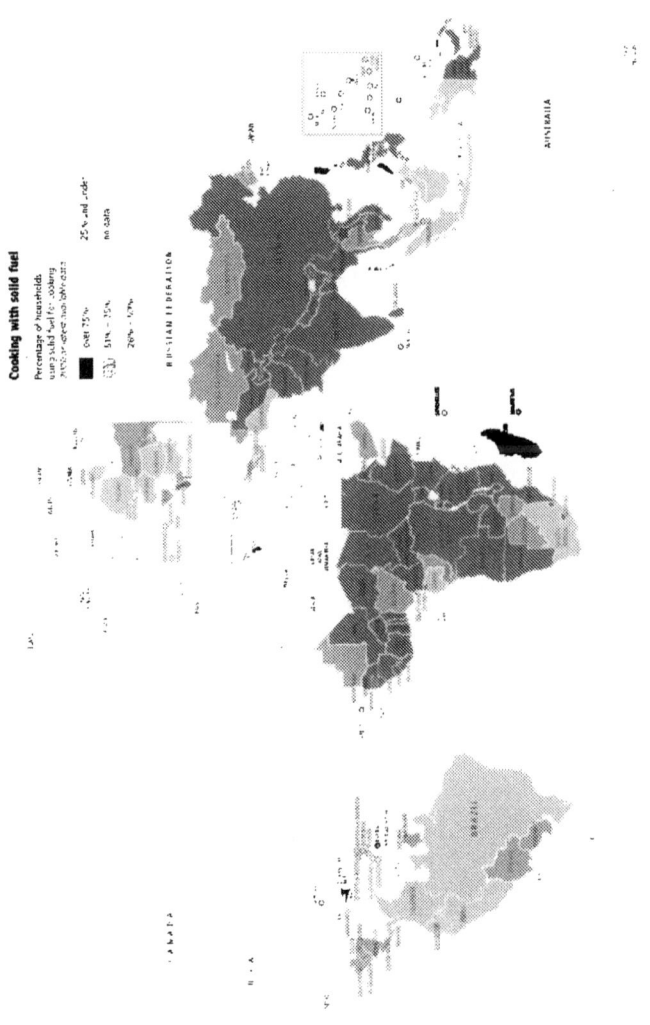

Fig. 16. Indoor air pollution: Percentage of households using solid fuel for cooking (from WHO, 2004c).

EHC 237: Principles for Evaluating Health Risks in Children

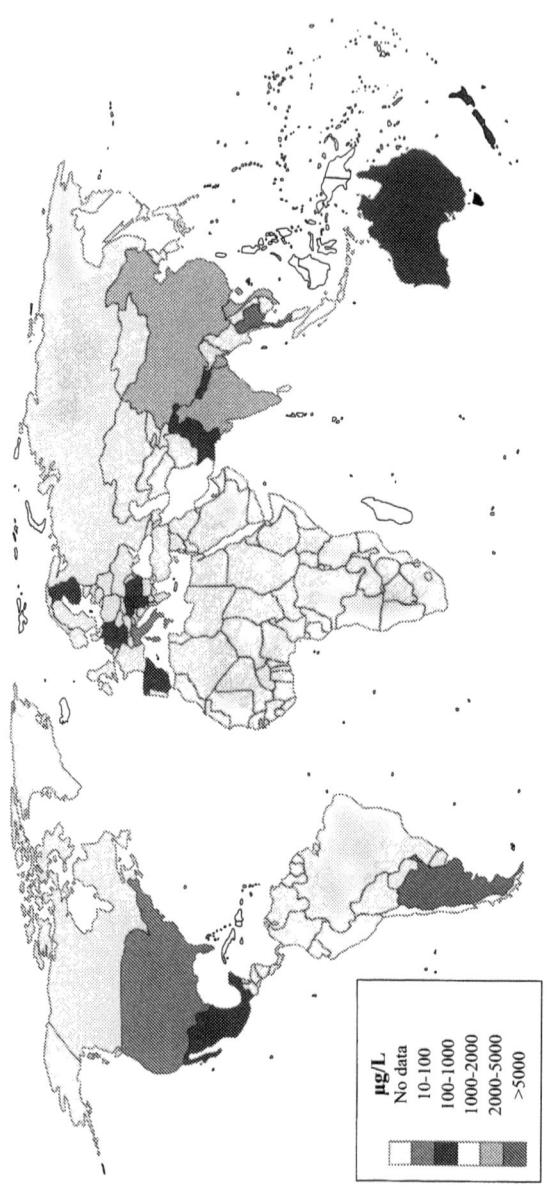

Fig. 17. Arsenic in water: Highest reported well water arsenic concentrations by country (from WHO, 2004c)

Exposure Assessment of Children

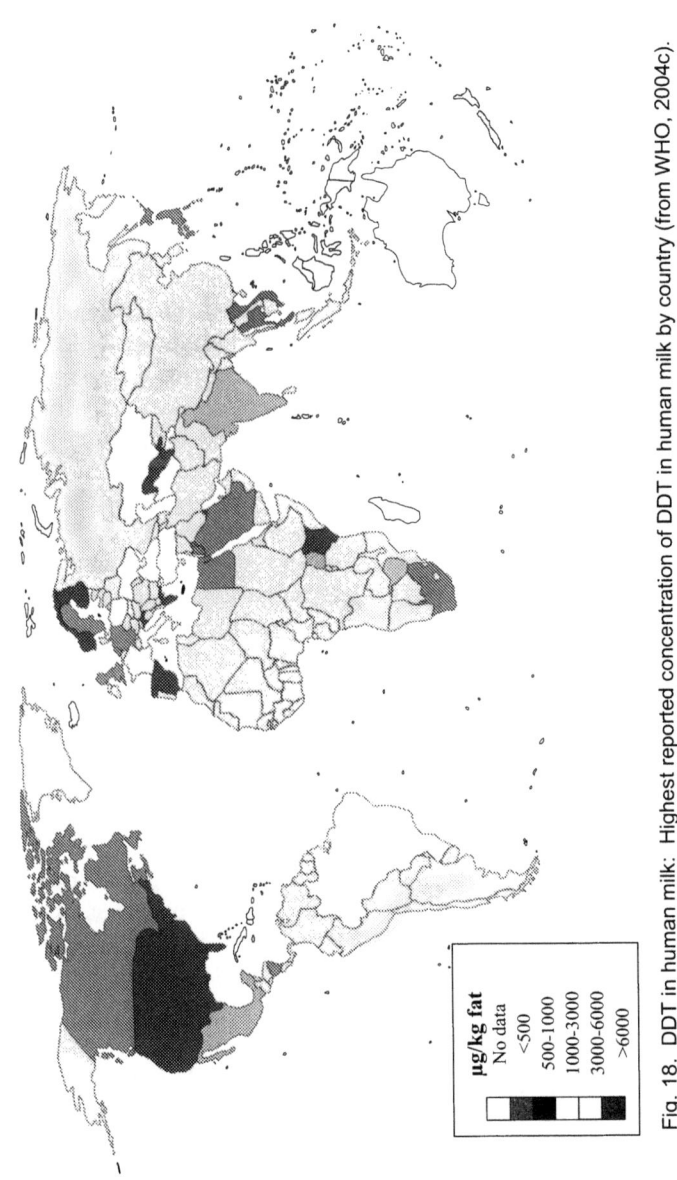

Fig. 18. DDT in human milk: Highest reported concentration of DDT in human milk by country (from WHO, 2004c).

1999); and Mexico City, Mexico (Borja-Aburto et al., 1998). In 22 developing countries, the World Resources Institute found 180 cities whose air quality did not reach the WHO guidelines (WRI, 2002).

5.5.2.2   *Indoor exposure pathways*

Indoor exposure pathways are very important. First, in many regions of the world, children spend more than 90% of their time indoors. Second, the indoor concentrations of many contaminants are much higher than those found outdoors. It is estimated that 70% of the poorest people in developing countries live in rural areas (World Bank, 2005). The indoor exposure pathway is especially important for these individuals (Figure 16). Approximately 50% of the world's population and up to 90% of rural households in developing countries still rely on coal or unprocessed biomass material in the form of wood, dung, and crop residues for fuel (Bruce et al., 2000). High levels of indoor air pollutants result from the use of either open fires or poorly functioning stoves to burn biomass or coal (Ezzati & Kammen, 2001). Women, especially those responsible for cooking, are the ones most heavily exposed. Young children who spend their time close to their mothers also have high exposures (Bruce et al., 2000). Many of the substances in smoke from either biomass or coal burning can be hazardous to humans. The most important are suspended particulate matter, carbon monoxide, nitrous oxide, sulfur oxides (coal), formaldehyde, and PAHs (Bruce et al., 2000; Smith et al., 2000).

ETS is an indoor air pollutant that is a major concern. WHO estimates that there are about 1.1 billion smokers in the world, or about one third of the global population who are 15 years of age or older. Of these, 800 million are in developing countries (WHO, 2005b). Especially in developing countries, people smoke indoors where they live and work, thus resulting in a high percentage of homes with ETS pollution and high inhalation exposures for children.

Several studies have identified house dust as an important route of exposure for many chemical contaminants (Butte & Heinzow, 2002; USEPA, 2004b). House dust is a sink for semivolatile organic compounds and particle-bound matter (Butte & Heinzow, 2002). House dust and compounds adsorbed to it may enter the body by inhalation of suspended and resuspended particles, through non-dietary ingestion of dust, through ingestion of particles adhering to food, to surfaces in the homes, and to the skin, as well as by absorption through the skin (Butte & Heinzow, 2002). Various levels of pesticides, PCBs, PAHs, plasticizers (phthalates, phenols), flame retardants, other organic xenobiotics, and inorganic constituents have been reported in house dust (Butte & Heinzow, 2002; USEPA, 2004b). High lead levels in house dust have been found in houses with deteriorating lead-based paint (USEPA, 2004c). High lead levels in house dust have also been found in mining areas (Yáñez et al., 2003) and in the vicinity of smelters (Díaz-Barriga et al., 1993). Ingestion of house dust through hand-to-mouth activities is the most likely pathway of lead exposure. Studies addressing the bioavailability of contaminants present in dust are needed to evaluate the relative importance of this pathway.

Indoor concentrations of pesticides in proximity to pesticide-treated farmland have been measured (Fenske et al., 2002). For example, it has been shown that pesticide exposure in children could potentially be increased if they live in homes in close proximity (60 m) to pesticide-treated farmland (Fenske et al., 2002). Clothing and cars of farm workers can also be a source of pesticide exposures for children. Usually, applications of insecticides and herbicides in and around the home are a more likely source for children's exposures.

The indoor environment can serve as an important pathway for exposures to fungal moulds as well as chemical contaminants. Moulds can be found almost anywhere; they can grow on virtually any organic substance, as long as moisture and oxygen are present. There are moulds that can grow on wood, paper, carpet, foods, and insulation. It is impossible to eliminate all moulds and mould spores in the indoor environment. Controlling moisture indoors is the most effective mitigation strategy. Moisture problems in portable classrooms and other temporary structures have frequently been associated with mould problems (USEPA, 2005c). Fungal toxins (e.g. aflatoxin) contaminate food and are a particular problem in African and South-east Asian countries (Egal et al., 2005).

5.5.2.3 Water exposure pathway

Ingestion of contaminants is the primary exposure pathway for drinking-water. Dermal absorption and inhalation of contaminants during bathing are other common pathways. When contaminated surface waters serve as recreational areas for children, accidental ingestion (water or sediment) and dermal contact become additional pathways for exposure. Finally, aquatic organisms can bioaccumulate contaminants in surface waters, which can lead to dietary exposure through the food-chain.

Industrial effluent, agricultural runoff (pesticides), and oil and mining wastes are important sources for surface water contamination. Hazardous waste sites are a recognized source of groundwater contamination. In many countries, the natural pollution of aquifers with metals such as fluoride and arsenic is an important source of contamination. High levels of fluoride in water sources have been identified in at least 25 countries, 23 of which are undeveloped nations, such as Mexico, Argentina, China, India, Pakistan, Bangladesh, Uganda, Kenya, and Tanzania (Ando et al., 1998; Grijalva-Haro et al., 2001; UNICEF, 2001b). In Mexico, approximately five million people live in areas where the fluoride levels in drinking-water are higher than the national guideline of 1.5 mg/l (Díaz-Barriga et al., 1997a). In India, 62 million people, including 6 million children, are exposed to elevated levels of fluoride in the drinking-water (Susheela, 1998).

High natural water levels of arsenic (Figure 17) have been found in developing countries, including China, India, Bangladesh, Cambodia, Thailand, Viet Nam, Mexico, Argentina, Chile, and Romania (UN, 2001b; Smedley & Kinniburgh, 2002). In these countries, around 45 million individuals are exposed to arsenic through drinking-water (UN, 2001b; Smedley & Kinniburgh, 2002). In Bangladesh, 80% of the population is estimated to be at risk of arsenic-related diseases. Arsenic-contaminated water poses a risk for millions of people globally (IPCS, 2001c).

Accessibility to safe drinking-water and management of wastewater are important health issues in developing countries. It is estimated that 2.4 billion people, including the poorest in the world, lack access to basic sanitation, and 1.1 billion people lack access to even improved water sources. In the less developed countries, only

54% of the population in rural areas is using improved drinking-water sources (World Bank, 2001).

5.5.2.4 Soil exposure pathway

Contaminated soils may expose children to multiple contaminants at levels of health concern (ATSDR, 1994). Ingestion of contaminated surface soil is a primary exposure route. Inhalation of contaminated dusts and direct dermal contact with contaminated soils can also lead to elevated exposure.

Worldwide, the most important sources of metals in soil are mine tailings, smelter wastes, and atmospheric fallout (Nriagu & Pacyna, 1988). Poor waste management practices in the mining industry have important implications for exposures around the world. Less than 1% of mined ore produces metals; the remainder is waste (UNEP, 2000). The amount of waste produced is enormous, given that world production of metals in 1999 was around one billion tonnes (UNEP, 2000). The United Nations Development Programme estimates that there are 6 million artisanal miners worldwide, with a further 30 million or more people dependent on these miners for their living (UNDP, 1999). If we assume that around 40 million individuals are working in the mining industry, then millions of children (including the children of the miners) may be directly exposed to environmental contaminants produced during mining. Most studies on children living in mining or smelter sites are limited to exposure assessments (Díaz-Barriga et al., 1997b; Hwang et al., 1997; Murgueytio et al., 1998). Few of them have described biological effects in the exposed children (Counter et al., 1997; Calderón et al., 2001). Further studies that evaluate exposures and link them with health effects are needed.

Organochlorine pesticides and other POPs, once applied, will remain in the soil, thus providing the potential for children's exposure through the soil pathway. In 1955, WHO started a global malaria control programme using organochlorine pesticides. By 1958, 75 countries had joined; at the peak of the campaign, 69 500 tonnes of pesticides, mainly DDT, were applied to 100 million dwellings each year (Wijeyaratne, 1993). For the control of malaria, houses were sprayed twice a year with DDT wettable powder to kill mosquitoes. Today, DDT has been substituted in many countries with agents such as pyrethroids, but it is still used in special instances for vector control in a small number of countries. Owing to past or present household spraying, levels higher than background concentration have been detected in both outdoor and indoor soils throughout the world (Yáñez et al., 2002a; Díaz-Barriga et al., 2003). DDT is one of the 12 POPs being phased out under the Stockholm Convention on Persistent Organic Pollutants (UNEP, 2004).

5.5.2.5 *Food-chain exposure pathway*

Many contaminants in the environment are concentrated up the food-chain and result in dietary exposure. Both on- and off-site hunting, fishing, foraging, and farming activities may bring people into contact with those contaminants. Some substances, particularly fat-soluble substances and heavy metals, may reach concentrations in animal tissues that are thousands of times higher than those found in water, soil, and sediment (Damstra et al., 2002). This pathway includes the exposure to chemicals by means of drinking animal milk or eating animal milk–based products.

Mercury is a good example of a metal for which the food-chain exposure pathway is important. Although much of the mercury in the environment is in the less toxic inorganic form, some microorganisms (plant and animals) can convert this to methylmercury, which accumulates up the food-chain (UNEP, 2002). People are then exposed, for example, by eating contaminated fish. Environmental mercury contamination from mining practices that rely on mercury amalgamation for gold extraction is widespread (Eisler, 2004). Contamination is very high in the immediate vicinity of active gold extraction and refining operations. Very high environmental concentrations of mercury from this source have been measured in Canada, the United States, Africa, China, the Philippines, Siberia, and South America (Eisler, 2004). In parts of Brazil, for example, mercury concentrations in abiotic materials, plants, and animals collected near ongoing mercury amalgamation gold mining sites were far in excess of allowable mercury levels promulgated by regulatory agencies for the protection of human health and natural resources (Eisler, 2004). In industrial countries, sources of mercury contamination include smelting processes, coal-fired power plants, incinerators, and chlorine production (UNEP, 2002; USEPA, 2004a). Mercury, especially in the form of water-soluble methylmercury, may be transported to pristine areas by rainwater, water currents, deforestation, volatilization, and other vectors (Eisler, 2004).

POPs are persistent organic chemicals that can be transported globally. POPs have been found in the tissues of humans and a number of wildlife species, even in areas distant from their source. They find their way into terrestrial, marine and freshwater food-chains. Ingestion of POPs via the food-chain pathway is particularly important for a number of native populations. The First Nations people in the Arctic have markedly high levels of POPs in their diet (Health Canada, 2003). Studies in Canada have shown that average intakes are generally higher in the Baffin Inuit population as a result of a diet involving large amounts of marine mammals and fish, while the Sahtu Dene/Métis peoples who consume mainly caribou and fish have lower intakes (Health Canada, 2003).

Children can be exposed to biological as well as chemical contaminants through the food-chain. For example, approximately 1.5 billion episodes of diarrhoea occur globally each year, resulting in the deaths of three million children under five years of age (mainly in developing countries) (WHO, 1999). It is estimated that 70% of these annual cases of diarrhoea worldwide have been caused by biologically contaminated food (WHO, 1999). Foodborne parasitic diseases also present a major public health problem. For example, foodborne trematodes affect 40 million people, with more than 10% of the world's population at risk of infection (WHO, 1999).

5.5.2.6 *Human to human exposure pathways*

1) Maternal exposure pathway

Most chemicals are able to cross the placental barrier, and others are excreted through breast milk. Therefore, during the fetal or neonatal stages, exposed mothers can be a source of exposure for their offspring. There are multiple settings in which the potential of contaminated breast milk is relevant. These include mining areas (metals), agricultural fields (pesticides), industrial areas (metals and organic compounds), rural areas (indoor pollution, such as PAHs), urban areas (chemical mixtures, such as gasoline), the Arctic (POPs), and endemic malaria areas (DDT, pyrethroids).

As an example of this pathway, Figure 18 shows the worldwide importance of human milk as a source of DDT. Although ingestion of breast milk can be a pathway for exposure to chemicals, it is essential to state that, overall, breastfeeding provides substantial benefits to both children and mothers. It significantly improves child survival by protecting against diarrhoeal diseases, pneumonia, and other potentially fatal infections, while it enhances quality of life through its nutritional and psychosocial benefits. Breastfeeding also contributes to maternal health in various ways, including prolonging the interval between births and helping to protect against ovarian and breast cancers. Therefore, the benefits of breastfeeding clearly outweigh the risks of exposure to chemicals through this pathway (Pronczuk et al., 2004).

2) Occupation-related exposure

Since many women in both developed and developing countries work outside the home, maternal occupational exposures that may result in ingestion, inhalation, or dermal absorption can be an important pathway for many chemicals. In some occupations (i.e. agriculture, mining, and manufacturing), both mothers and fathers can transport chemical contaminants into the home environment on their skin and clothing. The child can then become exposed through contact with the parent or through contact with surfaces that the parent has contaminated.

5.5.3 *Settings/microenvironments*

Most children spend their time in a few specific microenvironments, including the home, school, and recreational areas (playgrounds). A study of these microenvironments or settings is critical to an understanding of exposure patterns in children. For children's exposure, there are factors specific to each microenvironment. However, these settings are also modified by external factors, such as those related to geographical areas or to environmental equity factors. Finally, some children are exposed to chemicals in special settings, such as in child labour situations, in refugee camps, or on the street. These settings will be discussed further in the following sections.

5.5.3.1   Residential

Home is the most important setting for infants and young children. They often eat, play, and sleep in the same area. Examples of sources of exposure to pollutants include building materials (e.g. wood treated with arsenic-based pesticides), lead-based paints, insecticides that are sprayed indoors, fuel (e.g. coal and wood) for indoor cooking, disposal practices for domestic waste (e.g. incineration), household chemicals (e.g. solvents), and small-scale enterprises at the family residence (e.g. brick producers who operate low-technology combustion kilns and makers of pottery using lead-based paints).

5.5.3.2   School

School is an important setting for many children and adolescents. Many of the residential factors described above can apply to the school setting. However, there may be additional sources of chemicals that are associated with laboratories, activity rooms, or school equipment. For example, exposure to volatile compounds has been reported in art buildings (Ryan et al., 2002); polybrominated diphenyl ethers, used in flame retardants, were detected in teaching halls containing 20 computers (Sjodin et al., 2001); mercury intoxication resulting from use of school barometers has been reported in a number of countries (Koyun et al., 2004); and in Mexico, lead levels were higher in children who habitually bite coloured pencils (López-Carrillo et al., 1996).

5.5.3.3   Child-care centres

In the United States, The First National Environmental Health Survey of Child Care Centers was conducted in licensed child-care centres that serve children under the age of six (DHUD, 2003). An estimated 14 200 or 14% of licensed child-care centres have significant lead-based paint hazards. Centres in older buildings are more likely to have significant lead and asbestos hazards than those in newer buildings. In the United States, day-care centres where the majority of children are African American are likely to have significantly higher lead exposures and exposure to allergens than those where a majority of the children are Caucasian. Less than 22% of day-care centres had detectable levels of any of the allergens measured. Data on child-care centre exposures from most countries are generally unavailable, and, due to cultural factors, exposures may vary considerably.

5.5.3.4 Recreational

Playground environments provide opportunities for children's exposure to pollutants. Like any other setting, children will be exposed to contaminants that are present at the site. Thus, playgrounds built near hazardous waste sites, mining waste sites, or agricultural fields may be contaminated and, hence, provide a pathway for exposure. In addition, children will have more direct contact with the contaminated environment through their play activities, making exposures in recreational areas greater. In addition to exposures to contaminants present in the natural environment, there are two other risks associated with playgrounds: playground hazards, and materials used in playground equipment or in playground cover. A strong association between childhood injuries and the use of inappropriate surface materials under and around playground equipment has been described (Mowat et al., 1998). Significantly more hazards per play area were identified in playgrounds near low-income areas compared with those near high-income areas.

Several materials commonly used on playgrounds may provide a health risk. Chromated copper arsenate is a wood preservative that has been registered to protect wood from dry rot, fungi, moulds, termites, and other pests (USEPA, 2003c). Chromated copper arsenate–treated wood is most commonly used in outdoor settings for decks, walkways, fences, gazebos, boat docks, and playground equipment (USEPA, 2003c). New regulations have been put in place that will reduce the potential exposure risk to arsenic. Other materials that are used in playgrounds need further assessment. For example, "Kieselrot" (red slag), a by-product of copper production, is contaminated with leachable residues of PCDDs/PCDFs. This material has been used as surface cover for more than 1000 sports fields, playgrounds, and pavements in Germany and neighbouring countries (Wittsiepe et al., 2001). Children can ingest this material directly by hand-to-mouth activities or soil-pica behaviour. Transfer of leachable residues to the skin could result in dermal absorption of the residue on the skin or indirect ingestion through hand-to-mouth activities. The bioaccessibility of PCDDs/PCDFs in this material was estimated in an "in vitro" assay to be more than 60% when using a model with higher bile content and in the presence of whole milk powder (Wittsiepe et al., 2001).

Exposures to chemical and biological organisms through ingestion, inhalation, and dermal absorption can occur as a result of swimming in contaminated water. Swimming pools typically use chlorine for disinfection, resulting in high concentrations of chloroform and other disinfection by-products. Faecal contamination and contamination with microorganisms may be a problem for swimming pools and spas, as well as beaches and other natural swimming areas (WHO, 2003b, 2006). Industrial discharges, mine tailings, and untreated wastes all provide opportunities for contaminating recreational waters, which can then lead to children's exposures to these contaminants.

5.5.3.5 *Special settings*

Some children in various parts of the world are exposed to toxic chemicals or to hazardous environments in unique circumstances. Globally, millions of children are exposed as a result of special socioeconomic and cultural settings. Examples are described briefly below.

1) Child labour

An estimated 246 million children between 5 and 14 years of age are engaged in child labour worldwide (UNICEF, 2004). Of those, 171 million work in hazardous situations or conditions, such as in mines or agriculture. In addition, many children do not have access to education, are not provided adequate health care or nutrition, are abducted, abused, and/or beaten, and are essentially reduced to slave labour. Information is limited, but includes the following:

- Over 19% of children (127.3 million) in the Asian and Pacific regions are engaged in child labour.

- Sub-Saharan Africa has an estimated 48 million child workers. Almost one child in three (29%) below the age of 15 works.

- Latin America and the Caribbean have approximately 17.4 million child workers.

- Fifteen per cent of young children in the Middle East and northern Africa are engaged in child labour.

2) Street children

A street child is any girl or boy who has not reached adulthood, for whom the street (in the broadest sense of the word, including unoccupied dwellings, wasteland, etc.) has become his or her habitual abode and/or source of livelihood, and who is inadequately protected, supervised, or directed by responsible adults. Pollution, poverty, violence, discrimination, inadequate family support, and disease threaten the life, growth, and development of children living in the streets (UNICEF, 2001c). Their settings are unsafe environments, with limitations on good-quality basic health services, clean water, and sanitation. In the end, the opportunities for recreation, learning, social interaction, psychosocial development, and cultural expression are minimal. Furthermore, drug use may be high among this group. The well-being of street children is an important public health concern, and the magnitude of the problem is only expected to increase. Cities are expanding at a rapid pace, and the developing world is becoming increasingly urban. From 2000 to 2025, the number of people living in urban areas in the developing world will double from two billion to four billion (UNICEF, 2001c). Currently, one third of urban dwellers in the developing world live in substandard housing or are homeless, and this is not expected to improve. It is estimated that by 2025, 6 out of every 10 children will live in urban areas (UNICEF, 2001c). Based on these statistics, it is anticipated that there may be a large increase in the number of street or homeless children over the next 20 years.

3) Refugee children

Ample evidence exists to demonstrate that large-scale dislocation of people (characteristic of many recent refugee crises) creates adverse environmental impacts (UNHCR, 2001). The scale and suddenness of refugee flows can rapidly change a situation of relative abundance of natural resources to one of acute scarcity. Where the hosting environment is already under stress, as it is, for instance, in many arid regions of Africa and Asia, an influx of refugees can seriously threaten the integrity of local ecosystems, the economic activities dependent on them, and the welfare of local communities. Although deforestation tends to be the most apparent negative environmental feature of refugee situations, other visible impacts may include soil erosion, loss of wildlife and non-timber products, and loss of biodiversity (UNHCR, 2001). Indoor and outdoor air pollution caused by concentrated biomass burning, depletion or contamination of aquifers, and an altered pattern of transmission of certain diseases can be a serious threat to refugee health (UNHCR, 2001). Children, including adolescents under the age of 18, make up 45% of refugee populations worldwide (UNHCR, 2002). The estimated number of refugees in 2003 was 20 million (UNHCR, 2003). In order to assess the environmental exposure of these children in an integral way, we have to take into account the six most salient and sometimes interrelated concerns facing refugee children today: separation of families; sexual exploitation, abuse, and violence; military recruitment; lack of education; detention; and lack of documentation (UNHCR, 2003).

5.5.4 *Environmental equity factors (vulnerable communities)*

Today, most poor people live in rural areas and face risks associated with agriculture and other aspects of rural life. However, a rapid transition is occurring: many of the poor are moving to large urban areas and entering the informal sector of the economy, which may be accompanied by new kinds of toxic hazards. Poverty is often accompanied by high rates of morbidity and mortality from most diseases. However, poor people in developing nations are also more likely to be exposed to toxic chemicals (Yáñez et al., 2002b). It has been estimated that five to six million people die each year in developing countries due to waterborne diseases and air pollution (World Bank, 2005). Those who are poorly nourished and who have concurrent disease may be more susceptible to environmental exposures. For example, lead is known to be more toxic to children whose diets are deficient in calories, iron, and calcium (Mahaffey, 1995). Environmental pollution can also contribute to poverty by making resources unproductive. In eastern Europe, for example, short-term decisions to allow high levels of toxic pollution in a developing economy led to devastating economic impacts within just a few decades.

With regard to environmental justice, it has been shown that there are clear differences among racial groups in terms of disease and death rates; furthermore, racial minority and low-income populations experience higher than average exposures to selected air pollutants, hazardous waste facilities, contaminated fish, and agricultural pesticides in the workplace (USEPA, 1992b).

5.6 Special considerations for children's exposure: case-studies

5.6.1 Influence of activities

5.6.1.1 Arsenic

In the communities surrounding the Rocky Mountain Arsenal, a Superfund site in Colorado, USA, pathways for exposure to arsenic were evaluated through analysis of residence history, occupation, hobbies, dietary habits, water supply, housing, and activity patterns (Reif et al., 1993). Children of Hispanic origin or non-Caucasian children who drank less than three glasses of water daily and children who spent more time outdoors had an increased risk of having more than 10 µg/l of arsenic in their urine (Reif et al., 1993).

5.6.1.2 Insecticides

In a study done in an endemic malaria area in Oaxaca, Mexico, it was found that children were exposed to deltamethrin (an insecticide used in the control programme for malaria) (Yáñez et al., 2002b). Moreover, a negative correlation between urinary 3-phenoxybenzoic acid (a biomarker for deltamethrin) and age was found in these children (Yáñez et al., 2002b). The results can be explained considering that deltamethrin was sprayed on the ceilings and walls, both indoors and outdoors, contaminating household dust and external surface soil; levels of deltamethrin in surface soil and household dust in Oaxaca were higher than background levels. In tropical areas, these sites are important recreational zones for infants, since they have a lower temperature (Yáñez et al., 2002b).

5.6.1.3 Environmental tobacco smoke (ETS)

A Canadian study examined activity patterns and exposure to ETS in non-smoking respondents relative to age, sex, socioeconomic status, and prevalence of asthma (Leech et al., 1999). Children experienced the most exposure at home, primarily between 4 p.m. and midnight. For children, the living room (22%) and the bedroom (13%) were the most common locations (Leech et al., 1999). Determining characteristic time and location patterns for ETS exposure is critical for developing educational strategies to help non-smokers avoid ETS exposure (Leech et al., 1999).

5.6.1.4 Lead

A study of preschool children in New Jersey, USA, examined seasonal changes in residential dust lead content and its relationship to blood lead (Yiin et al., 2000). Blood and dust samples (floors, windowsills, and carpets) were collected to assess lead exposure. The geometric mean blood lead concentrations were 10.77 and 7.66 µg/dl for the defined hot and cold periods, respectively (Yiin et al., 2000). The regression analysis, including the three representative dust variables in the equations to predict blood lead concentration, suggests that the seasonality of blood lead levels in children was related to the seasonal distribution of dust lead in the home (Yiin et al., 2000). In addition, the outdoor activity patterns indicate that children are likely to contact high-leaded street dust or soil during longer outdoor play periods in summer (Yiin et al., 2000). Therefore, at least some of the seasonal variation in blood lead levels in children was probably due to increased exposure to lead in dust and soil.

5.6.2 Hazardous waste sites

The Agency for Toxic Substances and Disease Registry in the United States has confirmed from more than 10 years of public health assessments, toxicological investigations, epidemiological studies, and reviews by expert working groups that children living near hazardous waste sites may have higher exposures to environmental chemicals, which may result in a greater potential for health problems (ATSDR, 1997).

In the United States, an estimated three to four million children live within 1.6 km of at least one hazardous waste site (ATSDR, 2003). Furthermore, on the basis of data from 1255 hazardous waste sites, there were 1 127 563 children under six years of age living within 1.6 km of the borders of the sites, or about 11% of the potentially affected population. Women of child-bearing age account for about 24% of the population near waste sites (ATSDR, 2003). Some hazardous waste sites are located in highly populated, largely minority or low-income areas, while other hazardous waste sites are located in unpopulated areas (Atlas, 2001). According to other publications, hazardous waste sites are more likely to be found in tracts with Hispanic groups, primarily in regions with the greatest percentage of Hispanics (Anderton et al., 1994). A multivariate analysis of hazardous waste site distribution and a hazard regression analysis of the site prioritization process in the United States suggest that communities with a higher percentage of black residents are less likely to receive National Priorities List designation, delaying potential remediation (Anderton et al., 1997).

5.6.3 Aggregate exposure

Many chemicals, both natural and human-made, are released into the environment and, through dispersion and transport processes, may find their way into food, water, indoor and outdoor air, soil, and other environmental media. It has become increasingly clear in recent years that for some chemicals, significant exposures may occur by more than one route (ingestion, inhalation, dermal absorption) and from more than one pathway. Thus, the concept of aggregate exposure refers to the total exposure of humans to a single chemical or to a mixture of chemicals through all relevant pathways and routes. Three examples that show the importance of assessing aggregate exposure in children in order to design risk reduction programmes are described below.

5.6.3.1 Chlorpyrifos

A United States study examined the aggregate exposures of preschool children to chlorpyrifos and its degradation product, 3,5,6-trichloro-2-pyridinol (TCP) (Morgan et al., 2005). Samples that were collected included duplicate diet, indoor and outdoor air, urine, solid and liquid food, indoor floor dust, play area soil, transferable residues, and surface wipes (hand, food preparation, and hard floor). Generally, levels of chlorpyrifos were higher than levels of TCP in all media, except for solid food samples. For these samples, the median TCP concentrations were 12 and 29 times higher than the chlorpyrifos concentrations at homes and day-care centres, respectively. The median urinary TCP concentration for the preschool children was 5.3 ng/ml, and the maximum value was 104 ng/ml. The median potential aggregate absorbed dose of chlorpyrifos for these preschool children was estimated to be 3.0 ng/kg of body weight per day. The primary route of exposure to chlorpyrifos was through the diet, followed by inhalation.

5.6.3.2 Smelter areas

Children living near lead smelter areas in Torreon, Mexico, were exposed to lead by inhalation (lead in air particles), ingestion of soil, and ingestion of food cooked in lead-glazed ceramics (García Vargas et al., 2001; Albalak et al., 2003; Pineda-Zavaleta et al., 2004). Furthermore, in the smelter area, lead levels in household dust were higher than levels in control areas; thus, inhalation and ingestion of dust particles were additional pathways of exposure. Similar results were found for arsenic, in children living in the vicinity of a copper smelter in San Luis Potosi, Mexico (Díaz-Barriga et al., 1993; Carrizales et al., 2006).

5.6.3.3 Malarious areas

In order to control malaria, DDT was used in Mexico until the year 2000. As a result, DDT contamination was widespread, and it has been shown that children can be exposed to this insecticide by soil ingestion, household dust ingestion/inhalation, fish consumption, and human milk (Díaz-Barriga et al., 2003; Herrera-Portugal et al., 2005). In these areas, DDT levels in blood in children are higher than those in adults (Díaz-Barriga et al., 2003).

5.6.4 Cumulative exposure

Cumulative risk is the combined risk resulting from exposures that accumulate over time, pathways, sources, or routes for a number of agents or stressors. This concept of cumulative risk addresses the fact that individuals are not usually exposed to a single environmental contaminant by means of a single exposure pathway. Multiple contaminants are released from sources as chemical mixtures. Environmental fate and transformation processes affect the nature, pathways, and extent of human exposure. Exposures by different pathways may result in differential absorption, metabolism, and toxic response, even for the same chemical. Cumulative risks are difficult to assess, and methods are still under development (USEPA, 2003b). Most assessments for cumulative risk start with the receptor population and determine which chemicals, stressors, or other risk factors are affecting them. This is a particularly important and relevant concept when considering children's exposures and risks, especially in developing countries. Many of the examples presented here consider specific groups of children who may be exposed to high pollutant concentrations, poor nutrition, and poor sanitation at the same time; thus, they may have a differential risk compared with populations that are influenced by only a single stressor.

A much narrower concept of cumulative risk considers the risk from exposures to pesticides (e.g. organophosphate pesticides) that have a common mechanism of toxicity (USEPA, 2006b). Organophosphate pesticides are powerful inhibitors of carboxylic hydrolases, including acetylcholinesterase, and several studies in different countries have shown higher exposure to organophosphate pesticides in children than in adults (Wessels et al., 2003). Children of pesticide applicators, younger children within the zero- to six-year age range, children living closer to pesticide-treated orchards, children living in urban areas, and those living where pesticides are used inside or outside the home have all been shown to have higher levels of a urinary biomarker for organophosphate pesticides, suggesting higher exposures to either the pesticides or their breakdown products (Wessels et al., 2003).

5.7 Summary and conclusions

Because of differences in physiology, behaviours, body weight, and body surface area, the exposure levels in children may be different from and often higher than exposures in adults. Furthermore, in terms of risk, children may also be more susceptible to environmental pollutants because of differences in absorption, metabolism, and excretion. More information is needed about the behavioural and cultural factors that will influence the exposure to chemicals in children. Such factors may modify both the levels of exposure to chemicals and the nature and severity of health risks. Future studies must include in their analysis consideration of factors such as occupation, smoking, socioeconomic status, and nutritional conditions.

Some children are exposed to toxic chemicals or to hazardous environments in unique circumstances. There is a need to understand chemical exposures and other health stressors in special settings in the world (child labourers, street children, refugees). Globally, millions of children live under these conditions. Currently, data on children's exposures are inadequate to effectively assess multimedia and multiroute exposures in order to conduct child-protective risk assessments. The limited exposure data that are available have focused on children in developed countries, and information on the levels of chemical exposures in children in developing countries is generally lacking.

With the recognition of the special susceptibility of children, it is better to prevent than to treat environmental diseases in children. In developing countries, the most important issue may be to prioritize which exposure reductions will have the greatest overall impact with the limited resources that are available. It is important to identify the exposures that pose the greatest health risks, as well as the sources and pathways for these exposures. This information can then be used to make choices that lead to health benefits for children around the world.

Increased research is needed to assess levels of exposure to environmental chemicals on a global scale, particularly in developing countries. Additional studies are also needed for the development and improvement of methods for monitoring children's exposure and for the availability of improved biomarkers of exposure.

6. METHODOLOGIES TO ASSESS HEALTH OUTCOMES IN CHILDREN

6.1 Introduction

6.1.1 *Methodological approaches for children's health studies*

Children's health status is an important population marker of environmental threats to human health. Children are often a sensitive subgroup of the population (IPCS, 1984, 1986b; Etzel, 2003; Brent et al., 2004), necessitating the need for monitoring sentinel health end-points followed by purposeful research for areas of concern. Only recently have investigators focused on methodologies designed specifically to address the unique characteristics of children and the need, more generally, to consider exposures in the context of life stages. Essentially the same methodologies used for assessing adult health status in relation to environmental factors can be used for children, but they must be adapted to reflect the rapid rate of growth and development characteristic of infants and children. Added attention must be given to other unique aspects of children, as discussed in previous chapters. Measurements of exposure and outcomes may need to be more frequent than in adults and timed to reflect the key stages of human growth and development: i.e. embryonic, fetal, neonatal, infant, childhood, adolescence, and adulthood (see Table 1). Ideally, prospective follow-up of human conceptuses through adulthood (18–21 years of age) would permit a complete capture of health end-points and exposures that may vary during the follow-up interval. When characterizing exposures among children, investigators may need to rely on proxy reports from parents, caregivers, or teachers, especially for younger children who may be unable to accurately recall and report exposures such as diet or play. Data collection may need to rely on proxy reporting if children are unable to provide information in a valid and reliable manner. For example, an investigator interested in assessing dietary phytoestrogens may need to interview parents as a proxy for children. Proxy parental reporting may be prone to recall bias. However, there are strategies that permit empirical evaluation of bias and methodologies that may correct measurement bias (Thurigen et al., 2000; Sturmer et al., 2002). Appropriate study design benefits from the involvement of a multidisciplinary team of experts (e.g. epidemiologists and biostatisticians) to capture methodological nuances unique to paediatric study populations.

Examples of commonly used clinical tools or tests that may be appropriate for children's health issues are summarized in Table 8. This table underscores the utility in evaluating children's overall health status rather than restricted focus on specific organ systems, except for circumstances when a particular exposure or health concern exists for a defined study population.

Table 8. Examples of global clinical assessment tools, by organ system, amenable for epidemiological investigation of environmental influences on children's health

Organ system	Clinical assessment tool
Immune	• Blood tests: Antibody response to immunization (humoral immunity); serum concentrations of immunoglobulin subtypes (humoral immunity)
	• Skin testing for common allergens (cell-mediated immunity)
	• Frequency and duration of common infections
Respiratory	• Lung function: Spirometry and pulmonary function testing (measurements of lung volumes and flow rates); peak expiratory flow rate measurements (can be done in field with inexpensive hand-held meters)
	• Diffusing capacity for carbon monoxide (measurement of alveolar gas exchange)
Haematopoietic	• Blood tests: Complete blood count (red and white blood cell indices and platelets); measurement of clotting factors, prothrombin time, partial thromboplastin time
Cardiovascular	• Blood tests: Serum lipids (cholesterol, triglycerides)
	• Electrocardiograms: heart rate and rhythm
	• Anthropometric: Body mass index (weight in kilograms/height in metres squared); skinfold thickness or other methods
	• Blood pressure: individual or continuous monitoring of blood pressure using portable monitors

Table 8 (Contd)

Organ system	Clinical assessment tool
Liver	• Blood tests: Liver enzymes (alanine aminotransferase, aspartate aminotransferase, alkaline phosphatase, gamma-glutamyl transferase, bilirubin, lactate dehydrogenase) • Ultrasonography (portable units for field studies)
Kidney	• Blood tests: Serum creatinine, blood urea nitrogen • Urine collection: 24-h or spot for protein, glucose, creatinine clearance
Musculoskeletal	• Strength testing, flexibility testing using standardized instruments or clinical examination
Endocrine and metabolic	• Blood tests: Serum concentrations of pituitary horrmones (TSH, LH, FSH, ACTH, growth hormone, prolactin, vasopressin); serum concentrations of other hormones (insulin parathyroid hormone, glucagon, calcitonin, vitamin D); and serum electrolyte concentrations (sodium, potassium, calcium, magnesium) • Challenge tests: Releasing hormone challenge tests to test pituitary responsiveness to hypothalamic hormones (GnRH, corticotropin releasing hormone, thyroid releasing hormone) • Oral glucose tolerance test
Neurodevelopment	• At birth, newborn assessments (e.g. suckling, Babinski, and startle reflexes) • At and after birth, growth trajectories (e.g. weight, length, head, abdominal circumference) • After birth, standardized assessment tools (by trained professionals, parents, or other raters) for growth and development inclusive of cognition, language, learning, vision, auditory, behaviour

ACTH, adrenocorticotropic hormone; FSH, follicle stimulating hormone; GnRH, gonadotropin releasing hormone; LH, luteinizing hormone; TSH, thyroid stimulating hormone

Note: Some of above clinical assessment tools are age and/or sex dependent.

6.1.1.1 Epidemiological methods

Use of epidemiological methods can ensure the validity and reliability of study results. Briefly, this includes formulation of a research question or testable hypothesis, selection of an appropriate study design with respect to the research question and type of study covariates, selection of an appropriate sample (determining whether a representative or population-based sample is needed), standardized data collection instruments, and development of an analytical plan appropriate for the design and level of measurement of study covariates. While several study designs are available for assessing environmental factors and child health, each has its own strengths and limitations that need to be weighed in making a final decision about research methodology. Study designs can be interchanged across health outcomes, depending on the research aims, characteristics of the exposure, incidence (new cases) or prevalence (new and existing cases) of the study outcome, fiscal considerations, and logistical issues, as described below. Study design can tremendously impact the weight of evidence for a particular exposure and outcome (NRC, 2001), with analytic studies adequately designed and statistically powered to test hypotheses weighing more heavily than descriptive studies (e.g. cross-sectional or linkage studies). Study findings need to be evaluated within an established paradigm for assessing causality. With regard to infants and children, biological plausibility underlying the timing and dose of exposure at critical developmental windows needs careful attention in both designing the study and interpreting the results (IPCS, 2002).

6.1.1.2 Comparison of study designs

Table 9 presents a comparison of basic epidemiological study designs for assessing child health outcomes by their inherent methodological strengths and limitations. While experimental study designs are included for completeness, none is appropriate for the evaluation of environmental influences on children's health when the exposure(s) cannot be randomized within acceptable research practices.

Descriptive and analytic study designs are observational in nature, in that children cannot be randomly assigned to receive the environmental exposure (e.g. chemical). Analytic study designs are

Table 9. Comparison of epidemiological study designs by strengths and limitations

Study design	Description	Strengths	Limitations
Descriptive[a]			
Ecologic	Assessment of group exposures and health outcomes, thereby gauging impact of a particular exposure in a defined population	Hypothesis generating	Cannot link exposure to diseases or study outcomes among individuals Residual confounding may threaten validity
Cross-sectional	Design that simultaneously ascertains exposures and outcomes Appropriate for exploring research questions as a first attempt or to generate hypotheses for analytic study designs	Can be completed in a relatively short period of time, often at reduced cost Useful initial approach for evaluating human health risks	Disease prevalence only Cannot assess causality or the temporal relation between exposure and health outcome Residual confounding may threaten internal validity
Linkage	Physical merging of health and exposure data sets to explore research questions and conduct ecological analyses	Can be completed in a relatively short period of time, often at reduced research cost Useful as initial approaches for evaluating human health risks for a particular exposure Useful for population-based monitoring, such as the detection of spatial or temporal trends and patterns	Completeness of case ascertainment varies by type (active versus passive) of surveillance Residual confounding may threaten internal validity Not applicable for many health outcomes without available registry data

Methodologies to Assess Health Outcomes in Children

Table 9 (Contd)

Study design	Description	Strengths	Limitations
Analytic			
Case–control	Design that begins with disease status; cases refer to individuals, families, or households with a particular health outcome, while controls are similar to cases in every way save for the study health outcome	Well suited for 1) rare outcomes (<5% prevalence in population), such as birth defects, neurodevelopmental impairments, or childhood cancer, or 2) outcomes arising following a long latency	Typically, only one end-point can be studied (although multiple exposures can be addressed)
	Potential confounders, if known, can be addressed by restricting study subjects in the design phase or through multivariate modelling techniques in the analytic phase	If conducted properly, summary statistics approximate those from cohort studies	Response rates may vary by disease status, with cases often more likely to participate than controls, thereby introducing potential bias
	For disease outcome, cases need to comprise incident (newly diagnosed) cases, and controls need to be selected from population at risk of developing the disease of interest		Recall bias may stem from systematic differences in recollection and/or reporting of exposures by disease status
			Selection of inappropriate control group or low overall response rates can lead to biased results
Case only	Design modified from the traditional case–control study that is intended for the investigation of gene–environment interactions	Relatively simple and efficient approach for estimating gene–environment interactions	Requires population-based selection of cases
	No external controls used	Estimates multiplicative (not independent) effects of environmental factors and genes	Stringent assumption that environmental factor and genes are independent; if violated, can produce biased estimates

173

Table 9 (Contd)

Study design	Description	Strengths	Limitations
Cohort	Longitudinal design that begins with ascertainment of exposure(s) for cohort members with follow-up for occurrence of health events Such studies can be designed as historic (identification of a pre-existing cohort whose exposure has been identified) or prospective (current exposure ascertainment) with prospective follow-up for occurrence of health events The cohort study offers two additional strategies for analysis — case–cohort and nested case–control study designs: the case–cohort comprises all individuals in the cohort with a particular disease and a random sample of unaffected individuals from the cohort; the nested case–control design includes cohort members with a particular disease (cases) and unaffected individuals (controls) matched on relevant study covariates	Less subject to selection bias Can establish a temporal order between exposure and outcome Able to consider multiple exposures and outcomes within single design Can incorporate time-varying covariates	Loss to follow-up may bias results Depending upon length of follow-up needed, can be costly

Methodologies to Assess Health Outcomes in Children

Table 9 (Contd)

Study design	Description	Strengths	Limitations
Experimental			
Randomized trial	Experimental trial in which the investigator randomly assigns study participants to receive or not receive a study treatment or intervention; hence, every study participant has an equal chance of being assigned to the experimental treatment or intervention Investigators can be blinded to randomization process, dependent upon the characteristics of the study outcome	Random assignment of study participants to groups, thereby minimizing confounding by ensuring comparable groups Design given most weight in establishing causality or treatment efficacy	Not appropriate for study of most environmental agents External validity of general findings may be limited to referent population

[a] Excludes case-reports and case-series.

typically used when the etiologic relation between an exposure(s) and health outcome is of interest. While experimental study designs remain the best approach for establishing causality or identifying effective disease prevention strategies, such designs are unethical for most environmentally oriented research. To this end, only observational designs are discussed further in this chapter.

Choice of study design is dependent upon a number of factors. The decision will lie primarily with the research question (for descriptive study designs) or hypothesis (for analytic study designs) to be assessed in the context of budget and other feasibility issues (e.g. the ability to ascertain data on relevant study factors regardless of whether the data already exist or need to be collected). Unlike study design options for experimental animals, there are no universally recognized protocols (or set of guidelines) for assessing organ system–specific toxicity; rather, an epidemiological study design such as a case–control or cohort study is tailored to the particular study exposure, age of the children, and health outcome to be considered. Such a design may be entirely devised for implementation in the field, within a clinical setting, or a combination of the two settings. Choice of study design should be sensitive to the voluminous body of literature supporting the clustering of human pregnancy outcomes (e.g. pregnancy loss, birth defects, preterm and low-birth-weight infants). This clustering or correlation needs to be addressed in designing the study and the accompanying analytic plan. Failure to appropriately address the underlying correlation may result in incorrect statistical conclusions and inferences (Buck Louis et al., 2006). Currently, modelling techniques are available that are responsive to this issue (e.g. generalize estimating equations, hierarchical models).

6.1.1.3 Descriptive designs

Descriptive studies are designed to generate hypotheses or assess research questions (not hypothesis testing per se) for subsequent testing. Case-reports and case-series may also be categorized as descriptive studies; however, these approaches summarize data on an individual or a small group of individuals with a common set of symptoms or health condition. Since neither of these approaches utilizes an appropriate comparison group for whom the investigator attempts to delineate a common exposure, no further discussion of these approaches is offered. Key descriptive study design options include 1) ecologic design, 2) cross-sectional design, and 3) linkage studies. These designs have been powerful in identifying patterns of disease occurrence and in identifying potentially at risk subgroups.

Ecologic studies examine factors in relation to health outcome at the population level given the absence of individual-level data on these factors. While cautious interpretation of data is needed given the limited availability of information on potential confounders, important health concerns for children have been identified with such designs. For example, biomonitoring data for populations (e.g. ambient air monitoring) have been linked to live birth registries to assess the impact of air pollution on infant birth size (Wilhelm & Ritz, 2003), gestation (Ritz et al., 2000), or birth defects (Ritz et al., 2002). Similarly, geographic proximity to hazardous waste sites (Marshall et al., 1997) and the consumption of PCB-contaminated fish (Mendola et al., 2005) have been associated with birth defects using a state birth defects registry.

Cross-sectional designs collect information on study exposure and outcome at the same point in time so that a temporal ordering between the two cannot be established, and often exposures at critical windows for various life stages cannot be captured. Cross-sectional studies typically employ survey research methodologies, especially if the study sample is to be population based or representative of the targeted study population. Various registries routinely collect information that can be analysed to globally assess changes in the distribution or frequency of health end-points such as infant birth weight and gestation, plurality of birth, secondary sex ratios, fetal deaths, stillbirths, birth defects, or childhood cancers. In some populations, hospital (in- and outpatient) visits and diagnoses can be used to monitor changes in the prevalence of diseases that may be affected by environmental influences (e.g. asthma). Cross-sectional surveys simultaneously collect information on exposure and health status and may reveal associations in need of formal hypothesis testing, such as those suggesting a relation between blood lead levels and pubertal delays in girls in the United States (Selevan et al., 2003; Wu et al., 2003). Examples of other large cross-sectional studies in the United States are the National Children's Health and Nutrition Examination Survey (CDC, 2003a), the National Survey of Family Growth (NCHS, 1997), and the National Reports on Human Exposure to Environmental Chemicals (CDC, 2003b).

Linkage studies can be performed by linking routinely collected registry information with existing health information to the extent such information exists in a formal registry or established data system. Such information can be analysed to assess global changes in the distribution or frequency of health end-points such as infant birth weight and gestation, plurality of birth, secondary sex ratios, fetal deaths, stillbirths, birth defects, or childhood cancers. In some populations, hospital (in- and outpatient) visits and diagnoses can be used to monitor changes in the prevalence of diseases that may be affected by environmental influences (e.g. asthma). Often, one or more registries can be linked to assess childhood mortality and morbidity, such as the use of linked birth and death certificate files or the linkage of birth registries to birth defects or cancer registries.

6.1.1.4 Analytic designs

Analytic studies are designed to test formal hypotheses requiring methodologies to establish a temporal ordering between the study exposure and health outcome. There are two major types of observational analytic designs: case–control and cohort studies. Hybrid designs also exist, such as the case–cohort design, which can be useful for analysing rare failure events within a cohort study (Wacholder, 1991; Barlow et al., 1999). The determining factor is whether the investigator will ascertain study participants on the basis of disease (case–control design) or exposure (cohort). There are many practical considerations that impact the final choice of design, such as prevalence of the exposure or health outcome in a population, presumed latency period between exposure and outcome, and the estimated benefit of a cohort design over a case–control design (e.g. ability to look at a spectrum of outcomes). Case–control studies target incident (or newly diagnosed) cases of a particular disease in a specific population in time, and individuals free of that disease will serve as controls. Selection of a control group is extremely difficult and a process that requires careful consideration with respect to what is known about the exposure. Controls come from the same target population as cases and are similar to them in every way except for the presence of disease. Investigators attempt to ensure the comparability of controls with regard to cases by matching them on potential confounders in the design phase (i.e. matched case–control study) or in the analytic phase (i.e. multivariate modelling).

Prospective cohort studies are the design of choice when investigators can define a particular exposure or set of exposures in a population and follow individuals over time for disease incidence or newly occurring cases. Of particular note, the cohort study can be adapted to collect a multitude of data and biospecimens at critical windows or life stages along with the collection of other relevant study covariates (e.g. potential confounders). This aspect of exposure health outcome temporality is highly informative when assessing findings in relation to causality. A prospective cohort design can capture a spectrum of health end-points and outcomes (e.g. onset and progression of puberty). Follow-up of study participants can be a challenge, especially for subgroups of the population that may be hard to follow (e.g. transient, young, mobile, or individuals with name changes). Name changes for children may present a particular challenge, and investigators would do well to plan for such changes and to ascertain other information useful for tracking over long periods of time.

Retrospective cohort studies identify a historic exposure and focus on following up the study population to ascertain health status. An example of such a study is the identification of adults who were exposed to DES in utero to assess reproductive impairments or reproductive cancers. Prospective cohort studies ascertain exposure and follow the cohort for a defined time period and present a unique option for assessing child health, in that the latency period tends to be short (even shorter for intrauterine exposures and infant outcomes). For example, investigators interested in determining if endocrine disrupting chemicals adversely impact fetal growth could recruit couples at risk for pregnancy prior to conception, measure serum concentrations of endocrine disrupting chemicals at baseline and throughout pregnancy, measure fetal growth at relevant time periods, and obtain birth size measurements. Preconception recruitment of women and couples has been shown to be feasible (Buck et al., 2004), and the short latency period underscores the utility of cohort studies for answering related questions.

Cohort studies can be designed to commence with birth, with follow-up of offspring until targeted developmental ages relevant for assessing growth and development (e.g. through 36 months), minor neurodevelopmental impairments (e.g. through 60 months), or onset and progression of puberty (e.g. through 16 years). Cohort studies, however, are impractical when the disease of interest is rare, since a large cohort would be needed for ensuring a sufficient number of cases. Cohort studies may also be unfeasible in the context of limited resources, and other study designs (e.g. case–control studies) may be needed. These are addressed in subsequent paragraphs.

Given the increased recognition that diseases, including adverse pregnancy outcomes, may arise from the multiplicative effects of environmental factors and genes, variations of the traditional case–control study have been developed. The implications of gene–environment interactions for human reproduction and development have been reviewed (Cummings & Kavlock, 2004). Polymorphisms of genes have been associated with differential susceptibility to environmental exposures, underscoring the need for studies specifically designed to estimate gene–environment interactions and child health (Cummings & Kavlock, 2004). Case-only designs are responsive to this avenue of research and overcome methodological limitations associated with an inability to recruit population-based controls from the target population. Increasingly, it is difficult to find suitable controls or to enrol them in sufficient numbers in research, necessitating the need to develop designs not dependent on external comparison groups (Piegorsch et al., 1994; Khoury & Flanders, 1996). A case-only design is one such approach that uses cases of a particular disease (e.g. birth defect) to assess the association between an environmental factor and genes. Underlying this design is a strong assumption that the environmental factor and genes are independent.

6.1.1.5   *Unique methodological considerations*

Regardless of the epidemiological study design selected, key issues facing analytic studies include errors associated with the measurement of exposure(s), completeness of ascertaining health outcomes, capture of relevant covariates, and the validity of the assumptions underlying choice of statistical model (i.e. role of exposure, intermediate variables, and effect modifiers). Interpretation of study results with respect to potential biases or other sources of error is needed to rule out alternative explanations for the observed findings. For example, the validity of case–control studies is threatened by the potential for selection and recall bias. Systematic attrition also threatens the validity of cohort studies, such as in studies focusing on asthma in children utilizing hospital treatment

Methodologies to Assess Health Outcomes in Children

data, which have been reported to overestimate morbidity and utilization of health services.

6.1.2 Methodological approaches for animal studies

Many different experimental methods exist for investigating toxic effects of chemicals on reproduction and development in animals. Many of these methodologies incorporate standardized procedures for which guidelines have been issued by governmental agencies and international organizations, such as the USEPA, the United States Food and Drug Administration, the International Conference on Harmonisation of Technical Requirements for Registration of Pharmaceuticals for Human Use, the EU, and the OECD, while others are still undergoing scientific evaluation. In the following sections, methods internationally acceptable to regulatory authorities (i.e. the OECD test guideline methods) are discussed, with emphasis on effects induced during the prenatal and postnatal periods. Table 10 summarizes these methodologies: i.e. the Prenatal Developmental Toxicity Study (OECD Test Guideline 414), One- and Two-Generation Reproductive Toxicity Studies (OECD Test Guidelines 415 and 416), Reproductive/Developmental Toxicity Screening Tests (with or without the Combined Repeat Dose Toxicity Study) (OECD Test Guidelines 421 and 422), and the Developmental Neurotoxicity Study (draft OECD Test Guideline 426).

Other tests can reveal effects indicative of potential reproductive toxicity. Examples include the dominant lethal test, fertility assessment by continuous breeding, repeated-dose toxicity testing, and cancer studies where the gonads are subjected to pathological examination. These tests, however, provide information only on effects after dosing adult animals and are therefore not addressed below.

A number of assays, such as the uterotrophic assay, the Hershberger assay, male and female pubertal assays, and others, are currently being developed for detecting potential endocrine disrupting activity and effects of chemical substances on juvenile or young animals. The uterotrophic and Hershberger assays seem reliable for identifying chemicals with (anti)estrogenic and (anti)androgenic activity, respectively, and can also detect non-receptor-related estrogen or androgen effects. The pubertal assays provide knowledge on

Table 10. Overview of in vivo OECD test guidelines for reproductive toxicity testing

Test	Design	End-points	Advantages/limitations
OECD TG 414 Prenatal Developmental Toxicity Study (OECD, 2001a)	At least from implantation to 1 or 2 days before expected birth 3 dose levels plus control n = 20 pregnant females	Implantation, resorptions Fetal growth Morphological variations and malformations	+ malformations are assessed in all fetuses − the dosing period includes only the prenatal period − the effects assessment includes only effects in fetuses
OECD TG 415 One-Generation Reproductive Toxicity Study (OECD, 1983)	Exposure before mating for at least one spermatogenic cycle until weaning of 1st generation 3 dose levels plus control n = 20 pregnant females	Fertility Growth, development, and viability Histopathology and weight of reproductive organs, brain, and target organs	+ exposure covers most of the sensitive periods − no exposure from weaning to sexual maturation − not updated to include similar end-points as in the two-generation study
OECD TG 416 Two-Generation Reproductive Toxicity Study (OECD, 2001b)	Exposure before mating for at least one spermatogenic cycle until weaning of 2nd generation 3 dose levels plus control n = 20 pregnant females	Fertility Estrus cyclicity and sperm quality Growth, development, and viability Anogenital distance if triggered Sexual maturation Histopathology and weight of reproductive organs, brain, and target organs	+ exposure covers all sensitive periods + effect assessment in F1 and F2 + includes assessment of semen quality and estrus cyclicity − anogenital distance assessed in F2 only if triggered − areola/nipple retention is not assessed − malformations of reproductive organs investigated only in 1 per sex per litter

Table 10 (Contd)

Test	Design	End-points	Advantages/limitations
OECD TG 421 and TG 422 Reproduction/Developmental Toxicity Screening Test (with or without the Combined Repeat Dose Toxicity Study) (OECD, 1995, 1996)	From 2 weeks prior to mating until at least day 4 postnatally 3 dose levels plus control n = 8–10 pregnant females	Fertility Pregnancy length and birth Fetal and pup growth and survival until day 3	+ short-term test – limited exposure period – limited number of end-points – limited sensitivity due to number of animals
OECD TG 426 Developmental Neurotoxicity Study (OECD, 2003a)	At least from implantation throughout lactation (PND 20) 3 dose levels plus control n = 20 recommended, less than 16 not appropriate	Birth and pregnancy length Growth, development, and viability Physical and functional maturation Behavioural changes due to CNS and PNS effects Brain weights and neuropathology	+ exposure covers most of the sensitive periods – no exposure before mating and from weaning to sexual maturation – mating and nursing behaviour are not assessed

CNS, central nervous system; PND, postnatal day; PNS, peripheral nervous system; TG, Test Guideline effects during the juvenile phase, and some of the end-points included are similar to those in the two-generation study. Generally, clear effects observed in these assays indicate a potential for developmental toxicity in the two-generation study (Hass et al., 2004). The methodologies are summarized in Table 11.

During recent years, many in vitro test systems have been proposed as alternatives to animal testing for developmental toxicity. These tests may be useful for screening of closely related chemicals and for pinpointing mechanisms underlying developmental effects; however, they cannot replace animal testing, because of factors such as the limitations regarding metabolic activation of chemicals, developmental stage–specific vulnerabilities, and the multiple number of mechanisms leading to developmental toxicity. Consequently, they are not considered in the following sections.

6.1.2.1 Developmental stage susceptibility, dosing periods, and assessment of effects

The susceptibility windows for developmental toxicity effects start prior to conception and continue during prenatal development and during postnatal development to the time of sexual maturation (see Table 1). Developmental toxicity effects may become manifest at any time point in the lifespan of the organism. Figure 19 illustrates the vulnerable periods and the exposure periods covered in the OECD guidelines, while Figure 20 illustrates the timing of assessment of effects. Table 12 gives an overview of the outcomes assessed in offspring in OECD test guideline studies.

The two-generation study is unique, as it is the only study in which the animals are exposed during all of the susceptible time periods. The study requires that growth and survival of the offspring, sexual maturation, fertility, semen quality, and estrous cyclicity be investigated in young adult animals. In the one-generation study, the exposure of the offspring is stopped at weaning; consequently, juvenile animals are not exposed. The assessment of effects stops at weaning.

The exposure period in the developmental neurotoxicity study is during gestation and lactation, but not during the juvenile period until sexual maturation. The brain still undergoes development during the juvenile period, but effects induced during this period are

Table 11. Assays for detecting endocrine disrupting activity in juvenile or young animals (examples)

Test	Design	End-points	Advantages/limitations	Guideline(s)
Uterotrophic assay, detection of (anti)estrogens	3 days s.c. or p.o. to intact immature or adult ovariectomized female rats n = 6	Mandatory end-points: Body weight and weight of estrogen-responsive tissue, i.e. uterus wet weight and blotted weight	+ Used since 1935 + Simple, robust, and reproducible	The first and second phase of the validation of the uterotrophic assay within OECD is completed (OECD, 2003b) The guideline preparation is in progress within OECD
Hershberger assay, detection of (anti)androgens	10 day p.o. to immature castrated male rats n = 6	Mandatory end-points: Body weight and weight of ventral prostate, seminal vesicles, plus coagulating glands, levator ani/bulbocavernosus muscle, Cowper's glands, glans penis	+ Used since 1940 + Simple, robust, and reproducible + More sensitive than the pubertal assay to androgen receptor ligands − Inhibition of steroidogenesis not detected − Surgical castration	The first and second phases of the validation of the Hershberger assay are completed (OECD, 2003c) The third phase is in progress within OECD

Table 11 (Contd)

Test	Design	End-points	Advantages/limitations	Guideline(s)
Pubertal female assay	Daily dosing by oral gavage on PND 22–42 At least 2 dose levels plus control n = 15	Growth, serum T4 and TSH, age at vaginal opening, vaginal cytology, ovarian and uterus weight and histology, weight of liver, kidney, pituitary, adrenals	+ Sensitive to modulators of the HPG axis and the thyroid + End-points the same as in the generation studies − Does not detect 5α-reductase and some aromatase inhibitors − Growth and nutritional status may influence vaginal opening	Recommended by EDSTAC to be part of a Tier 1 in vivo screening battery together with the uterotrophic and the Hershberger assay
Pubertal male assay	Daily dosing by oral gavage on PND 23–54 At least 2 dose levels plus control n = 15	Growth, age at balano-preputial separation, serum T4 and TSH, weight of seminal vesicles, levator ani/bulbocavernosus muscle, and ventral prostate Thyroid, testis, and epididymal weight and histology	+ Sensitive to modulators of the HPG axis and the thyroid + End-points the same as in the generation studies − Does not detect all aromatase inhibitors − Growth and nutritional status may influence preputial separation	EDSTAC has also considered an alternative Tier 1 in vivo screening battery, which includes the pubertal male assay and the uterotrophic assay

EDSTAC, Endocrine Disruptor Screening and Testing Advisory Committee; HPG, hypothalamic–pituitary–gonadal; PND, postnatal day; p.o., per oral (by mouth); s.c., subcutaneous; T4, thyroxine; TSH, thyroid stimulating hormone

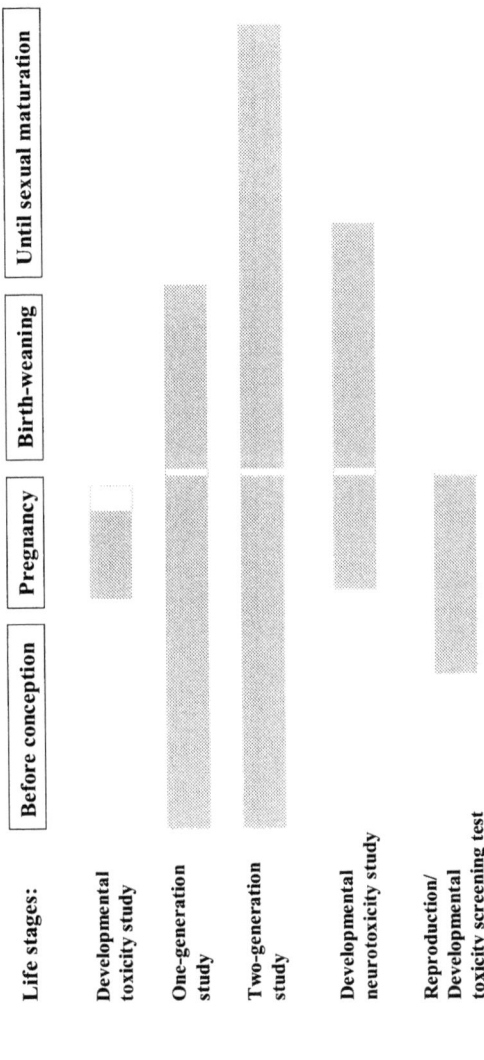

Fig. 19. Exposure periods in the OECD test guidelines

EHC 237: Principles for Evaluating Health Risks in Children

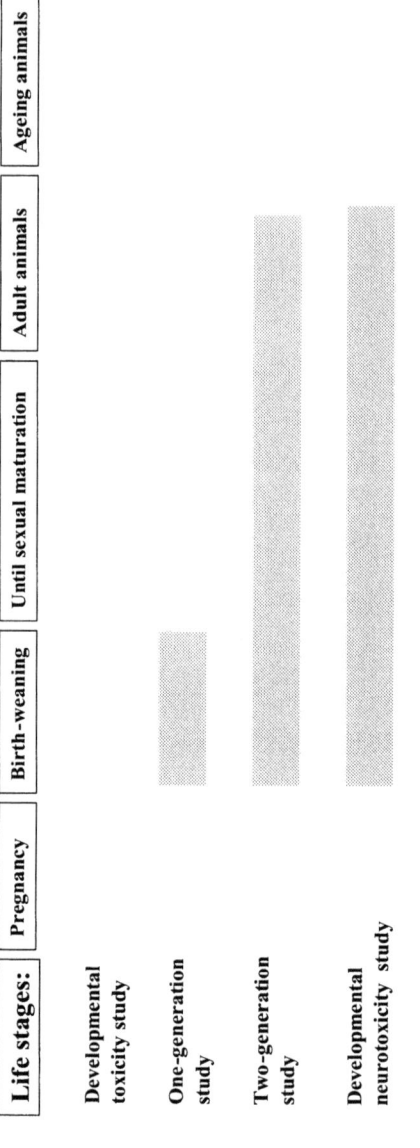

Fig. 20. Assessment of effects in the OECD test guidelines

not covered in the guideline. The assessment of effects in the study continues after exposure until around the age of two to four months.

Table 12. Outcomes assessed in offspring in OECD guideline studies

End-points	TG 415	TG 416	TG 421 & 422	Draft TG 426
Birth weight	+	+	+	+
Survival — perinatal period	+	+	+	+
Survival — lactation period	+	+	–	+
Survival — adult	–	+	–	+
Growth — perinatal period	+	+	+	+
Growth — lactation period	+	+	–	+
Growth — adult (adolescence!)	–	+	–	+
Physical development — sexual maturation	–	+	–	+
Functional development	–	(+)	–	+
Behaviour	–	(+)	–	+
Neuropathology	–	+	–	+
Reproductive functions	–	+	–	–
Other functions (e.g. immune)	–	–	–	–

TG, Test Guideline; + required; (+) optional; – not assessed

The prenatal developmental toxicity study was originally designed to investigate malformations, and the pregnant animals are sacrificed on the day prior to the expected birth. The background for this is that the dams may eat malformed offspring. As such, the prenatal developmental toxicity study covers only effects induced during prenatal development and visible at term.

Limited preliminary information is available on reproductive and developmental toxicity from the screening information data sets for high production volume chemicals.

In summary, among the current OECD test guidelines for reproductive toxicity, all susceptible periods of development are covered only in the two-generation study design. Late effects are partly covered in young adults, especially in relation to reproductive function and developmental neurotoxicity. Effects manifested during ageing are not included in any guidelines for reproductive toxicity.

6.1.2.2   Dosing of fetuses and pups

The dosing of the animals in reproductive toxicity studies is mainly oral. Oral dosing by gavage normally includes only the dams — i.e. the fetuses and pups are assumed indirectly dosed via placenta or maternal milk. Oral gavage may be stressful for the animals, especially around the time of birth; consequently, the animals are normally not dosed from the day before expected birth until a few days after birth. During the third week of the lactation period, the pups gradually change from maternal milk to their rat diet, and the exposure of the pups will therefore decline during this period. This means that although the dosing period in the one- and two-generation studies comprises the pregnancy and lactation period, the fetuses and pups are not exposed for some days around the time of birth, and the pups are exposed only to a limited extent during the third week of the lactation period. When using oral dosing via diet or drinking-water, the dams are normally dosed during the time of birth. When the pups gradually change from maternal milk to rat diet during the third week of lactation, they will still be dosed, although the dose level may differ depending on the levels in maternal milk.

For some chemicals, inhalation exposure may be the relevant route. During the postnatal development of the pups, the exposure may be of both the dam and the pups or of the dam only. Direct dosing of preweaning animals may be needed to ensure adequate exposure of the offspring during critical stages of development (e.g. when assessing effects on the developing nervous or immune system) and/or to quantify exposure of pups. Details concerning methodologies and design issues in relation to direct exposure of pups are available from the International Life Sciences Institute (Zoetis & Walls, 2003).

6.2   Growth and development

6.2.1   *Human studies*

The timed and highly interrelated processes underlying human development are important considerations when designing epidemiological research focusing on growth and developmental endpoints. The same exposure (or mixture of exposures) at varying gestational ages may manifest in different outcomes, as discussed above. To this end, exposures need to be considered in relation to life stages relevant for human populations. Prospective pregnancy studies are perhaps the best design for addressing timing and concentration of an exposure along with other attributes (e.g. acute versus chronic; intermittent versus constant) and a spectrum of outcomes at developmentally relevant critical windows. Such information is especially informative when assessing study results with respect to causality between exposure and effect. The short interval between conception and birth and the opportunity to consider a range of exposures within a single design further argue for use of prospective cohort designs.

By definition, growth and development in humans are dynamic processes involving numerous bodily functions. While some critical windows have been identified for structural birth defects (Wilson, 1965) and other health outcomes, such as neurodevelopment (Selevan et al., 2000; Morford et al., 2004), critical gaps exist for many other health end-points relevant for children's health. Established embryonic critical windows typically begin with early pregnancy or approximately two weeks post-conception. Unfortunately, investigators are often unable to capture exposures during this interval, because women may not recognize their pregnancy or seek medical care. Hence, retrospective collection of information is required, which assumes that women know and can accurately report exposures in the periconception period. The ability to recognize postimplantation pregnancy via the hCG biomarker affords investigators an opportunity to define periconception critical windows using prospective cohort designs (Wilcox et al., 1988; Wang et al., 2003). A theoretical description of critical windows during this interval has recently been described (Morford et al., 2004). The periconception critical window is unique in that it is consistent with the couple-dependent nature of human reproduction and the potential for maternal, paternal, and/or parental exposures (Chapin et al., 2004). Measuring conception and capturing exposures from periconception through implantation remain a challenge, but field-based technologies are arising and offer promise for future investigations.

Once exposures are identified and measured, it is necessary to determine how best to measure growth and development. If pregnant women comprise the study population, repeated fetal measurements will be needed at standardized intervals. Growth requires a minimum of three measurements during pregnancy, preferably at established intervals. While this might readily translate into one measurement per trimester of pregnancy, the study hypothesis should drive the timing of growth measurement. For example, the peak velocity for length is in the second trimester, and that for weight is in the third trimester (especially the last month of pregnancy). Infants born short and lean may have had chronic exposure extending throughout pregnancy, whereas infants born long and lean may reflect acute exposures late in pregnancy. Thus, symmetry of growth can provide insight into the possible timing and duration of an exposure. Such measurements are possible with ultrasonography, and standardized protocols for assessing numerous indices of fetal growth are clinically available and adaptable for field research. Birth size measurements are frequently used to characterize fetal growth. Birth weight is also a frequently used end-point when considering in utero exposures and fetal growth. When available, measurements on birth length, head and abdominal circumference, and other anthropometric indicators provide insight about the rate of fetal growth and possible timing of exposure. While these measures may be prone to measurement error, none is likely to be biased, given the absence of plausible reasons for systematic differences in the measurement process with respect to many exposures.

For infants and children, a number of well defined anthropometric methodologies are available that require the use of standardized scales and tape measurements by trained personnel, along with skinfold measurements (Dibley et al., 1987; NCHS, 1998). Summary measures of adiposity include the ponderal index for infants and the body mass index for children. Both indices provide a measure of how lean/fat the infant or child is for his/her birth length and height, respectively. Simpler methods have also been utilized in the field for measuring growth, such as measuring standing height and arm or leg circumference with standardized strings.

Growth charts can be used as a global assessment of infant or child size-for-age and are well suited for temporal surveillance (tracking) and identification of at-risk children. Typically, growth charts are available for weight, height, and head circumference, so that infants and children can be ranked in terms of age-specific percentiles (NCHS, 2003). Growth charts can also be tailored with regard to infant sex, plurality of birth, and race/ethnicity in recognition of differences across subgroups of the population. The appropriateness of birth size for gestational age can be summarized as small (<5th or 10th percentile), large (>5th or 10th percentile), or appropriate for gestational age. Infants born at the extremes of birth size for gestation may be at risk for mortality or morbidity.

The effects of exposures to environmental chemicals on human development are of global concern (see chapters 4 and 5). Developmental effects can be assessed at any life stage using a variety of approaches. Each approach addresses a variety of end-points relevant for studying human disabilities (WHO, 1980). Paediatricians use a clinical definition of neurodevelopmental disability, which assumes an etiology before birth. However, the terms developmental disability, developmental effects, and impaired development, as used in this document, encompass effects resulting from exposures to environmental chemicals from preconception through adulthood. Major neurodevelopmental impairments include cerebral palsy, mental retardation, blindness, deafness, and multiple impairments. An added dimension to assessing these outcomes is functional status of affected children. Vohr & Msall (1997) noted increasing survival for extremely low birth weight infants (<1000 g) without a concomitant increase in major neurodevelopmental impairments. However, an increasing percentage of children may have functional limitations associated with diminished birth weight. For example, approximately 20% of extremely premature infants born were found to have major impairments at age four years, yet all but 5% could function or perform the activities of daily living (i.e. walk unassisted, feed, dress, and toilette oneself). Thus, most investigators encompass neurodevelopmental impairments and function into assessment protocols. Minor neurodevelopmental impairments include deficits (not impairments per se) in vision, motor, perception, and cognition. Typically, these impairments cannot be reliably diagnosed until preschool or school ages. Various options exist for population-based research (Krasnegor et al., 1992; Msall et al., 1993; Msall, 1996), although some require administration by trained clinicians. The choice of instrument is largely dependent upon the study hypothesis (exposure and outcome), infant/child's chronological age (or mental age for children with cognitive impairments), and whether the instrument needs to be administered by a trained psychologist (e.g. Bayley, 1993) or can be administered by a parent (Bricker & Squires, 1995) or a teacher (Leviton et al., 1993). Standardized prospective follow-up of children's growth and health status between birth and age two years as captured with monthly diaries completed by mothers along with in-home assessments of children at 12 and 24 months of age were found to be feasible and acceptable to parents (Senn et al., 2005).

Unlike adults (Hutchinson et al., 1992), there is no universally accepted methodology for measuring infant and child development in relation to environmental exposures. The selected approach must be age, gender, and culturally appropriate. A number of evaluation tools exist for measuring targeted aspects of infant or child development, especially motor, cognitive, or sensory domains. Many instruments can be jointly administered to ensure assessment of various aspects of development.

6.2.1.1 Puberty

Onset and progression of puberty can be used for both boys and girls to measure the influence of exposures on this developmental milestone. This approach includes assessing normal progression and deviations, such as early or delayed onset. Puberty can be measured with a variety of instruments, such as self-rating schemes, anatomical markers for staging pubertal development performed by highly trained health-care practitioners, such as the Tanner Scales (Marshall & Tanner, 1969), and longitudinal hormonal assessments to capture changes in concentrations. Approaches for assessing puberty (including the applicability to specific subgroups of the population, such as adolescents with chronic illness or developmental disabilities) along with promising new biomarkers, such as spermarchy in (pre)adolescent boys, have been summarized by Rockett et al. (2004). Hormonally active environmental chemicals (e.g. PBBs, endocrine disrupting chemicals) can potentially impact precocious puberty (defined as the onset of secondary sex characteristics before eight and nine years of age in females and males, respectively) (Bates, 1998; Blanck et al., 2000). With regard to pubertal delays, authors have assessed delays in attaining specific pubertal milestones at specific chronological ages and in terms of the rate of progression between pubertal stages such as Tanner's stages (Selevan et al., 2003; Wu et al., 2003).

6.2.1.2 Birth defects

Approximately 3–4% of infants are diagnosed with a major birth defect in the first year of life, although birth defect prevalence varies according to many factors, including maternal age, race, and medical history, such as presence of insulin-dependent diabetes (Edmonds et al., 1981; Lynberg & Edmonds, 1996) (also see chapter 4). Birth defect registries are available for some populations and are a useful tool for etiologic research. Capture of major malformations is more complete when active surveillance of defects is utilized, compared with passive systems that rely on the reportings by physicians or health-care providers. In addition, many registries do not include minor malformations (e.g. hypospadia), resulting in an inability to monitor these defects on a population basis. Also, birth defect registries typically do not capture data on relevant study covariates (e.g. maternal diet, lifestyle factors such as cigarette smoking, use of medications or herbs), including the exposure of interest. Additional studies may be needed to capture such data.

Given the rarity of major malformations, the design of choice remains a case–control study. The choice of control group is exceedingly important to minimize the risk of over- or understating an effect. Recall bias, stemming from the systematic difference in reporting exposures between mothers of affected (cases) and unaffected (controls) children, is a well recognized threat to validity and needs to be considered when interpreting study findings. The case-only design offers promise for assessing gene–environment interactions, although strong assumptions must be made about the independent relation between the environmental factor and genes. A second consideration in designing studies focusing on birth defects is the need to capture exposures during critical windows of human development (Wilson, 1965; Selevan et al., 2000).

6.2.2 Animal studies

6.2.2.1 Body weight and postnatal growth

Fetal body weight is recorded in the Prenatal Developmental Toxicity Study (OECD Test Guideline 414), where the fetuses are killed the day before expected birth. Birth weight and postnatal growth are recorded in all other OECD reproductive toxicity test guidelines. It is important in the evaluation of the data to consider variations due to different litter sizes or different sex distribution in the litters. A change in offspring body weight is a sensitive indicator of developmental toxicity, in part because it is a continuous variable. In some cases, weight reduction in offspring may be the only indicator of developmental toxicity in a generation study. While uncertainty remains as to whether weight reduction is a permanent or transitory effect, little is known about the long-term consequences of short-term fetal or neonatal weight changes.

6.2.2.2 *Pre-, peri-, and postnatal death*

Prenatal developmental toxicity studies (e.g. OECD Test Guideline 414) are very suitable for the demonstration of intrauterine death resorption after implantation. In studies where dosing is started before implantation, preimplantation loss may also be assessed by comparing the number of corpora lutea in the ovaries of the pregnant animals with the number of implantations. Uteri that appear non-gravid should be further examined.

There are some limitations of generation studies concerning stillbirth and early postnatal death, since the commonly used laboratory animals may eat their dead or seriously malformed pups immediately after birth. An effect may, therefore, be indicated only indirectly by a smaller litter size. If only a few pups are affected, the reduction in litter size will be small compared with the normal variation in litter size and may, therefore, go undetected or not reach statistical significance. Preimplantation losses and resorption are also indicated in an indirect way as a decreased litter size, and the sensitivity for these effects may be rather low.

6.2.2.3 *Physical and functional developmental landmarks*

The physical development of the offspring is normally monitored by registration of body weight several times during the preweaning period and once every second week after weaning. Other physical and functional parameters are monitored by registration of so-called developmental milestones or developmental landmarks. These observations often show "when" rather than "if" the various landmarks first appear and are used to assess delayed or accelerated developmental time courses for the specific parameters being studied (Lochry et al., 1985). These tests evaluate the presence or absence of each parameter, usually over a period of successive days, beginning prior to or approximately on the day of expected development.

Examples of frequently suggested physical developmental landmarks are ear unfolding, first coat, upper and lower incisor eruption, eye opening, full coat, and onset of puberty. The reliability of observing six physical landmarks (ear unfolding, first coat, upper incisor eruption, lower incisor eruption, eye opening, and full coat) by different observers was assessed in a study. As a result of this evaluation, the three reliable physical parameters (i.e. ear unfolding, upper incisor eruption, and eye opening) were selected for use. Registration of these physical landmarks is not required in OECD Test Guideline 416 or 426, but should be considered when appropriate.

Functional development can be assessed by, for example, registration of the time of emergence of the surface righting reflex, negative geotaxis reflex, auditory startle reflex, and air righting reflex. The draft OECD Test Guideline 426 requires that two measures be registered equally spaced over the preweaning period. Registration of functional end-points requires some training in order to ensure that the animals are scored similarly each time. For that reason, it is also preferable that the assessment be performed by one person (or a few persons) using similar criteria each time. Early handling during inspection of physical or functional landmarks may influence the behaviour of the animals later in life. Therefore, litters from all groups (exposure and control) should be investigated similarly so as to avoid confounder bias.

The age of the offspring may be decided from the time of birth (i.e. postpartum age) or from the time of mating (i.e. gestational age). Studies have shown gestational age to be a better predictor of time of appearance of developmental landmarks in the preweaning period than postnatal age, especially if the length of gestation periods differs among groups (Raimondo & Draghetti, 1990). Gestational age has been used in several studies of developmental neurotoxic effects (Kelly et al., 1988; Hass et al., 1994, 1995).

6.2.2.4 Birth defects and malformations

The Prenatal Developmental Toxicity Study (OECD Test Guideline 414) is designed to detect malformations. The sensitivity of the test for detection of rare malformations is limited, owing to the use of a relatively small number of animals. With the normal group sizes of 20 pregnant rats, it is not possible to identify any increase in major malformations unless high dose levels are administered or the substance studied is highly embryo/fetotoxic (Palmer, 1981). To assess the developmental toxicity of a chemical, it is therefore important to include information on other developmental effects, such as minor anomalies, skeletal variations, fetal death, and growth. The development of some organs, such as the reproductive organs and the brain, continues after birth, and malformations of these organs may not become manifest until the animal is sexually mature (see sections 6.3.2 and 6.4.2).

The Committee on International Harmonization of Nomenclature in Developmental Toxicology of the International Federation of Teratology Societies has developed and published a glossary of internationally accepted common nomenclature to use when describing observations of fetal and neonatal morphology (Wise et al., 1997). The purpose of this effort was to advance the harmonization of terminology and to reduce confusion and ambiguity in the description of developmental effects, particularly in submissions to regulatory agencies worldwide. Familiarity with the International Federation of Teratology Societies terminology for external, visceral, and skeletal observations and appropriate use of the terminology in data collection, reporting, and review are encouraged. It is recognized, however, that although the common nomenclature developed by this effort has been widely available and internationally accepted, there is no guarantee that the terminology has been uniformly used by all laboratories conducting studies for chemical hazard assessment.

6.3 Reproductive development and function

6.3.1 *Human studies*

Study of human reproductive health necessitates appreciation of the highly interrelated and timed series of events underlying successful human reproduction (Källén, 2006). In assessing the reproductive toxicity of an environmental agent, two broad categories of outcomes can be studied — fecundity and fertility. Fecundity refers to the biological capacity of men and women for reproduction, whereas fertility refers to the ability of a woman to give birth to a liveborn infant or a man to have fathered a liveborn infant (Wood, 1994). Fecundity can be "proved" only when the couple has a liveborn infant. A live birth is the biomarker of fertility.

The ability to identify structural abnormalities or deficiencies (e.g. cryptorchidism, hypospadia, endometriosis) in the reproductive organs of children, men, and women often requires purposeful clinical examination and invasive diagnostic procedures, such as pelvic laparoscopy in women. Often this is done in response to health concerns or signs/symptoms indicative of underlying disease. Epidemiological studies that incorporate clinical populations frequently are limited with regard to both internal and external validity, making it difficult to systematically evaluate organ-specific abnormalities. Choice of comparison group or the selectness of individuals who seek medical care can potentially impact study findings. For example, exposure to dioxins and PCBs has been linked with an increased risk of endometriosis in a few studies. However, diagnosis requires pelvic laparoscopy or laparotomy to confirm the presence or absence of disease. Choice of sampling framework to explore environmental causes is difficult, because study participants cannot be asked to undergo laparoscopy in the absence of signs/symptoms for research purposes only. To this end, women with pelvic pain or infertility for whom a laparoscopy is medically indicated are often selected as the comparison group, as are women undergoing tubal sterilization procedures. Studies on the former groups of women may fail to reflect an association between an exposure and disease if the exposure affects a spectrum of gynaecological effects (not just endometriosis). Conversely, use of fertile women may exaggerate an association if exposure concentrations have been affected by pregnancy or lactation patterns.

Fecundity can be estimated or approximated by assessing reproductive hormonal profiles of men and women, semen quality in men, or menstruation in women or by measuring time to pregnancy for couples interested in becoming pregnant. Time to pregnancy can be measured in calendar months or menstrual cycles, depending upon the study population, and has been shown to be a reasonable estimate of cycle-specific probability of conception when comparing exposed and unexposed women or couples (Baird et al., 1986). Time to pregnancy can be dichotomized as conception delay, defined as requiring more than six menstrual cycles for conception, or as infertility or the absence of pregnancy despite 12 or more months of regular unprotected intercourse. Women with conception delays are reported to be at increased risk of delivering a preterm or low-birth-weight infant (Olsen et al., 1983; Williams et al., 1991; Joffe & Li, 1994; Henriksen et al., 1999), although no effect was seen in another study after controlling for potential confounders (Cooney et al., 2006).

Fecundity end-points are not necessarily adverse health states and may also include puberty, sexual libido, gynaecological or urological disorders (e.g. endometriosis and erectile dysfunction), fecundity impairments (e.g. early pregnancy loss), and premature reproductive senescence. The need to consider fecundity end-points is supported by a possible relation between PCB exposure and endometriosis (Mayani et al., 1997; Buck Louis et al., 2004) and between consumption of PCB-contaminated fish and diminished fecundability (Axom et al., 2000; Buck et al., 2000). Male fecundity impairments have been associated with both birth defects and chronic disease. For example, cryptorchidism has been associated with impairments in male fecundity and testicular cancer. This constellation of ecological patterns (declining semen quality, rising rates of hypospadias, cryptorchid testes, and testicular cancer) has been referred to as the testicular dysgenesis hypothesis, for which an environmental origin has been hypothesized (Skakkebaek et al., 2001) (see also chapter 4).

Use of fertility monitors offers promise for capturing information about hormonal patterns during the menstrual cycle, including information on ovulation and, more precisely, information about time required for conception. The Clearblue Easy fertility monitor tracks changes in estrone-3-glucuronide, a metabolite of estradiol, and LH, using urine collected via special test sticks. After the woman has urinated on the test stick, two blue lines appear in the test stick window; the monitor optically measures the intensity of these lines to track changes in estrone-3-glucuronide and LH. The monitor is reported to be highly accurate (99%) in detecting the LH surge and in predicting peak fertility (91%) in comparison with ultrasonography (Behre et al., 2000). After 5 min, the monitor displays the woman's fertility status for the current day (e.g. low, high, or peak fertility) and can store up to 40 days of detailed information and up to six months of summary data that can be downloaded to a personal computer with the help of a card reader. The accuracy of the Clearblue Easy monitor has been evaluated, and it has been determined that the monitor supports the WHO criteria for detecting the LH surge or impending ovulation (WHO, 1983).

Pregnancy loss comprises three groups: losses occurring prior to implantation of the conceptus in the endometrium, following implantation and identified with hCG testing, or after clinical recognition of pregnancy. hCG pregnancies are referred to as early or clinically unrecognized pregnancies, in that most women will not be aware they are pregnant unless measuring hCG, such as with home pregnancy test kits. The incidence of early pregnancy loss has been estimated with active monitoring of hCG in only a few prospective cohort designs where couples have been enrolled prior to attempting pregnancy. Of these studies, approximately one third of all hCG-confirmed pregnancies were spontaneously lost, especially in the first few weeks following implantation (Wilcox et al., 1988; Wang et al., 2003). Specifically, two thirds of these pregnancy losses were hCG-detected pregnancies, and the remaining one third were clinically recognized pregnancies. These figures underscore the importance of capturing hCG and not just clinically recognized pregnancies to avoid underascertaining pregnancy losses. An important point to keep in mind is that studies starting with pregnant women or newborns are not designed to capture hCG-confirmed pregnancy loss, necessitating the need to consider other developmental outcomes. As such, an exposure that causes embryonic death may not be linked to deficits in children. This notion is referred to as competing risk and is important to keep in mind when assessing developmental outcomes and interpreting study results that rely only on clinically recognized pregnancies. The design of choice for assessing embryonic and fetal loss is a prospective pregnancy study design to estimate as accurately as possible the number of conceptions. Losses occurring later in pregnancy include spontaneous terminations of pregnancy, fetal deaths, and stillbirths, which typically occur in the few weeks prior to delivery or any time following gestational ages deemed viable. Fetal death registries exist in many countries and can be used for ascertaining cases for defined populations with respect to time. However, a number of methodological issues face use of vital registries, such as varying criteria for defining fetal losses (e.g. by gestation, birth weight, or both) and poor quality of data, including cause of death (Lammer et al., 1989; Kirby, 1993).

Fertility end-points include live births, plurality of birth, and secondary sex ratio, or the ratio of male to female live births. Xenobiotics that selectively impact the X or Y chromosome may result in decrements of the sex ratio, possibly due to differences in rates of conception or pregnancy loss. In fact, investigators have used this ratio as a sentinel marker of male fecundity (Davis et al., 1998), with declines reported in some populations (Allan et al., 1997; Scialli et al., 1997) and increases in others (Astolfi & Zonta, 1999). WHO has established protocols for the evaluation of semen quality (male fecundity) and infertile couples.

6.3.2 Animal studies

6.3.2.1 Malformations of reproductive organs

Examination of structural changes of the reproductive organs is included in all OECD guideline studies except draft Test Guideline 426. Malformations of reproductive organs include, for example, persistent nipples, hypospadias, and cryptorchidism in male offspring. OECD Test Guideline 414 is designed especially to investigate major malformations, and the pregnant animals are killed prior to the expected day of delivery (gestation day 21 in the rat). The test guideline specifies that investigations of the fetuses should pay particular attention to the reproductive tract. These techniques may not be sensitive for detecting all malformations among organs that are not fully developed at birth.

In studies performed according to OECD Test Guideline 414, Prenatal Developmental Toxicity Study, before the test guideline was updated (OECD, 1981), the animals were dosed only during the major organogenesis (i.e. gestation days 6–15 in the rat). As important parts of the development of the reproductive organs happen after gestation day 15, the potential for effects on the development of the reproductive organs cannot be assessed in such studies. In the updated OECD Test Guideline 414, Prenatal Developmental Toxicity Study, the exposure period is extended until a few days before birth (OECD, 2001a). However, the development of the reproductive organs continues after birth, and some effects may not become manifest until the animal is sexually mature. Consequently, OECD Test Guideline 414 is not suitable for detection of some important malformations of the reproductive organs.

Malformations of the reproductive organs, such as hypospadias and cryptorchidism, can potentially be identified in the generation studies, since the offspring is investigated until young adulthood. However, only one animal per sex per litter is selected at weaning for the next generation, in contrast to the assessment of malformations using OECD Test Guideline 414, where all fetuses are investigated. As malformations normally are rare effects, the generation studies have a limited sensitivity for detecting such effects; therefore, malformations in the reproductive organs occurring at low rates may not reach statistical significance. The short-term studies (i.e. OECD Test Guidelines 421 and 422) include a limited number of litters, and the animals are immature when investigated on postnatal day 3 or 4. Therefore, the potential for malformations of reproductive organs can be assessed only to a very limited extent in these studies.

6.3.2.2 *Anogenital distance*

Visual inspection of the anogenital distance in fetuses and newborn pups is used for deciding the sex of the animals, as the anogenital distance normally is twice as long in males as in females. In the two-generation study, anogenital distance should be measured at postnatal day 0 in the pups in the second generation, if triggered by alterations in the sex ratio or timing of sexual maturation in the first generation. There is a relation between the anogenital distance and the size of the pup; therefore, the body weight of the pup is normally used as a covariate in the analysis of the data. However, if body weight is significantly influenced by exposure, this may actually mask effects on anogenital distance. In general, a statistically significant change in the anogenital distance (adjusting for size of the pups) would be considered adverse. Several studies have shown that hormones and exposure to endocrine disrupting chemicals may change the anogenital distance. This is especially true for antiandrogens, where decreased anogenital distance has been shown for some phthalates, procymidone, and vinclozolin (Gray et al., 1999; Mylchreest et al., 1999; Ostby et al., 1999).

6.3.2.3 Nipple/areola retention

Assessment of nipple or areola (dark area around the nipple bud) retention in male offspring is not included at present in any OECD test guideline. In female offspring, 12 areolas normally become visible around postnatal day 13, while very few or none are visible in male offspring. As the development of fur in the animals makes it difficult (impossible) to see the areolas a few days later, it is important to establish the correct time for the assessment in the animals used for the study. Often, only the presence or absence is registered in the males; however, the number of areolas in each male may provide a more sensitive assessment. In general, a statistically significant increase in the number of nipples/areolas in male pups would be considered adverse. This is especially the case if it is shown that some of these nipples are persistent (i.e. they are also present in the adult males).

6.3.2.4 Sexual maturation and puberty

Assessment of the timing of sexual maturation is included in OECD Test Guideline 416 and as an optional end-point in draft OECD Test Guideline 426. Assessment of the onset of puberty in females is done by inspection of the vaginal opening. In rats, this occurs around postnatal days 30–35. In males, testicular descent and balano-preputial separation, which occur around postnatal days 21–30 and 42–48, respectively, may be used as indicators of puberty. Observation of testicular descent relies on how the animal is handled during inspection, and testicular descent is rather difficult to assess. Balano-preputial separation corresponds to puberty in male rats (Korenbrot et al., 1977) and is the end-point included in the developmental neurotoxicity study and the Two-Generation Reproductive Toxicity Study (OECD Test Guideline 416). Both the age and the body weight of the animal at sexual maturation need to be recorded, as there is a relationship between these end-points. In general, significant changes in the timing of sexual maturation that are not explained by body weight effects should be considered to indicate a potential adverse effect in humans.

6.3.2.5 Fertility

Assessment of fertility is included in generation studies and in the reproductive screening tests. Assessment of fertility in exposed offspring is possible only in the two-generation study. Fertility is generally expressed as indices that are ratios derived from the data collected. For example, the mating index is used as a measure of the male's or female's ability to mate and is defined as the number of animals with confirmed mating in the total number of animals cohabiting. The fertility index is a measure of the ability to achieve pregnancy and is defined as the number of males impregnating a female or the number of pregnant females per total number of animals cohabiting. The effects on fertility may be related to effects induced either before mating or thereafter, but before implantation (i.e. preimplantation losses). The data will not necessarily be similar for studies in which there is more than one mating per generation or more than one mating generation. The interpretation of fertility data should consider the duration of treatment and the number of animals investigated. The males are not dosed during the total of the spermatogenic cycle in the reproductive screening tests, and the studies use a limited number of animals. Therefore, it is unlikely that reproductive effects are manifested in the fertility data.

Reduced fertility has been found for a number of chemicals, but often at relatively high exposure levels. However, it has to be considered that the rat is the most commonly used experimental animal and that a male rat can generally still produce normal progeny after having its sperm production reduced to 10% of the normal level (Aafjes et al., 1980). Thus, fertility data from rat studies alone can be a rather insensitive end-point. Human males may not have a similar sperm reserve capacity as rodents, and therefore the two-generation study has recently been updated to include assessment of sperm quality. It is unknown whether female rats (compared with human females) are also less sensitive to effects on fertility, but the two-generation study has recently been updated in that aspect by the inclusion of assessment of estrous cyclicity.

The assessment of sperm quality includes measures of sperm number, anomalies, and motility, but the ability of the sperm to fertilize the ovum is not assessed. In order to increase the sensitivity for detection of fertility effects, investigation of in vitro fertilization could be considered. Another potentially more sensitive option may be the continuous breeding protocol, where the animals produce several litters instead of only one litter per pair.

Effects manifesting during the ageing process are not included in any guideline for reproductive toxicity. For example, the reproductive span of females is limited from the time of sexual maturation to reproductive senescence. The time of sexual maturation may be assessed in the two-generation study, but reproductive senescence is not assessed. Consequently, effects on the reproductive span of females are not covered in the reproductive toxicity test guidelines.

6.3.2.6 *Histopathology of reproductive organs*

Histological examination of reproductive organs is included in the generation studies and the in vivo reproductive toxicity screening studies (i.e. OECD Test Guidelines 421 and 422). The two-generation study that specifies dosing of the male for the entire spermatogenic cycle combined with analysis of sperm quality requires less extensive histopathological examination than the studies in which the dosing regime is shorter and no sperm analyses are conducted (e.g. OECD Test Guidelines 421 and 422).

The postlactational ovary should contain primordial and growing follicles as well as the large corpora lutea of lactation. In the two-generation study, the histopathological examination includes assessment of qualitative depletion of the primordial follicle population in the parental animals. A quantitative evaluation of primordial follicles should be conducted for F1 females; the number of animals, ovarian section selection, and section sample size should be statistically appropriate for the evaluation procedure used. Examination should include enumeration of the number of primordial follicles, which can be combined with small growing follicles, for comparison of treated and control ovaries.

Histopathological findings are generally classified according to qualitative criteria, and the data are presented as the number of animals affected within a dose group. There may not be an obvious relation between histopathological findings and fertility. For short-term studies (i.e. OECD Test Guidelines 421 and 422) in which the animals are treated for less than the duration of the spermatogenic cycle, an effect on spermatogenesis may not have had adequate time to become evident as reduced sperm counts. In general, any dose-related significant histopathological finding would be considered to indicate a potential adverse effect in humans.

6.3.2.7 Sperm quality and estrous cyclicity

These end-points are included in the revised two-generation study, but not at present in the one-generation study. However, the one-generation study could be updated to include assessment in the parental animals without significant changes in the design. Assessment of these end-points in exposed offspring is possible only in the two-generation study design. However, it would be possible to include the end-points in the one-generation study if the study period were extended to around postnatal day 90 instead of postnatal day 21.

The end-points included for assessment of sperm quality are sperm number, sperm morphology, and sperm motility. Testicular lesions of sufficient magnitude can impact sperm quality, but normal sperm quality is dependent on a number of other factors. Therefore, changes in sperm end-points should not be discounted in the absence of histological lesions. For example, sperm changes could be due to effects on the epididymis. In general, a statistically significant change in sperm parameters would be interpreted as indicating a potential effect on human fertility.

Vaginal cytology is evaluated to determine the length and normality of the estrous cycle in P and F1 females in the two-generation study. The data can provide information on cycle length, persistence of estrus or diestrus, and incidence of pseudopregnancy. An effect on the estrous cycle can affect reproductive performance, but this will depend on the nature and the magnitude of the effect. In general, a statistically significant change in the length of the cycle or prolonged estrus or diestrus would be considered potentially adverse.

6.4 Neurological and behavioural effects

6.4.1 Human studies

Environmental agents have been associated with neurotoxic effects in infants and children (IPCS, 1986a, 2001b). Given the ability of agents to impact various target sites or pathways (e.g. autonomic, peripheral, or central nervous system), a diverse range of outcomes should be considered. To this end, clinical assessment coupled with a battery of standardized assessment tools are likely to be needed. With respect to behaviour, gender-specific tools should be considered, if not implemented. Both DES and PCB exposures have been associated with alterations in gender-specific behaviour (Collaer & Hines, 1995; Guo et al., 1995; Longnecker et al., 2003). Standardized clinical assessments are available for newborns and paediatric populations, which can be tailored to meet particular research goals, taking into account the characteristics or physical/ biological properties of the exposure under investigation.

6.4.2 Animal studies

A guideline for a developmental neurotoxicity study was issued by the USEPA in 1991 (USEPA, 1991), and a revised United States guideline was proposed in 1995 (USEPA, 1998). During recent years, a draft OECD Test Guideline 426, Developmental Neurotoxicity Study, has been developed based on the United States guideline (OECD, 2003a). Developmental neurotoxicity studies are designed to develop data on the potential functional and morphological hazards for the nervous system arising in the offspring from exposure of the mother during pregnancy and lactation. The OECD draft test guideline is designed as a separate study, but the observations and measurements can also be incorporated into a two-generation study. The neurological evaluation consists of assessment of reflex ontogeny, motor activity, motor and sensory function, and learning and memory; and evaluation of brain weights and neuropathology during postnatal development and adulthood. The behavioural testing includes assessment of the individual animal for a number of relevant behavioural functions, but none of the tests assesses two or more animals together. This means that some behavioural end-points of potential relevance (e.g. sexual behaviour, play behaviour, social interaction among animals, and aggression) are not assessed using the current test guidelines.

6.4.2.1 Motor activity

According to the draft OECD Test Guideline 426, motor activity should be monitored using an automated recording apparatus at least once for each of the preweaning, post-weaning, and young adult periods. The open field and the hole-board have generally been used to measure short-term activity, whereas automated devices (photo cells) such as the figure 8 maze, radial arm maze, and cages similar to home cages have been used for measuring activity over longer time periods. The recommendations given in the draft OECD Test Guideline 426 relate mainly to the testing of longer-term activity (e.g. 30 min) and should provide data for evaluating the potential for effects on motor activity and habituation.

6.4.2.2 Motor and sensory functions

According to the draft OECD Test Guideline 426, motor and sensory function should be examined in detail at least once for the adolescent period and once during the young adult period. Neuromotor abilities are often evaluated in regard to the ontogeny of particular reflexes or coordinated movements. Measures of reflex and motor development are the most widespread of all functional end-points assessed in behavioural teratology studies (Buelke-Sam & Kimmel, 1979; Adams, 1986). The procedures for most of the commonly used measurements have been described in several reviews (Barlow & Sullivan, 1975; Adams, 1986). Until recently, measures of sensory function in developmental toxicity studies have been quite gross — measuring the presence or absence of response rather than the magnitude of the response. During the last decade, however, more sophisticated automated behavioural techniques allowing quantitative assessment of function have been developed.

6.4.2.3 Learning and memory

In the draft OECD Test Guideline 426, testing of learning and memory is required post-weaning and for young animals. The use of different tests or different animals is recommended, because repeated testing in the same test animal may decrease the sensitivity of the test. The time of post-weaning testing could be shortly after the end of exposure (i.e. at days 24–28) and just before termination of the study, around days 60–80. The test for cognitive function (i.e. learning and memory) should be based on associative learning and should include the possibility of assessing changes across repeated learning trials as well as memory function.

A number of different tests have been used for assessing effects on learning and memory. Many of these are based on the animals moving and using their senses; therefore, an impaired performance in a learning test may reflect behavioural effects other than learning abilities. The radial arm maze and the Morris maze have been used to demonstrate the effects of several positive control substances. Schedule controlled operant conditioning in Skinner boxes may detect very subtle effects, but may also be too time-consuming for the initial testing of learning and memory.

6.4.2.4 Evaluation of effects

Developmental neurotoxicity can be indicated by behavioural changes or morphological changes in the brain. The severity and nature of the effect should be considered. Generally, a pattern of effects (e.g. impaired learning during several consecutive trials) is more persuasive evidence of developmental neurotoxicity than one or a few unrelated changes. In the standard developmental neurotoxicity study design, treatment is stopped following postnatal day 10 or postnatal day 21, while neurobehavioural testing is conducted around the time of weaning, during the time of puberty, and again just before termination, at approximately postnatal day 60. Apparent reversibility in adult offspring of effects observed early in life may be related to compensatory developmental or behavioural processes and not represent a true recovery per se. Likewise, findings observed in adult offspring that had not been previously observed in young test subjects should not be discounted for lack of concordance, since they may represent the latent expression of early alterations in neurological development. Effects observed during the beginning of a learning task but not at the end should not be interpreted as a reversible effect. Rather, the results may indicate that the speed of learning is decreased.

The experience of offspring, especially during infancy, may affect their later behaviour. For example, frequent handling of rats during infancy may alter the physiological response to stress and behaviour in tests for emotionality and learning. In order to control for environmental experiences, the conditions under which the offspring are reared should be standardized within experiments with respect to variables such as noise level, handling, and cage cleaning. The performance of the animals during behavioural testing may also be influenced by factors such as time of day and the stress level of the animals. The most reliable data are obtained in studies where control and treated animals are tested alternately and environmental conditions are standardized.

Most developmental neurotoxicity studies have focused on general impairment of behaviour, but some studies have also found evidence for effects on sexual dimorphic behaviour. Hormones play a central role in central nervous system development, including the sexual differentiation of the brain. Studies on hormones and various endocrine disrupting chemicals (particularly those with estrogenic or antiandrogenic effects) have shown that the developing brain may be susceptible to disturbances in sexual behaviour. Therefore, effects on one sex but not the other should not be dismissed, but must be evaluated in the context of effects on sexual differentiation of the brain.

Of critical concern is the possibility that developmental exposure may result in an acceleration of age-related decline in function. Animal studies have demonstrated that developmental exposure to neurotoxicants such as methylmercury, methylazoxymethanol, and ethanol may cause few or no neurotoxic effects in young animals, but marked effects in ageing animals. Investigations of effects in ageing animals are not included in regulatory guidelines.

6.5 Cancer

6.5.1 *Human studies*

Given the relative rarity of childhood cancers, case–control study designs are primarily utilized for assessing environmental carcinogens. For many countries, cancer registries will be used for ascertaining cases for a defined population in time. Selection of controls may include the use of siblings, neighbours, schoolmates, or children seeking medical care from clinics, hospitals, or private physician offices. The need for matching on known confounders may exist, or at the very least the matching may capture data on potential or unknown confounders.

Linkage studies are sometimes used for assessing possible new exposures. For example, a recent linkage study combined live birth and cancer registries to assess whether children born from assisted reproductive technologies were at risk for childhood cancer in comparison with children born without such technologies (Brinton et al., 2004). This linkage study was a population-based attempt to further explore an earlier report linking in utero hormonal exposure to neuroblastoma (Michalek et al., 1996; Olshan et al., 1999). Linkage studies may be limited by the completeness of data on the exposure (e.g. specific type of assisted reproductive technology) and other etiologic factors impacting the couple's fecundity. The methodological challenges underlying the separation of an assisted reproductive technology effect from underlying couple infecundity have recently been reviewed (Buck Louis et al., 2004).

6.5.2 Animal studies

Studies for assessing the carcinogenicity of chemicals after developmental exposure are not included in any regulatory test guidelines. Transplacental carcinogenesis has been demonstrated in rats, mice, hamsters, rabbits, pigs, dogs, and monkeys for about 60 chemicals (IPCS, 1984). All the transplacental carcinogens that have been studied were already known to be carcinogenic in adult animals. It appears that the action of chemical carcinogens may be stronger or weaker after passing through the placenta. Based on current knowledge, it is not possible generally to estimate if peri-pubertal exposure is more or less important than adult exposure. Negative results in testing for transplacental or perinatal carcinogenic effects should be evaluated with caution, because the period of development in experimental animals is relatively short compared with human development, and some chemicals may require more prolonged exposure in order to induce tumours.

6.6 Immune system effects

6.6.1 Human studies

Environmental agents including chemicals have been shown to affect the immune system in a number of ways (IPCS, 1999b). However, there are no universally established guidelines for assessing immune function in children in relation to environmental agents. Diagnostic approaches used by clinicians can be adapted for research purposes and may include alterations in B and T lymphocytes or T helper/T suppressor cell ratios. Age-appropriate assessments should recognize the ongoing development of the immune system during fetal development and childhood (Holladay & Smialowicz, 2000).

6.6.2 *Animal studies*

Studies of immunotoxicity after developmental exposure are not included in any regulatory test guidelines. Organogenesis of the immune system occurs during the prenatal and early postnatal periods (Holladay & Smialowicz, 2000). Consequently, the perinatal period is a time of high susceptibility to immunotoxicants that can cross the placenta or expose the neonate via lactation. Postnatal immunotoxic effects from exposure during the initial establishment of the immune organs may be both more severe and more persistent than those that occur in adult animals exposed at similar levels. Chemical agents that induce developmental immunotoxicity in rodents are diverse and include halogenated aromatic hydrocarbons, PAHs, hormonal substances, therapeutic agents, heavy metals, and mycotoxins (Holladay & Smialowicz, 2000; Luebke et al., 2006).

6.7 Respiratory system effects

6.7.1 *Human studies*

The mature respiratory system evolves throughout fetal life, childhood, and early adulthood. Exposure to environmental chemicals can affect a number of respiratory processes, such as cellular differentiation and lung growth, underscoring the need to select health end-points appropriate for the age of infants or children (Fanucchi et al., 1997; Smiley-Jewell et al., 1998). There are no universally established guidelines for assessing respiratory function in children following environmental exposures, necessitating the need for clinical assessment and capture of acute end-points (e.g. respiratory infections in a specific period of time) or chronic end-points (e.g. bronchitis, asthma). Symptom inventories (e.g. wheezing, cough, phlegm) can also be used, along with field-based spirometry to assess lung function (American Thoracic Society, 1987). Diagnostic approaches used by clinicians can be adapted for research purposes.

6.7.2 *Animal studies*

Studies of effects on the respiratory system after developmental exposure are not included in any regulatory test guidelines. Exposure during critical periods of lung development may have effects that would not be seen if the same exposure were to occur in adulthood (Dietert et al., 2000).

6.8 Haematopoietic/cardiovascular, hepatic/renal, skin/musculoskeletal, and metabolic/endocrine system effects

6.8.1 Human studies

There are no established universally accepted guidelines or study protocols for assessing the organ-specific health end-points included in this section.

6.8.2 Animal studies

Studies of these specific organ system outcomes are not included in any regulatory test guidelines.

6.9 Summary and conclusions

Child health status can be measured very narrowly by focusing on one or two related end-points or globally by being inclusive of all organ systems, recognizing the highly interrelated processes underlying the dynamic state of children and child development. To date, there is no universally defined or accepted methodology for assessing children's overall health status in relation to a multitude of environmental factors, although efforts are currently under way to address this gap. For many aspects of child health, such as growth and development, a number of assessment tools are available, and many can be implemented in field-based research; in contrast, no assessment tools for other organ systems, such as the endocrine system, are available.

Given that children, by definition, are in a state of continual growth and development, methodologies for the assessment of child health should be responsive to all organ systems. Prospective studies are particularly relevant, since they permit the capture of time-varying exposures and other relevant covariates for children's health. The short interval between many exposures and outcomes (e.g. in utero exposures and infant birth size) further supports the use of prospective studies.

Challenges remain regarding the impact of the environment on children's health during development. One such challenge is the need to identify critical windows, including those before, during, or shortly after conception, for the spectrum of health end-points relevant for child health. Recruitment of couples prior to first attempting pregnancy offers promise for identifying new critical windows and the ability to assess maternally, paternally, and parentally mediated effects on child health. Use of home fertility monitors, in light of our inability to measure conception, may help to time conception and, hence, exposures in relation to conception and gestation. While standardized methodologies exist for measuring some aspects of children's health status, such as growth and development, few standardized approaches exist for many other organ-specific end-points. Methodologies that can build upon clinical assessment of children as a part of well-baby or well-child visits with health providers may offer utility and feasibility for capturing exposures in relation to acute health effects (e.g. air pollution and asthma attacks or upper respiratory infections), while ensuring methodologies for tracking children's health trajectories in a standardized fashion. The absence of registries for assessing most health outcomes facing children other than cancer or birth defects makes it difficult to assess secular or regional trends in children's health. Use of in- and outpatient discharge diagnoses may crudely provide information on receipt of care for medical diagnoses. However, the absence of identifying information in such registries makes it impossible to remove clustering of outcomes stemming from our inability to remove repeated diagnoses for the same person.

Methodologies can be tailored to the unique characteristics of the study exposure(s) or other population/host factors that might impact study conclusions. Efforts aimed at identifying a minimal data set essential for the analysis of most environmental exposures and health outcomes would be informative for investigators and allow for regional comparisons. All new methodologies will need to be sensitive to cultural, gender, and racial/ethnicity-related issues.

Reproductive toxicity studies in animals provide important information for evaluating the potential developmental toxicity in children. Developmental toxicity effects assessed in reproductive toxicity studies include fetal growth retardation, malformations, fetal loss, decreases in peri- and postnatal growth and survival, retarded postnatal physical and functional development, and effects on reproductive organs and the brain. Among the current OECD test guidelines for reproductive toxicity, all vulnerable periods of development are covered only in the two-generation study design. Late effects are partly covered in young adults, especially in relation to reproductive function and developmental neurotoxicity. Potentially important areas of concern for children, such as immunotoxicity and functional effects on the respiratory system, are not assessed in regulatory test guidelines.

Potential developmental toxicity effects of endocrine disrupting chemicals is an area of concern. In most cases, such effects can be revealed only in the two-generation study. A number of in vivo assays for detecting endocrine effects are currently being developed. In addition, clear effects in these assays give a strong indication for developmental toxicity of the chemical. Further development of the in vivo assays for detecting endocrine effects with the aim of using the results for regulatory purposes could reduce the need for performing the relatively long-lasting and expensive two-generation studies. A major data gap in test guidelines is the inability to monitor effects of early exposures that do not appear until older ages.

7. IMPLICATIONS AND STRATEGIES FOR RISK ASSESSMENT FOR CHILDREN

7.1 Introduction

The preceding chapters have provided ample evidence that children may have different vulnerabilities at different developmental stages, with respect to both exposure and health outcomes. Poor, neglected, and malnourished children often living in parts of the world where there is increased environmental pollution and environmental degradation are at greatest risk.

This chapter will address the implications of the data presented in previous chapters for assessing the risks from environmental chemical exposures. WHO/IPCS has defined risk assessment as an empirically based paradigm that estimates the risk of adverse effects from exposure of an individual or population to a chemical, physical, or biological agent. As shown in Figure 21, it includes the components of hazard identification (Is there an adverse effect?), dose–response assessment (How severe is it?), exposure assessment (What is the level of exposure?), and risk characterization (What is the risk?) (NRC, 1983; IPCS, 2000).

This model has been extensively used to assess all human health risks, including reproduction and developmental toxicity (USEPA, 1991; IPCS, 1999a, 2001d) and neurodevelopmental toxicity (USEPA, 1998; IPCS, 2001b). The importance of the interactions of risk assessment with risk management and risk communication has been recognized (NRC, 1994; Renwick et al., 2003).

In the current document, this risk assessment model is being extended to cover potentially vulnerable life cycle stages such as pregnancy, childhood, and adolescence (see Box 2). This risk assessment approach builds upon previous IPCS EHCs and upon the activities of other organizations (e.g. USEPA) that address approaches for assessing risks from exposures during critical developmental stages (IPCS, 1984, 1986b, 2001b, 2001d). A conceptual framework that focuses on the uniqueness of early life stages is under development by the USEPA and is based on an International

Life Sciences Institute workshop (Olin & Sonawane, 2003; USEPA, 2005a). This framework provides a systematic approach to the consideration of a variety of factors, particularly the timing of exposure, that may influence risk during development from conception through adolescence. This framework and frameworks developed by IPCS and other agencies now incorporate the concept of problem formulation (Suter et al., 2003).

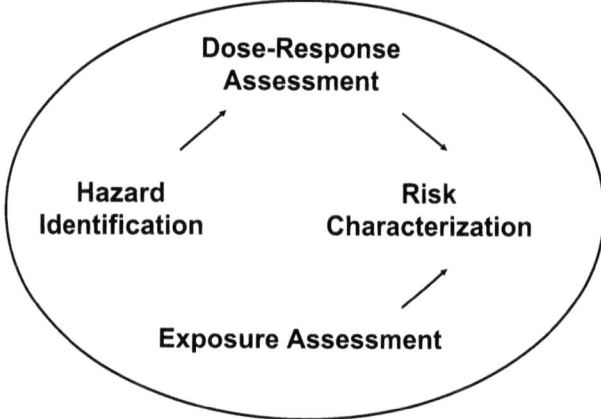

Fig. 21. Risk assessment paradigm for human health.

Box 2. Considerations in children's risk assessment[a]

Characterization of the overall risk assessment

Define the purpose of the risk assessment, including the regulatory and/or public health need.

Consider the historical perspective and whether other assessments of the same or comparable exposures have been carried out.

Define the life stages of interest.

Characterization of the health hazard

Characterize the entire database that provides information on the potential for health concerns in children. Specifically, describe:

- the quantity and quality of the data;
- whether the data are from human or laboratory animal studies (single or multiple species);

Box 2 (Contd)

- the appropriateness of the life stages studied and how inclusive the end-points are with respect to defining alterations in development for a given life stage;
- the potential for not only immediate, but also delayed, effects following an exposure.

With specific reference to the available human data, describe:

- the types of data used (e.g. ecologic, case–control, or cohort studies; or case-reports or case-series);
- the degree to which developmental stages are addressed;
- the degree to which exposures are detailed;
- the degree to which confounding/modifying factors are accounted for;
- the degree to which other causal factors are excluded.

Characterize the dose–response nature of the effects of an exposure, including:

- the data used;
- any model(s) used to develop the dose–response curve(s) and the rationale and chemical-specific information supporting the choice(s).

Describe the assumptions and uncertainty factors used for the qualitative and quantitative aspects of the assessment, including the impact of extrapolation from the observed data to environmental exposures.

Describe the route, level, stage, and duration of exposure as compared with expected human exposures, including available toxicokinetic data used to extrapolate across routes of exposure.

Describe what is known about the mechanism of action/toxicity of the exposure and any toxicokinetic considerations that may influence the toxicity of the exposure at specific life stages.

Characterization of exposure

Characterize the sources, duration, and pattern of exposures at the appropriate life stages. Describe:

- the most significant sources of environmental exposure;
- the relative contribution of different sources of exposure;
- the most significant environmental pathways for exposure.

Describe the populations assessed, including:

- children in general, highly exposed groups, and highly susceptible groups;
- whether all ages or only specific life stages will be at risk for exposure.

> **Box 2 (Contd)**
>
> Describe the basis for the exposure assessment, including:
>
> - any monitoring, modelling, or other analyses of exposure distributions;
> - the range of exposures for the "average" child and subgroups of children (e.g. ethnic, racial, or socioeconomic subgroups);
> - the factors and/or methods used in developing the central tendency estimate and the high-end estimate;
> - the results of different approaches, i.e. modelling, monitoring, probability distributions, including the limitations of each and the range of most reasonable values;
> - the potential for cumulative or aggregate exposures.
>
> [a] Adapted from USEPA (1996), IPCS (2000), and Daston et al. (2004).

7.2 Problem formulation

Problem formulation (Olin & Sonawane, 2003; Renwick et al., 2003) is the first step in any risk assessment, including those carried out for the purpose of determining the potential risk from childhood exposures. This step brings together risk assessors and risk managers to define the problem to be addressed in the risk assessment. The problem formulation step also establishes the goals, breadth, and focus of the assessment and identifies the major factors and regulatory/policy context to be considered. Although the major components of problem formulation are no different for assessments of childhood or adult exposures, some of the specific considerations will be different. Problem formulation is an interactive process that provides the foundation for the technical approach to be used in the assessment. A risk assessment on the health effects of chemical exposures to children should focus on the identification of life stages, the timing of and response to the exposures, and the integral relationship among them. Children's health risk assessment can bring together a number of interests and areas of expertise, and these need to be considered in the problem formulation phase. For example, the potential increased vulnerability of children and the possibility of their unique exposure pathways must be addressed. Historically, assessments of health hazard and chemical exposure are generally carried out independently in a risk assessment by individuals with different expertise. However, the timing and level of chemical exposure are important factors in both hazard assessment and exposure assessment and, thus, need to be integrated into a common framework. Problem formulation should serve as a qualitative screen to identify the exposure scenarios that need to be considered (including settings unique to children) and whether or not there is a potential for higher exposures or greater susceptibility in children. The identification of exposure scenarios can help pinpoint specific populations of interest (e.g. school children, pregnant women, children in developing countries), as well as exposure characteristics with respect to medium (e.g. air, water, soil), route, duration, frequency, and life stage.

From the risk management perspective, there may be regulatory, judicial, economic, and societal considerations that may influence the timing and breadth of the assessment. For example, a specific regulatory requirement, a community need, a health crisis, or some other factor may drive the risk assessment. The reason the assessment is being performed, as well as factors that may influence risk management options and the schedule for developing the assessment, must be clear to all concerned, including the public. Consequently, from the risk communication perspective, the interaction of the risk assessment and risk management groups with input from all interested parties during the problem formulation phase is critical.

Problem formulation should result in a conceptual model, based on the qualitative characterization of hazard and exposure (Olin & Sonawane, 2003; Daston et al., 2004; USEPA, 2005a). The conceptual model should identify key components critical to the overall risk assessment, including exposure scenarios, exposed life stage groups, and the chemical and toxicological characteristics of the exposure that may contribute to an increased risk in children. Box 2 provides guidance on the type of considerations that should be made during problem formulation and carried through the analytical and characterization phases of the risk assessment.

7.3 Hazard identification

Hazard identification, as defined by IPCS, is the identification of the inherent capability of a substance to cause adverse effects when an organism, system, or (sub)population is exposed to that substance (see Figure 21). The challenge in life stage risk assessment is not only to identify the hazard but to determine, in the later stage of risk characterization, whether any adverse effects place a disproportionate risk of harm on potentially susceptible subpopulations, such as the developing child. Children may differ both qualitatively and quantitatively in how they are affected by exposure to xenobiotics. Effects from exposures during specific periods of development can be observed at any time in the life of the exposed individual and may even cross generations. In addition to the potential for harm during critical periods of development, the long-term consequences of early exposure as precursors for later onset of adult disease must be considered.

In characterizing the database, a number of assumptions are applied when data are not available or are incomplete (USEPA, 1991; IPCS, 2005; Kimmel et al., 2006). These include uncertainties about toxicokinetics, mechanism of action, low-dose–response relationships, and human exposure patterns. Each of these assumptions is supported to some extent by the scientific literature. The following assumptions are generally accepted in risk assessment strategies:

- It is assumed that an agent that produces an adverse effect following exposure during development in experimental animals will potentially pose a risk to humans following sufficient exposure during childhood.

- It is assumed that all four manifestations of developmental toxicity (death, structural abnormalities, growth alterations, and functional deficits) are of concern.

- It is assumed that the types of effects seen in animal studies are not necessarily the same as those that may be produced in humans.

- It is assumed that in the absence of adequate human data or data from an identified "most appropriate" animal species, the most sensitive species is appropriate for use.

- It is assumed that for health effects other than cancer, a threshold or non-linear dose–response relationship exists. This is based on known compensatory and adaptive mechanisms that protect against the toxic effects of childhood exposures, as well as on repair mechanisms at the molecular, cellular, and tissue levels. (It should be noted that for a number of chemicals, such as endocrine disrupting chemicals, the existence of thresholds for certain non-cancer health effects is beginning to be challenged. Conversely, a non-linear dose–response relationship is being postulated for some chemicals that induce cancer by non-genotoxic mechanisms.)

7.3.1 End-points and critical periods of exposure

For the purpose of this document, childhood is considered to encompass the life stages summarized in prenatal and postnatal periods from conception through adolescence. Within each of these stages and the comparable stages of laboratory animal development, there are many end-points that can be used to assess manifestations of childhood exposures. A critical period is a specific phase during which a developing system is particularly vulnerable. Exposure during a critical period can lead to an immediate effect on the developing system or may not result in an observable effect until much later in life. There are many critical periods within each of the stages of development, as described in chapters 3 and 4 and in Selevan et al. (2000). Since not all systems are at the same point in their maturity at any particular time in development, the critical period for one organ system will not necessarily coincide with the critical periods of other developing systems, even within the same developmental stage.

From a risk assessment perspective, the tests that are used to define the potential toxicity of an exposure must cover a wide range of developmental end-points and critical periods of susceptibility. Chapter 6 summarizes the test protocols and the outcomes that are currently covered by the different OECD test guidelines. However, there are gaps in coverage, not only of certain life stages, but also in the evaluation of certain end-points (e.g. the cardiovascular and immune systems) (USEPA, 2002b; OECD, 2004). Consequently, it is important to consider the points noted in Box 2 regarding the appropriateness of the life stages and inclusiveness of the end-points with respect to defining alterations in development within a given life stage. Moreover, the potential for not only immediate, but also delayed, effects following an exposure must be considered.

7.3.2 Human studies

Human data are preferred for determining the potential health effects of exposure. However, human studies are often limited by ethical issues in collecting data and by their complexity in establishing exposure conditions and associated effects. Consequently, it is important to understand the various human study designs and their strengths and limitations (see chapter 6).

The application of human data in risk assessment for children has been detailed in a number of publications (USEPA, 1991; Richter-Reichhelm et al., 2002; IPCS, 2005; Kimmel et al., 2006). In general, the risk assessor should evaluate each human study for its power and potential bias. The power of the study is the study's ability to detect an effect. It is dependent on the size of the study population, the frequency of the effect or the exposure in the population, and the level of risk to be identified. The greater the population size and the effect or exposure frequency, the greater the power of the study. In studies of low power, it is generally not possible to establish the lack of an association between an exposure and an effect, and even positive findings may be difficult to support. Meta-analysis, which combines populations from different studies, may increase the power of the overall database, but the potential for the combination of dissimilar populations must be considered in any risk assessment.

Study bias may be selection bias or information bias. Selection bias may occur in the choice of subjects for the study (e.g. exclusion of individuals who are not fluent in a particular language). Selection bias may also result from an individual's reluctance to participate in a study owing to concerns over a perceived exposure, resultant health effect, or educational and socioeconomic status of the participants. Parents who perceive that an exposure in their child's environment may have resulted in an adverse health effect may feel responsible for not "protecting" their child. Information bias may result from inappropriate classification of the individual study participants or from the information provided. For example, interview bias may result when an interviewer is not "blind" to the exposure of the test population. Recall bias may result when participants with specific exposures or effects respond differently from those without the specific exposures or effects.

7.3.3 Relevance of animal studies for assessing potential hazards to children

While human data are preferable for risk assessment, most assessments rely primarily on data from controlled experimental animal studies. Chapter 6 details the various animal tests that are employed in defining the potential for adverse health effects from environmental chemical exposures. During development, all mammalian organisms move from a state of *pluripotency* (ability to develop into many different tissue types) to one of *differentiation* (acquiring particular structural and functional modes of operation) (Morford et al., 2004). Table 13 shows the approximate ages that correspond to specific events or life stages in laboratory animals, compared with those in humans (USEPA, 2002b). Because of a much compressed developmental period and different rates of maturation of specific functional systems in experimental animals, it is often difficult to conduct temporal extrapolations between developing humans and developing experimental animals. Nevertheless, toxicity testing in experimental animals plays a key role in identifying and characterizing developmental hazards for children. Many studies of animal/human concordance in developmental toxicology and neurotoxicology have been carried out over the past 50 years; for most chemicals known to cause developmental effects in humans, at least one animal species has been found to exhibit similar effects.

Morford et al. (2004) summarized much of the work that has been carried out on the ability of animal models to predict human risk for developmental toxicity. In one particular comparison of experimental animal studies and epidemiological studies that met stringent design criteria, it was concluded that concordance of developmentally adverse effects exists when all of the measures of developmental toxicity (i.e. death, structural alterations, growth alterations, and functional deficits) are considered (Holson et al., 1981, 2000; Kimmel et al., 1984). These authors noted that although strict anatomical concordance is not always present, an alteration is a signal that development may be perturbed. Testing for concordance of identical anatomical aberrations requires detailed knowledge of comparative stages of organ system development and toxicokinetic information so that similar target organ doses at equivalent stages of development can be compared. If such detailed knowledge were

Table 13. Approximate age at equivalent life stages in several species[a]

Rat		Mouse		Rabbit		Beagle dog		Human	
Life stage	Age	Life stage	Age	Life stage	Age	Life stage	Age	Life stage	Age
Embryonic	GD 0–16	Embryonic	GD 0–15	Embryonic	GD 0–19	Embryonic	GD 0–30?	Embryonic	GD 0–58
Fetal[b]	GD 16–22 (22–23 days)	Fetal	GD 15–20 (18–22 days)	Fetal	GD 19–32 (30–32 days)	Fetal	GD 30–63 (53–71 days)	Fetal	GD 58–267
Neonate[c]	PND 0–14	Neonate	PND 0–14	Neonate	PND 0–21?	Neonate	PND 0–21	Neonate	PND 0–30
Weaning[d]	PND 21	Weaning	PND 21 (19–28)	Weaning	PND 42 (42–56)	Weaning	PND 42	Infancy	PND 30–1 year
								Toddler	2–3 years
Young	PND 22–35	Young	PND 21–35	Young	PND 42–?	Young	1.5–5 months	Preschool	3–6 years
								Elementary school age	6–12 years
Puberty	PND 35–60	Puberty	PND 35–?	Puberty	3–8 months	Puberty	5–7 months	Adolescence	12–21 years
Sexual maturity	2.5–3 months	Breeding age	1.5–2 months	Breeding age	6–9 months	Breeding age	12 months	Young adult	21–40 years

Table 13 (Contd)

Rat		Mouse		Rabbit		Beagle dog		Human	
Life stage	Age	Life stage	Age	Life stage	Age	Life stage	Age	Life stage	Age
Mature adult	5–18 months	Mature adult		Mature adult		Mature adult		Mature adult	40–65 years
Old adult	18 months– 2+ years	Old adult		Old adult		Old adult	~15 years	Old adult	>65 years?

GD, gestation day; PND, postnatal day

a Taken from USEPA (2002b).
b Range of gestation length in parentheses.
c Some neonatal events in rodents occur in utero in humans.
d Range of weaning ages in parentheses.

available, it would be possible to test for the ability of an agent to elicit specific malformations. In a report on the relevance of developmental neurotoxicology end-points, Adams et al. (2000) noted that extrapolation of animal data from standard regulatory test batteries was stronger for effects on sensory and motor functioning than for cognitive or social functioning. They suggested that the testing paradigms and their concordance could be improved by the use of more contemporary and sensitive methods for evaluating behaviour and cognitive function.

Testing protocols for reproductive and developmental effects in laboratory animals are well established and include exposure at various time periods and assessment of a number of different outcomes. As with human study designs, it is important that the risk assessor understand the various experimental animal study designs and their strengths and limitations. An advantage of experimental animal studies is that they can be carried out under controlled conditions. In evaluating any study, the risk assessor should confirm that appropriate exposure groups and sufficient numbers of animals were used. As an example, it is highly unlikely that all females will become pregnant in a routine rodent developmental toxicity study. Consequently, the study design should initially incorporate more females than will be needed to assess the effect of an exposure at the end of the study. With regard to exposure groups, the risk assessor will need to consider the route of exposure, the timing and levels of exposure (often based on dose range–finding studies), and the randomization of the experimental animals among the different exposure groups.

During the prenatal and early postnatal periods (through weaning), it is important to evaluate the maternal animal. Changes in such end-points as maternal body weight and weight change, gestation length, food/water consumption, and clinical signs help characterize the effects of the exposure. As examples, changes in weight gain during the exposure period in a prenatal rodent study can be an indicator of general toxicity. Changes in weight gain (corrected for gravid uterine weight) can give an indication of whether a reduced weight gain is a consequence of intrauterine effects (e.g. reduced pup weights, reduced litter size) or results primarily from effects on the maternal animal, or a combination of the two.

Implications and Strategies for Risk Assessment for Children

Chapter 6 has reviewed the end-points used in assessing potential developmental effects in animal studies. Other sources also give detailed guidance on how the risk assessor should consider data on specific end-points in the overall risk assessment (IPCS, 1984, 1986b, 1999a, 2001b; USEPA, 1991; Schwenk et al., 2003). Ideally, all of the manifestations of development (viability, growth, and structural and functional integrity) should be assessed. However, this is seldom the case; consequently, the strength of the overall database may be limited by the absence of certain data. This is especially true of functional integrity, as this outcome is not routinely evaluated. As discussed below, a general sense of the dose–response relationship is important for the characterization of the health-related database.

A number of national and international efforts have focused on identifying the mode of action in evaluating the relevance of animal data in humans (Sonich-Mullen et al., 2001; Meek et al., 2002; Seed et al., 2005; USEPA, 2005a). Most of these efforts have focused on the importance of mode of action–based approaches in the risk assessment of carcinogens (Preston & Williams, 2005). Building on efforts initiated by the International Life Sciences Institute, a Human Relevance Framework has been developed for chemical carcinogens. This framework provides a structured approach for evaluating all data pertaining to the animal mode of action followed by all data relevant to the human mode of action. Recently, considerable efforts are also under way to develop mode of action approaches for toxic end-points other than cancer (Seed et al., 2005). The availability of mode of action information will improve the extrapolation of animal data and relevant human data in risk assessment approaches.

7.3.4 Reversibility and latency

Reversible effects are those that return to "normal" following cessation of exposure. With regard to risk assessment for children, it is important to understand that many "reversible" effects are related to or precursors of other adverse effects. For example, low birth weight may be "reversible" through catch-up growth postnatally, but it may also be related to developmental delays or other health outcomes that result from prenatal growth reduction/retardation. Conversely, an agent may produce relatively mild and reversible neurological effects in adults but produce permanent behavioural impairment following in utero exposure. Latency or the latency period is the time between exposure to an agent and manifestation or detection of a health effect of concern. Exposures during childhood will often result in latent effects. A classic example of latency is the appearance of clear cell adenocarcinomas in women who had been exposed in utero to DES (chapter 4). Reversibility and latency are only rarely evaluated directly. Yet either event could have a major impact on the hazard identification. Additional studies from less-than-lifetime exposures to evaluate latency to effect and reversibility of effect are a critical research need (Damstra et al., 2002; USEPA, 2002a).

7.3.5 Characterization of the health-related database

Following the review of the toxicity data in both humans and animals, the health-related database is characterized as being sufficient or insufficient to proceed further in the risk assessment process. The process for characterization of this database as well as a description of what constitutes sufficient/insufficient evidence are reviewed in several publications (USEPA, 2005a; Kimmel et al., 2006). Box 3 shows the criteria for characterization used by the USEPA for developmental toxicity (USEPA, 1991). In general, the characterization of hazard considers the context of exposure (e.g. dose, route, duration, and timing) relative to the life stage(s) during which exposure occurred. The strengths and weaknesses as well as the uncertainties of the data are described. It is important that all data, whether indicative of a potential hazard or not, are considered in this characterization. This process requires a great deal of scientific judgement and a multidisciplinary team of experts in specific areas of developmental and reproductive toxicity. When the database is considered sufficient, the risk assessment process continues with the dose–response evaluation.

7.4 Dose–response assessment

Identifying dose–response relationships is an important component of any risk assessment. This process establishes the exposure levels that produce effects, as well as those that produce no effects. As noted in Box 2, it is important to characterize what data were used, what model was employed to develop the dose–response curve(s), and whether chemical-specific information is available to support the observed dose–response relationship. While the risk assessment paradigm shown in Figure 21 separates hazard

> **Box 3. Categorization of the health-related database**[a]
>
> **Sufficient evidence**
>
> The "sufficient evidence" category includes data that collectively provide enough information to judge whether or not a human developmental hazard could exist within the context of dose, duration, timing, and route of exposure. This category may include both human and experimental animal evidence.
>
> **Sufficient human evidence**
>
> This category includes data from epidemiological studies (e.g. case–control and cohort) to provide convincing evidence for the scientific community to judge that a causal relationship is or is not supported. A case-series in conjunction with strong supporting evidence may also be used. Supporting animal data may or may not be available.
>
> **Sufficient experimental animal evidence — Limited human data**
>
> This category includes agents for which there is sufficient evidence from experimental animal studies and/or limited human data that provide convincing evidence for the scientific community to judge if the potential for developmental toxicity exists. The minimum evidence necessary to determine if a potential hazard exists would be data demonstrating an adverse developmental effect in a single appropriate, well conducted study in a single experimental animal species. The minimum evidence needed to judge that a potential hazard does not exist would include data from appropriate, well conducted laboratory animal studies in several species (at least two) that evaluated a variety of the potential manifestations of developmental toxicity and showed no developmental effects at doses that were minimally toxic to the adult.
>
> **Insufficient evidence**
>
> This category includes agents for which there is less than the minimum sufficient evidence necessary for assessing the potential for developmental toxicity, such as when no data are available on developmental toxicity, as well as for databases from studies in animals or humans that have a limited study design (e.g. small numbers, inappropriate dose selection/exposure information, other uncontrolled factors), or data from a single species reported to have no adverse developmental effects, or databases limited to information on structure/activity relationships, short-term tests, pharmacokinetics, or metabolic precursors.
>
> [a] From USEPA (1991).

identification and dose–response assessment, in reality these two components cannot be totally separated from one another. The potential for an exposure to result in an adverse effect is dependent not only on the agent to which a child is exposed, but on the dose, route, timing, and duration as well. The timing of exposure is particularly important in determining the nature and severity of health outcomes resulting from exposure during critical developmental periods.

7.4.1 Application of health outcome data

As noted previously, human data are preferable for determining the potential health effects of exposures in children. In order to characterize dose–response relationships, it is important to characterize the type of epidemiological study design, the range and detail of exposures measured, and the specific outcomes and populations monitored. Human studies are often limited in their power to establish an association between an outcome and the range of exposures (especially individual exposures) that have been measured. Moreover, childhood exposures may be greater during certain critical periods of development; even within a critical period, certain children may be more sensitive to certain exposures than others. A specific population that is monitored in a study may or may not be applicable to a particular risk assessment if the critical developmental periods of interest are not included. Thus, establishing a dose–response relationship based solely on human data is even more difficult than identifying a potential hazard using such data. As with the hazard assessment, experimental animal studies offer the advantage of being carried out under controlled conditions. This includes controlled exposure conditions of dose, route, duration, and timing of exposure.

The risk assessor should be sensitive to certain dose–response patterns that are often encountered in studies on developmental toxicity. For example, the lowest effective doses in adults and young are often similar or may be the same, but the type of effects may be very different; as well, the effects on the developing child may be permanent (or lead to latent effects), whereas the effects on the adult may be transient. Also, the end-points used in evaluating alterations in children's health may vary considerably. The difference between the maternal toxic dose and the developmental toxic dose may at times be related to the relative thoroughness with which end-points are evaluated. Also, the variability and level of severity within a particular end-point need to be defined, since end-point variability and level of severity can have a significant effect on the power of the study and the ability to establish an effect level. Approaches to carrying out dose–response assessments are described below.

7.4.2 Quantitative evaluation

The quantitative evaluation of the dose–response nature of a chemical exposure has evolved over the past 20 years, and current methodology has been reviewed in a number of publications (IPCS, 2004b, 2005; USEPA, 2005a; Kimmel et al., 2006). Traditionally, a threshold has been assumed for health outcomes (with the exception of cancer) resulting from childhood exposures (USEPA, 1991). In this context, a threshold is a level of exposure below which an adverse effect will not be observed. This assumption has been based on the known capacity of the developing organism to compensate for or repair damage at various levels of biological complexity. While this is beginning to be challenged as an across-the-board assumption, current quantitative methods described below continue to recognize this assumption.

7.4.2.1 Tolerable daily intake (TDI) and reference dose (RfD)/reference concentration (RfC) approaches

The dose–response evaluation of either human or animal data has traditionally been based on developing health-based guidance values such as a tolerable daily intake (TDI) or reference dose (RfD)/reference concentration (RfC). These values are derived by dividing the lowest-observed-adverse-effect level (LOAEL) or the highest exposure level at which no adverse effects are observed (no-observed-adverse-effect level, or NOAEL) by uncertainty factors. More recently, the use of chemical-specific adjustment factors has been introduced to provide a method for the incorporation of quantitative data on interspecies differences or human variability into the risk assessment process (Meek et al., 2002; IPCS, 2005). These approaches are generally applied to lifetime exposures and are not focused on exposures during specific life stages (Groeneveld et al., 2004). Modifications that account for less-than-lifetime exposures include developing acute and short-term reference exposure values and acute dietary levels (Solecki et al., 2005). Specific life stage dose–response methodology is limited, but there are approaches for developing drinking-water health advisories and for assessing the incidental non-dietary pesticide ingestion in toddlers that are thought to be protective of children (USEPA, 2002b).

Uncertainty factors are intended to account for animal-to-human extrapolation, variability within the human population, use of a

LOAEL where a NOAEL is not available, and database deficiencies. Lack of reproductive and developmental toxicity data is often used as a basis for including a database uncertainty factor. The default value for any one uncertainty factor is 10, but this may be reduced depending on the confidence in the data or information that provides assurance of reduced intra- or interspecies variability (Renwick et al., 2000). As noted above, chemical-specific data on toxicokinetics and toxicodynamics may be used to replace part or all of these uncertainty factors, and this strategy has been used by WHO/IPCS (IPCS, 1994, 2004b, 2005).

When such data are available, life stage considerations can be included in two general ways: intraspecies adjustments or interspecies extrapolation (USEPA, 2005a). In general, qualitative predictions of the relative difference in toxicokinetic processes between children and adults can be made using adult/child ratios for a toxicant that is metabolized by the same pathway. Quantitatively, adjustments to adult physiologically based toxicokinetic models can be used to develop an appropriate dose metric for a specific life stage in children. In an evaluation of child/adult pharmacokinetic differences based on the therapeutic drug literature, Ginsberg et al. (2002) reported that half-lives of drugs are three to nine times longer in neonates than in adults, the difference disappearing by two to six months of age. This range of longer half-lives exceeds the 3.16 uncertainty factor that is applied to account for interindividual pharmacokinetic variability. Other studies have further evaluated these differences and suggest that an additional factor may be necessary for newborns and neonates (Hattis et al., 2003; Ginsberg et al., 2004a,b). Consequently, the traditional uncertainty factor may be inadequate at this life stage. Additional data will have to be derived from animal studies. Unfortunately, the comparability of the developmental stages in test animals and humans is not always straightforward and will have to be determined (Beckman & Feuston, 2003; Marty et al., 2003; Zoetis & Hurtt, 2003a,b; Zoetis et al., 2003; Walthall et al., 2005). Moreover, quantitative comparisons will need to account for interspecies toxicokinetic differences at equivalent developmental stages. Obviously, the application of appropriate toxicokinetic and toxicodynamic data can increase the confidence in a life stage–specific risk assessment. However, the risk assessor must be cognizant of the models that are used and their uncertainties, so as not to substitute one uncertainty for another. Additional toxicokinetic considerations are noted in section 7.4.2.5.

As noted above, the lowest effective doses in adults and young are often similar. However, the type and severity of effects from an exposure may be very different. This becomes an important consideration, especially in evaluating prenatal animal studies. Because the developing embryo/fetus is exposed in the maternal animal, it has been argued that if maternal toxicity is observed, any developmental toxicity could be due to the compromised maternal system. However, several issues should be considered. The difference between the lowest maternally toxic dose and the developmentally toxic dose may at times be related to the relative thoroughness with which end-points are evaluated in dams and offspring, as well as to the sensitivity of the end-points. Moreover, the severity of the effects must be considered; the developmental effects may be permanent, while the maternal effects may be reversible. From a risk assessment perspective, developmental toxicity in the presence of maternal toxicity cannot be simply considered "secondary to maternal toxicity" and discounted (USEPA, 1991).

An assumption that has generally been made in the dose–response evaluation of end-points other than cancer is that there is a threshold relationship at low exposure levels. The TDI and RfD/RfC approaches described above are based on this assumption. However, as more becomes known about the cellular/molecular mechanisms of toxicity, the dichotomy in the approaches to cancer and all other end-points is coming into question. This has led to a move towards harmonization of risk assessment approaches (Bogdanffy et al., 2001; see also http://www.who.int/ipcs/methods/harmonization/). With regard to cancer, the concern for early-life susceptibility to environmental agents has led to the development of guidance for age-dependent adjustment factors for toxicants acting through a mutagenic mechanism of action (USEPA, 2005d). This guidance is based on limited data comparing adult with early-life exposures and the subsequent risk of carcinogenesis. With regard to end-points other than cancer, a recent major review of the RfD/RfC approach recognized the continued need for a default approach like the RfD/RfC approach, but stated that this approach "can and should be improved upon or replaced when more specific data on toxicokinetics and mode of action are available to allow the development of a chemical-specific or a biologically based dose–response model" (USEPA, 2002b).

7.4.2.2 Benchmark dose (BMD)/benchmark concentration (BMC) approach

When sufficient data are available, use of the benchmark dose (BMD) or benchmark concentration (BMC) approach is preferable to the traditional health-based guidance value approaches (IPCS, 1999a, 2005; USEPA, 2000; Sonich-Mullin et al., 2001). The BMDL (or BMCL) is the lower confidence limit on a dose (the BMD) (or concentration, BMC) that produces a particular level of response or change from the control mean (e.g. 10% response rate for quantal responses; one standard deviation from the control mean for a continuous response) and can be used in place of the NOAEL. The BMD/BMC approach provides several advantages for dose–response evaluation: 1) the model fits all of the available data and takes into account the slope of the dose–response curve; 2) it accounts for variability in the data; and 3) the BMD/BMC is not limited to one experimental exposure level, and the model can extrapolate outside of the experimental range.

Briefly, a mathematical model is selected, based on the data that are being analysed and the characteristics of the response. Generally, the more limited the database, the more simple the model. Databases with larger numbers of dose groups and a greater experimental complexity will be better suited for more complex models. The model is applied with the appropriate considerations for statistical linkage, parameter estimation, and response. As noted in IPCS (2004b), this approach will generate a BMD/BMC, but will also provide dose–response functions and/or extrapolated risk estimates. The BMD method includes the determination of the response at a given dose, the dose at a given response, and their confidence limits. Using extrapolation of the dose–response model below the biologically observable dose range, the response at specified (lower) dose levels as well as the dose corresponding to a specific response level can be estimated. For more detailed description and examples of this approach, see USEPA (2000) and IPCS (2004b).

7.4.2.3 Biologically based dose–response models

Biologically based dose–response models are considered a major advance for evaluating dose–response relationships (Shuey et al., 1994; IPCS, 2000). Although considerable work remains in developing such models, they should provide information on the potential for chemicals to alter critical signalling pathways, define

Implications and Strategies for Risk Assessment for Children

the toxicokinetic and toxicodynamic similarities and differences between animal models and humans, and provide a more accurate estimation of low-dose risk to humans.

7.4.2.4 Duration adjustment

Approaches to duration adjustment are reviewed in Kimmel et al. (2006). Prior to derivation of NOAELs, LOAELs, or BMDs/BMCs, the toxicity data are adjusted to a continuous exposure scenario. For oral studies, a daily exposure adjustment is made (e.g. a five days per week exposure is converted to seven days per week). For inhalation exposures, a concentration × time ($c \times t$) adjustment is made. Traditionally, the inhalation exposure adjustment has not been done, because of concerns about peak versus integrated exposure and the likelihood of a threshold for effects. However, a review of the RfD and RfC processes by the USEPA recommended that inhalation developmental toxicity studies be adjusted in the same way as for other end-points (USEPA, 2002b). Derivation of a human equivalent concentration for inhalation exposures is intended to account for pharmacokinetic differences between humans and animals.

A number of approaches have been developed for establishing short-duration (less-than-lifetime) exposure limits that are applied in specific exposure scenarios (Jarabek, 1995; Kimmel, 1995). A common feature of most of these approaches is the assumption that Haber's Law applies (i.e. the response depends on the cumulative exposure, the product of exposure concentration and duration). Recent reviews of this approach have begun to question its general applicability over wide ranges of concentration and duration (Pierano et al., 1995; Eastern Research Group, 1998). Evidence is accumulating that demonstrates that for several environmental chemical exposures, short, high-level exposures have a greater effect on development than cumulative equivalent long, low-level exposures (Tzimas et al., 1997; Weller et al., 1999; Kimmel et al., 2002).

7.4.2.5 Toxicokinetics

Toxicokinetic data provide information on the absorption, metabolism, distribution (including placental transfer), and/or excretion (including via breast milk) of an agent. Chapter 3 (section 3.5) reviews many of the issues that must be considered in relation to toxicokinetics and child development. When available, toxicokinetic data can provide estimates of internal dose, as well as the level and duration of an exposure at the target site (e.g. peak concentration). This can be useful for interspecies extrapolation, as well as for indicating the range of intraspecies variability (Gundert-Remy et al., 2002; De Zwart et al., 2004). From an exposure perspective, toxicokinetic information can help define similarities and differences among routes of exposure.

Daston et al. (2004) and Ginsberg et al. (2004b) reviewed the considerations that should be made in analysing toxicokinetic data and factoring the data into an assessment of children's health risks from exposure to environmental chemicals. Data that are particularly important include the absorption rate for the relevant exposure pathways, the distribution from the exposure sites and systemic distribution to the metabolizing or target organs, the type of storage and body compartments of interest (in utero, this would include maternal, placental, and embryo/fetal compartments), and the metabolic rates for both activation and detoxification pathways. To apply this in a life stage–specific assessment, chemical-specific data are needed to identify the main pathways of chemical activation, detoxification, and clearance as seen in adults or animal models, and then age-specific data are needed to adjust these factors for the particular childhood period of interest.

7.5 Exposure assessment

The exposure assessment characterizes the pathways, magnitude, frequency, and duration of human exposures from various sources. Chapter 5 provides an overview of these components and addresses the principles of exposure assessment in children. General principles of exposure assessment have been reviewed in a number of publications (USEPA, 1992a, 2005a; IPCS, 1999a, 2000; Needham et al., 2005). This chapter will focus on the considerations that are important when applying the exposure data to a children's health risk assessment (see Box 2).

7.5.1 Age-specific exposures

A child's anatomy, physiology, and metabolism change over time, as well as their behaviour and interaction with their

Implications and Strategies for Risk Assessment for Children

environment. The age/developmental stage of the child must be a primary consideration when conducting an exposure assessment. A breakdown of age/developmental stages and corresponding behavioural, physiological, and exposure characteristics are shown in Figure 14. All of these characteristics must be considered in trying to establish an estimated exposure of children during specific developmental stages. Socioeconomic, cultural, and physical conditions can also influence exposure levels.

The exposure pathway and physicochemical characteristics of a particular environmental chemical can provide useful information on the likelihood of childhood exposure (chapter 5). Age-specific exposure pathways of particular relevance include those during the prenatal and early developmental years postnatally (e.g. placental transfer, breast milk, toys, soil, indoor air/dust, child-care centres). Exposures to persistent environmental chemicals are of special concern, since the internal exposure may continue and result in a level sufficient to cause effects during critical developmental stages, even after the external exposure has ceased or been removed.

Exposure of either parent may affect the germ cells that will form the child. Prenatal and postnatal (via the breast milk) exposure occurs through the maternal system; the mother is exposed directly, and her developing child is generally exposed indirectly. The exposure assessment will have to consider maternal absorption, distribution, metabolism, and excretion, as well as placental/lactational metabolism and transfer. In utero, transit time will be influenced by the ability of the child to metabolize and/or excrete the chemical. Most chemical agents are able to reach the child in utero, and there may be accumulation in the embryo/fetus if there is conjugation and reduced embryo/fetal excretion. Assessment of exposure via breast milk should consider such physicochemical characteristics as fat solubility, since breast milk and maternal fat form a "sink" for fat-soluble compounds. The mother's exposure alone cannot be assumed to be a surrogate for the prenatal or nursing child. The exposure of the in utero/nursing child may not be the same as for the pregnant or lactating mother, and measurement of the agent in cord blood and in breast milk may give a better estimate of exposure.

At birth, the child is exposed to the environment directly. At this time, the child's respiration rate is rapid, food and water consumption are high, and the skin surface area to body weight ratio is larger. Children's metabolic pathways, especially in fetal life and in the first months after birth, are immature. If the child breastfeeds, the mother continues to be a source of exposure.

Infants/toddlers are small in stature, crawling or just beginning to walk, and prone to be in contact with rugs, floors, lawns, and compounds that layer at low levels. The limited variety of their diets may shield them from many exposures, but may make them particularly vulnerable to others. This is especially true if the exposure pathway of an agent is through particular foods that comprise a large portion of the diet, such as fruits and milk or milk products. This is also the stage at which hand-to-mouth behaviours may result in exposure.

By adolescence, the child has become increasingly independent. Physically, adolescents go through a new growth spurt accompanied by an increase in food and water consumption. Their environments are more varied, including home, school, and expanded social and occupational settings. Consequently, they will be exposed to a greater variety of chemicals and physical agents. As adolescents begin to take control of their own life decisions, their limited life experience and willingness to take risks may result in a greater disregard for exposures that may be harmful.

Default values have been published for use in estimating exposures — for example, from food and water consumption in adults and children, soil ingestion in children, and respiration rates in children and adults (USEPA, 1990). The Child-Specific Exposure Factors Handbook summarizes data on human behaviour and characteristics that affect children's exposure to environmental agents and recommends values to use for these factors (USEPA, 2002a).

7.5.2 Assessment methods

Guidelines for exposure assessment (USEPA, 1992a; OECD, 1999; IPCS, 2000) and a handbook of child-specific exposure factors (USEPA, 2002a) have been published. Both list a number of references that are applicable to the quantitative estimate of exposure. Generally, the methods used for the quantitative estimate of exposure are not different for children and adults. The magnitude of exposure is a product of the exposure concentration as a function of

Implications and Strategies for Risk Assessment for Children

time. Other IPCS documents (IPCS, 1999a, 2000) have reviewed this quantitative approach and discuss the integration of exposures for a given population and the determination of the applied dose. Doses are often presented as dose rates (i.e. the dose per unit time). For biological processes that are described in terms of lifetime probabilities (e.g. cancer), lifetime average doses are often presented.

The risk assessor should understand the type of methods and models used to determine exposure (i.e. direct, biomarkers, and modelling). Direct methods of assessment measure the contact of the child with the agent and can identify exposure concentrations in a particular medium over an identifiable period of time. In pregnancy, the measurement is not direct (except in cases of physical exposures, such as heat and radiation), and the maternal exposure generally serves as a surrogate for embryo/fetal exposure. The actual embryo/fetal exposure will depend on maternal absorption, distribution, metabolism, and excretion and on the placental transfer of the agent or its metabolites. Direct methods offer the advantage that the exposure is made at the point of contact and are likely to provide the most accurate estimate of exposure of the defined time period. When data from a large number of individuals are combined, the individual variability within the population can be estimated. Limitations that should be considered in the application of direct method data are 1) the accuracy and variability of the measurement devices and techniques used; 2) any assumptions that are made concerning the relationship between short-term sampling and long-term exposures; and 3) the fact that this method is not source specific (IPCS, 1999a).

Biomarkers of exposure are an indicator of absorbed dose and may present unique advantages in exposure assessment. Biomarkers demonstrate that internal exposure has occurred and can be used to estimate chemical uptake over time and help establish the relationship between exposure and effect. They are apical in nature, in that they account for and integrate over all sources of exposure. Specifically in relation to potentially sensitive subpopulations like children, biomarkers may be able to identify increased absorption or biological response in comparison with the general population. Biomarker data alone cannot be used to establish source and route of exposure and are limited in providing information on frequency, duration, and intensity. Moreover, metabolism of any chemical biomarker necessitates a clear understanding of the properties of the metabolites. Mathematical models can be used to quantify the processes leading to exposure (and internal dose). The general models that are used for estimating exposure are shown in Figure 13, and examples of specific models are referenced in Table 6.

7.6 Risk characterization

The final phase of the risk assessment process is risk characterization. Risk characterization involves the synthesis of critically evaluated information and data from exposure assessment, hazard identification, and dose–response considerations into an overall evaluation of the assessment that can be communicated to risk managers and public health officials. It should be based on the purpose for the risk assessment that was defined in the problem formulation stage. The risk characterization should incorporate all life stages that were identified in the problem formulation stage, and, if part of a larger risk assessment, it should place the vulnerability of the child in perspective with the other populations being considered. In addition, if important new information, not anticipated in the problem formulation stage, has been identified during the risk assessment process, that information should also be captured in the risk characterization.

It is important that both the qualitative and quantitative characterization be clearly communicated to the risk manager. The qualitative characterization includes the quality of the database, along with strengths and weaknesses, for both health and exposure evaluations; the relevance of the database to humans; the assumptions and judgements that were made in the evaluation; and the level of confidence in the overall characterization. The quantitative characterization also includes information on the range of effective exposure levels, dose–response estimates (including the uncertainty factors applied), and the population exposure estimates. Kimmel et al. (2006) reviewed many of the components of the risk characterization for reproductive and developmental effects and provided a comprehensive list of issues to be considered for each of the components of the risk assessment.

In general, integration of the health and exposure assessments should include statements regarding the relevance of the route, timing, and duration of exposure modelled from the experimental data to the expected human exposure modelled from the exposure assessment. The dose–response patterns (shape and slope), the method for dose–response analysis, and, where possible, the relevant toxicokinetics should be characterized. In addition to the route, timing, and duration of exposure, the size and characteristics of the exposed populations and the pattern of exposure and how it can influence the target end-point(s) should be described. Because of differences in vulnerability during critical windows of susceptibility, the timing and sequence of exposure should be characterized whenever possible. If similar effects can be expected in adults, the risk characterization should indicate this and whether the effects will occur at different exposure levels compared with adults.

The uncertainties and variability of the database, along with the judgements and assumptions that were made during the assessment, should be clear. The description should include the major strengths and weaknesses of the database and the limits of understanding of particular mechanisms of toxicity that may be involved in the effect(s). Whenever alternative views can be supported by the database, these should be addressed in the risk characterization. If the assessment favours one view over others, the rationale for choosing that view should be stated.

The use of Monte Carlo and other stochastic analytical methods to characterize the distribution of exposure and dose–response relationships is increasing (IPCS, 2001a). The Monte Carlo method uses random numbers and probability in a computer simulation to predict the outcome of exposure. These methods can be important tools in risk characterization to assess the relative contribution of uncertainty and variability to a risk estimate.

Three types of descriptors of human risk are especially useful and important in risk characterization (Kimmel et al., 2006). The first of these is related to interindividual variability — i.e. the range of variability in population response to an agent and the potential for highly susceptible subpopulations. The second is related to highly exposed individuals — i.e. individuals who are more highly exposed because of occupation, residential location, behaviour, or other factors. The third descriptor that is sometimes used to characterize risk is the margin of exposure (MOE) — i.e. the ratio of the NOAEL (or BMDL/BMCL) from the most appropriate or sensitive species to the estimated human exposure level from all potential sources. This means that the lower the MOE, the greater the risk. The MOE can be used to prioritize different contaminants, providing that a consistent approach has been adopted. The acceptability of an MOE depends on its magnitude and is ultimately a risk management decision (IPCS, 2004b). To aid that decision, the risk assessor should provide information on the nature and magnitude of uncertainties in both the toxicological and exposure data. Although the risk assessor should not provide an assessment of the acceptability of the MOE, guidance should be given on its adequacy, taking into account the inherent uncertainties and variability (IPCS, 1994; Kimmel et al., 2006).

Ultimately, the risk characterization results in a statement of the potential susceptibility of children for specific effects from specific exposures to environmental agents. This statement forms the basis, together with other considerations, on which regulatory or management decisions will be made. Often, the risk manager is not a specialist in children's health; thus, it is imperative that the risk characterization be clear, definitive, and unencumbered by scientific terminology that may be misunderstood or misinterpreted. The risk assessor must effectively communicate what is known, what is not known, and what is questionable, in order for the risk assessment to be appropriately factored into the overall risk management process.

7.7 Summary and conclusions

This chapter and the monograph as a whole should be a useful tool for public health officials, research and regulatory scientists, and risk managers in addressing the major scientific principles underlying the assessment of health risks from exposure to environmental chemicals in children during critical stages of development. Considerable progress has been made in developing risk assessment approaches that address the special developmental stage–specific vulnerabilities of children. Focused research has led to improvements in data collection and the breadth and depth of the overall database. There is an increased understanding of normal and abnormal development and the influence of age-specific conditions on a child's vulnerability. Nevertheless, life stage–specific risk assessments are only beginning to be incorporated into the overall risk assessment process, and many gaps in knowledge and in the appropriate application of data into child-protective risk assessment policies need to be addressed. These include the following:

- The development of new conceptual frameworks with a particular focus on the uniqueness of early life stages should be harmonized in order to focus the risk assessor on the critical elements of the risk assessment.

- Life stage–specific risk assessments are likely to require modification of the current toxicity testing and human health assessment paradigms.

- Considerable effort will be required to develop approaches to incorporating data from molecular studies and generated from new technologies (e.g. genomic) into a meaningful framework for children's health risk assessments.

- The addition of the problem formulation step to the risk assessment paradigm will assist in focusing the purpose for determining the potential risk from specific childhood exposures and foster an increased interaction between scientists, risk assessors, public health officials, and the public.

- A greater sensitivity to effective communication among individuals of varying backgrounds and points of view will be required.

- Risk assessors must be particularly sensitive to the potential for significantly higher exposures in areas of the world where hazardous environmental exposures are not sufficiently controlled. Compounding factors such as poverty, inadequate nutrition, and compromised health status must also be considered in problem formulation throughout the risk assessment process.

- Whenever possible, human data should be used/considered in the risk assessment. However, since risk assessments generally rely on test animal data, comparative studies into the toxicokinetics and toxicodynamics of animals and humans are important for extrapolating test animal data to the human situation. Moreover, in the case of children's risk assessment, it is important to define the comparative adult/child toxicokinetics and toxicodynamics at different life stages.

- Research on the impact of environmental factors on children's health has most often focused on an exposure to specific chemicals or particular organ systems or end-points. Additional emphasis should be placed on prospective longitudinal studies capturing multiple exposures over various life stages.

- Childhood exposures may lead to immediate effects, or there may be a long latency period between exposure and effects. Considerably more information from less-than-lifetime exposures needs to be collected in order to evaluate issues of latency and reversibility of effect.

- There is a continuing need for validated biomarkers of exposure that provide information on the frequency, duration, and intensity of an exposure, as well as a better understanding of distribution, metabolism, and excretion within the individual. Likewise, continued development of analytical methods (e.g. Monte Carlo) that provide a broad characterization of exposure and dose–response relationships should be encouraged.

REFERENCES

Aafjes JH, Vels JM, & Schenck E (1980) Fertility of rats with artificial oligozoospermia. J Reprod Fertil, **58**: 345–351.

Aarskog D (1970) Clinical and cytogenetic studies in hypospadias. Acta Paediatr Scand Suppl, **203**: 201–204.

Abel EL (1984) Prenatal effects of alcohol. Drug Alcohol Depend, **14**(1): 1–10.

Adams J (1986) Methods in behavioral teratology. In: Riley EP & Vorhees CV eds. Handbook of behavioral teratology. New York, Plenum Press, pp 67–97.

Adams J (1993) Structure–activity and dose–response relationships in the neural and behavioral teratogenesis of retinoids. Neurotoxicol Teratol, **15**(3): 193–202.

Adams J & Lammer EJ (1993) Neurobehavioral teratology of isotretinoin. Reprod Toxicol, **7**(2): 175–177.

Adams J, Barone S Jr, LaMantia A, Philen R, Rice DC, Spear L, & Susser E (2000) Workshop to identify critical windows of exposure for children's health: Neurobehavioral work group summary. Environ Health Perspect, **108**(Suppl 3): 535–544.

Akazawa H & Komuro I (2005) Cardiac transcription factor Csx/Nkx2.5: Its role in cardiac development and diseases. Pharmacol Ther, **107**: 252–268.

Albalak R, McElroy RH, Noonan G, Buchanan S, Jones RL, Flanders WD, Gotway-Crawford C, Kim D, Kignam T, Daley WR, Jarrett J, Eduardo E, & McGeehin MA (2003) Blood lead levels and risk factors for lead poisoning among children in a Mexican smelting community. Arch Environ Health, **58**: 172–183.

Alcorn J & McNamara PJ (2003) Pharmacokinetics in the newborn. Adv Drug Deliv Rev, **55**(5): 667–686.

al-Hazzaa SA & Krahn PM (1995) Kohl: A hazardous eyeliner. Int Ophthalmol, **19**(2): 83–88.

Allan BB, Brant R, Seidel JE, & Jarrell JF (1997) Declining sex ratios in Canada. Can Med Assoc J, **156**(1): 37–41.

Allebeck P & Olsen J (1998) Alcohol and fetal damage. Alcohol Clin Exp Res, **22**(Suppl 7): 329S–332S.

American Thoracic Society (1987) Standardization of spirometry, 1987 update. Am Rev Respir Dis, **136**: 1285–1298.

Amery A, Bossaert H, & Verstraete M (1969) Muscle blood flow in normal and hypertensive subjects. Influence of age, exercise, and body position. Am Heart J, **78**: 211–216.

Anderson HR & Cook DG (1997) Passive smoking and sudden infant death syndrome: Review of the epidemiological evidence. Thorax, **52**: 1003–1009.

Anderson LM, Jones AB, Riggs CW, & Ohshima M (1985) Fetal mouse susceptibility to transplacental lung and liver carcinogenesis by 3-methylcholanthrene: Positive correlation with responsiveness to inducers of aromatic hydrocarbon metabolism. Carcinogenesis, **6**(9): 1389–1393.

Anderson LM, Hagiwara A, Kovatch RM, Rehm S, & Rice JM (1989) Transplacental initiation of liver, lung, neurogenic, and connective tissue tumors by *N*-nitroso compounds in mice. Fundam Appl Toxicol, **12**(3): 604–620.

Anderson LM, Diwan BA, Fear NT, & Roman E (2000) Critical windows of exposure for children's health: Cancer in human epidemiological studies and neoplasms in experimental animals. Environ Health Perspect, **108**(Suppl 3): 573–594.

Andersson U, Bird AG, Britton BS, & Palacios R (1981) Humoral and cellular immunity in humans studied at the cell level from birth to two years of age. Immunol Rev, **57**: 1–38.

Anderton DL, Anderson AB, Oakes JM, & Fraser MR (1994) Environmental equity: The demographics of dumping. Demography, **31**: 229–248.

Anderton DL, Oakes JM, & Egan KL (1997) Environmental equity in Superfund. Demographics of the discovery and prioritization of abandoned toxic sites. Eval Rev, **21**: 3–26.

Ando M, Tadano M, Asanuma S, Tamura K, Matsushima S, Watanabe T, Kondo T, Sakurai S, Ji R, Liang C, & Cao S (1998) Health effects of indoor fluoride pollution from coal burning in China. Environ Health Perspect, **106**(5): 239–244.

Arms AD & Travis CC (1988) Reference physiological parameters in pharmacokinetic modeling. Washington, DC, United States Environmental Protection Agency, Office of Health and Environmental Assessment (NTIS PB 88-196019).

Armstrong TW, Hushka LJ, Tell JG, & Zaleski RT (2000) A tiered approach for assessing children's exposure. Environ Health Perspect, **108**(6): 469–474.

Ashby J, Tinwell H, Stevens J, Pastoor T, & Breckenridge CB (2002) The effects of atrazine on the sexual maturation of female rats. Regul Toxicol Pharmacol, **35**: 468–473.

Asklund C, Jorgensen N, Kold Jensen T, & Skakkebaek NE (2004) Biology and epidemiology of testicular dysgenesis syndrome. Br J Urol Int, **93**(Suppl 3): 6–11.

Astolfi P & Zonta LA (1999) Reduced male births in major Italian cities. Hum Reprod, **14**(12): 3116–3119.

Atlas MK (2001) Safe and sorry: Risk, environmental equity, and hazardous waste management facilities. Risk Anal, **21**: 939–954.

ATSDR (1994) Environmental data needed for public health assessments. A guidance manual. Atlanta, GA, United States Department of Health and Human Services, Agency for Toxic Substances and Disease Registry.

References

ATSDR (1997) Healthy children — toxic environments. Acting on the unique susceptibility of children who dwell near hazardous waste sites. Report of the Child Health Workgroup. Atlanta, GA, United States Department of Health and Human Services, Agency for Toxic Substances and Disease Registry.

ATSDR (1999) Toxicological profile for alpha-, beta-, gamma-, and delta-hexachlorocyclohexane. Atlanta, GA, United States Department of Health and Human Services, Agency for Toxic Substances and Disease Registry.

ATSDR (2003) Children living near hazardous waste sites. Atlanta, GA, United States Department of Health and Human Services, Agency for Toxic Substances and Disease Registry (http://www.atsdr.cdc.gov/child/ochchildhlth.html#dhac).

Avol EL, Gauderman WJ, Tan SM, London SJ, & Peters JM (2001) Respiratory effects of relocating to areas of differing air pollution levels. Am J Respir Clin Care, **164**: 2067–2072.

Axom A, Rylander L, Stromberg U, & Hagmar L (2000) Time to pregnancy and infertility among women with a high intake of fish contaminated with persistent organochlorine compounds. Scand J Work Environ Health, **26**: 199–206.

Baer JS, Sampson PD, Barr HM, Connor PD, & Streissguth AP (2003) A 21-year longitudinal analysis of the effects of prenatal alcohol exposure on young adult drinking. Arch Gen Psychiatry, **60**(4): 377–385.

Bailey LB, Rampersaud GC, & Kauwell GP (2003) Folic acid supplements and fortification affect the risk for neural tube defects, vascular disease and cancer: Evolving science. J Nutr, **133**(6): 1961S–1968S.

Baird DD & Wilcox AJ (1985) Cigarette smoking associated with delayed conception. J Am Med Assoc, **253**: 2979–2983.

Baird DD, Wilcox AJ, & Weinberg CR (1986) Use of time to pregnancy to study environmental exposures. Am J Epidemiol, **124**: 470–480.

Barlow SM & Sullivan FM (1975) Behavioural teratology. In: Berry CL & Poswillo DE eds. Teratology — Trends and applications. New York, Springer-Verlag, pp 103–120.

Barlow WE, Ichikawa L, Rosner D, & Izumi S (1999) Analysis of case–cohort designs. J Clin Epidemiol, **52**: 1165–1172.

Barnett J (1996) Developmental immunotoxicology. In: Smialowicz R & Holsapple M eds. Experimental immunotoxicology. Boca Raton, FL, CRC Press.

Barone S Jr, Das KP, Lassiter TL, & White LD (2000) Vulnerable processes of nervous system development: A review of markers and methods. Neurotoxicology, **21**(1–2): 15–36.

Barr DB, Weihe P, Davis MD, Needham LL, & Grandjean P (2006) Serum polychlorinated biphenyl and organochlorine insecticide concentrations in a Faroese birth cohort. Chemosphere, **62**(7): 1167–1182.

Barr M, DeSesso JM, Lau CS, Osmond C, Ozanne SE, Sadler TW, Simmons RA, & Sonawane BR (2000) Workshop to identify critical windows of exposure for children's health: Cardiovascular and endocrine work group summary. Environ Health Perspect, **108**(Suppl 3): 569–571.

Bates GW (1998) Normal and abnormal puberty. In: Carr BR & Blackwell RE eds. Textbook of reproductive medicine. Stanford, CT, Appleton & Lange, pp 93–111.

Bayley M (1993) The Bayley scales of infant development, 2nd ed. San Antonio, TX, The Psychological Corporation.

Beckman DA & Feuston M (2003) Landmarks in the development of the female reproductive system. Birth Defects Res B Dev Reprod Toxicol, **68**: 137–143.

Behre HM, Kuhlage J, Gassner C, Sonntag B, Schem C, Schneider HPG, & Nieschlag E (2000) Prediction of ovulation by urinary hormone measurements with the home use ClearPlan® Fertility Monitor: Comparison with transvaginal ultrasound scans and serum hormone measurements. Hum Reprod, **15**: 2478–2482.

Bellanti J, Malka-Rais J, Castro H, de Inocencio J, & Sabra A (2003) Developmental immunology: Clinical application to allergy-immunology. Ann Allergy Asthma Immunol, **90**(6 Suppl 3): 2–6.

Bellinger D, Leviton A, Allred E, & Rabinowitz M (1994) Pre- and postnatal lead exposure and behavior problems in school-aged children. Environ Res, **66**(1): 12–30.

Bellinger DC (2004) Lead. Paediatrics, **113**(Suppl 4): 1016–1022.

Ben-Jonathan N, Mershon JL, Allen DL, & Steinmetz RW (1996) Extrapituitary prolactin: Distribution, regulation, functions, and clinical aspects. Endocr Rev, **17**: 639–667.

Bennett GD & Finnell GD (1998) Periods of susceptibility to induced malformations of the developing mammalian brain. In: Slikker WJ & Chang LW eds. Handbook of developmental neurotoxicology. San Diego, CA, Academic Press, pp 189–208.

Bennett WD, Zeman KL, & Kim C (1996) Variability of the fine particle deposition in healthy adults: Effect of age and gender. Am J Respir Crit Care Med, **153**: 1641–1647.

Berthelsen JG & Skakkebaek NE (1983) Testicular cancer: Abnormal structure and function of the contralateral testis. Int J Androl, **6**: 209–211.

Biason-Lauber A, Konrad D, Navratil F, & Schoenle EJ (2004) A WNT4 mutation associated with Mullerian-duct regression and virilization in a 46,XX woman. N Engl J Med, **351**(8): 792–798.

Birnbaum L (1995) Developmental effects of dioxin. Environ Health Perspect, **103**(Suppl 7): 89–94.

Birnbaum LS & Fenton SE (2003) Cancer and developmental exposure to endocrine disruptors. Environ Health Perspect, **111**(4): 389–394.

References

Bishop CE, Whitworth DJ, Qin Y, Agoulnik AI, Agoulnik IU, Harrison WR, Behringer RR, & Overbeek PA (2000) A transgenic insertion upstream of sox9 is associated with dominant XX sex reversal in the mouse. Nat Genet, **26**: 490–494.

Blanck HM, Marcus M, Tolbert BE, Rubin C, Henderson AK, Hertzberg VS, Zhang RH, & Cameron L (2000) Age at menarche and Tanner stage in girls exposed in utero and postnatally to polybrominated biphenyl. Epidemiology, **11**: 641–647.

Blanck HM, Marcus M, Rubin C, Tolbert PE, Hertzberg VS, Henderson AK, & Zhang RH (2002) Growth in girls exposed in utero and postnatally to polybrominated biphenyls and polychlorinated biphenyls. Epidemiology, **13**(2): 205–210.

Bland ML, Desclozeaux M, & Ingraham HA (2003) Tissue growth and remodeling of the embryonic and adult adrenal gland. Ann N Y Acad Sci, **995**: 59–72.

Blaylock B, Holladay S, Comment C, Heindel J, & Luster M (1992) Exposure to tetrachlorodibenzo-*p*-dioxin (TCDD) alters fetal thymocyte maturation. Toxicol Appl Pharmacol, **112**: 207–213.

Blumberg BS (1997) Hepatitis B virus, the vaccine, and the control of primary cancer of the liver. Proc Natl Acad Sci U S A, **94**: 7121–7125.

Blyler G, Landreth K, & Barnett J (1994) Gender-specific effects of prenatal chlordane exposure on myeloid cell development. Fundam Appl Toxicol, **23**: 188–193.

Bo S, Cavallo-Perin P, Scaglione L, Ciccone G, & Pagano G (2000) Low birthweight and metabolic abnormalities in twins with increased susceptibility to Type 2 diabetes. Diabet Med, **17**: 365–370.

Bobak M & Leon DA (1999a) The effect of air pollution on infant mortality appears specific for respiratory causes in the postneonatal period. Epidemiology, **10**: 666–670.

Bobak M & Leon DA (1999b) Pregnancy outcomes and outdoor air pollution: An ecological study in districts of the Czech Republic 1986–8. Occup Environ Med, **56**: 539–543.

Bobak M, Richards M, & Wadsworth M (2001) Air pollution and birth weight in Britain in 1946. Epidemiology, **12**: 358–359.

Bogdanffy MS, Daston G, Faustman EM, Kimmel CA, Kimmel GL, Seed J, & Vu V (2001) Harmonization of cancer and non-cancer risk assessment: Proceedings of a consensus-building workshop. Toxicol Sci, **61**: 18–31.

Boice JD Jr, Land CE, & Preston DL (1996) Ionizing radiation. In: Schottenfeld D & Fraumeni JF Jr eds. Cancer epidemiology and prevention, 2nd ed. New York, Oxford University Press, pp 319–354.

Boisen K, Kaleva M, Main K, Virtanen H, Haavisto AM, Schmidt I, Chellakooty M, Damgaard I, Mau C, Reunanen M, Skakkebaek N, & Toppari J (2004) Difference in prevalence of congenital cryptorchidism in infants between two Nordic countries. Lancet, **363**: 1264–1269.

Bolognesi C, Rossi L, & Santi L (1988) A new method to reveal the genotoxic effects of N-nitrosodimethylamine in pregnant mice. Mutat Res, **207**(2): 57–62.

Borja-Aburto VH, Castillejos M, Gold DR, Bierzwinski S, & Loomis D (1998) Mortality and ambient fine particles in southwest Mexico City, 1993–1995. Environ Health Perspect, **106**(12): 849–855.

Bosley AR, Sibert JR, & Newcombe RG (1981) Effects of maternal smoking on fetal growth and nutrition. Arch Dis Child, **56**: 727–729.

Botto LD, Olney RS, & Erickson JD (2004) Vitamin supplements and the risk for congenital anomalies other than neural tube defects. Am J Med Genet C Semin Med Genet, **125**(1): 12–21.

Braback L, Breborowicz A, Julge K, Knutsson A, Riikjarv MA, Vasar M, & Bjorksten B (1995) Risk factors for respiratory symptoms and atopic sensitisation in the Baltic area. Arch Dis Child, **72**: 487–493.

Braun-Fahrlander C, Ackermann-Liebrich U, Schwartz J, Gnehm HP, Rutishauser M, & Wanner HU (1992) Air pollution and respiratory symptoms in preschool children. Annu Rev Respir Dis, **145**: 42–47.

Braun-Fahrlander C, Vuille JC, Sennhauser FH, Neu U, Kunzle T, Grize L, Gassner M, Minder C, Schindler C, Varonier HS, & Wuthrich B (1997) Respiratory health and long-term exposure to air pollutants in Swiss schoolchildren. Am J Respir Crit Care Med, **155**: 1042–1049.

Brechner RJ, Parkhurst GD, Humble WO, Brown MB, & Herman WH (2000) Ammonium perchlorate contamination of Colorado River drinking water is associated with abnormal thyroid function in newborns in Arizona. J Occup Environ Med, **42**: 777–782.

Brenner BM, Garcia DL, & Anderson S (1988) Glomeruli and blood pressure. Less of one, more of the other? Am J Hypertens, **1**: 335–347.

Brent RL & Beckman DA (1990) Environmental teratogens. Bull N Y Acad Med, **66**(2): 123–163.

Brent RL, Tanski S, & Weitzman M (2004) A pediatric perspective on the unique susceptibilities and resilience of the embryo and the child to environmental toxicants: The importance of rigorous research concerning age and agent. Paediatrics, **113**: 935–944.

Bricker D & Squires J (1995) Ages & Stages Questionnaires®: A parent-completed, child-monitoring system. Baltimore, MD, Paul H. Brookes Publishing Co.

Bridges JP & Weaver TE (2006) Use of transgenic mice to study lung morphogenesis and function. ILAR J, **47**(1): 22–31.

Briggs GG, Freeman RK, & Yaffe SJ eds (2002) Drugs in pregnancy and lactation: A reference guide to fetal and neonatal risk, 6th ed. Philadelphia, PA, Lippincott Williams & Wilkins.

Brinton LA, Kruger Kjaer S, Thomsen BL, Sharif HF, Graubard BI, Olsen JH, & Bock JE (2004) Childhood tumor risk after treatment with ovulation-stimulating drugs. Fertil Steril, **81**: 1083–1091.

Brophy VH, Hastings MD, Clendenning JB, Richter RJ, Jarvik GP, & Furlong CE (2001) Polymorphisms in the human paraoxonase (PON1) promoter. Pharmacogenetics, **11**: 77–84.

Brouwer A, Morse DC, Lans MC, Schuur AG, Murk AJ, Klasson-Wehler E, Bergman A, & Visser TJ (1998) Interactions of persistent environmental organohalogens with the thyroid hormone system: Mechanisms and possible consequences for animal and human health. Toxicol Ind Health, **14**: 59–84.

Brown RP, Delp MD, Lindstedt SL, Rhomberg LR, & Beliles RP (1997) Physiological parameter values for physiologically based pharmacokinetic models. Toxicol Ind Health, **13**(4): 407–484.

Bruce N, Perez-Padilla R, & Albalak R (2000) Indoor air pollution in developing countries: A major environmental and public health challenge. Bull World Health Organ, **78**: 1078–1092.

Brunekreef B, Janssen N, de Hartog J, Harssema H, Knape M, & van Vliet P (1997) Air pollution from truck traffic and lung function in children living near motorways. Epidemiology, **8**: 298–303.

Brustle O, Ohgaki H, Schmitt HP, Walter GF, Ostertag H, & Kleihues P (1992) Primitive neuroectodermal tumors after prophylactic central nervous system irradiation in children. Association with an activated K-ras gene. Cancer, **69**: 2385–2392.

Buck GM, Vena JE, Schisterman EF, Dmochowski J, Mendola P, Sever LE, Fitzgerald E, Kostyniak P, Greizerstein H, & Olson J (2000) Parental consumption of contaminated sport fish from Lake Ontario and predicted fecundability. Epidemiology, **11**: 388–393.

Buck GM, Lynch CD, Stanford JB, Sweeney AM, Schieve LA, Rockett JC, Selevan SG, & Schrader SM (2004) Prospective pregnancy study designs for assessing reproductive developmental toxicants. Environ Health Perspect, **112**(1): 79–86.

Buck Louis GM, Schisterman EF, Dukic VM, & Schieve LA (2004) Research hurdles complicating the analysis of infertility treatment and child health. Hum Reprod, **20**: 12–18.

Buck Louis GM, Weiner JM, Whitcomb BW, Sperrazza R, Schisterman EF, Lobdell DT, Crickard K, Greizerstein H, & Kostyniak PJ (2005) Environmental PCB exposure and risk of endometriosis. Hum Reprod, **20**(1): 279–285.

Buck Louis GM, Dukic V, Heagerty P, Louis TA, Lynch CD, Ryan LM, Schisterman EF, Trumble A, & Pregnancy Modeling Working Group (2006) Analysis of repeated pregnancy outcomes. Stat Methods Med Res, **15**(2): 103–126.

Buelke-Sam J & Kimmel CA (1979) Development and standardization of screening methods for behavioural teratology. Teratology, **20**: 17–29.

Bunn T, Marsh J, & Dietert R (2000) Gender differences in developmental immunotoxicity to lead in the chicken: Analysis following a single early low level exposure in ovo. J Toxicol Environ Health A, **61**: 677–693.

Bunn T, Parsons P, Kao E, & Dietert R (2001a) Exposure to lead during critical windows of embryonic development: differential immunotoxic outcome based on stage of exposure and gender. Toxicol Sci, **64**: 57–66.

Bunn T, Parsons P, Kao E, & Dietert R (2001b) Gender-based profiles of developing immunotoxicity to lead in the rat: assessment in juveniles and adults. J Toxicol Environ Health A, **64**: 101–118.

Bunn T, Dietert R, Ladics G, & Holsapple M (2001c) Developmental immunotoxicology assessment in the rat: age, gender, and strain comparisons after exposure to lead. Toxicol Meth, **11**: 1–18.

Burbacher TM & Grant KS (2006) Neurodevelopmental effects of alcohol. In: Davidson PW, Myers GJ, & Weiss B eds. Neurotoxicity and developmental disabilities: individual differences in personality and motivational systems. San Diego, CA, Elsevier Academic Press.

Burke JM, Zufall MJ, & Ozkaynak H (2001) A population exposure model for particulate matter: Case study results for $PM_{2.5}$ in Philadelphia, PA. J Expo Anal Environ Epidemiol, **11**: 470–489.

Burr ML, Limb ES, Maguire MJ, Amarah L, Eldridge BA, Layzell JC, & Merrett TG (1993) Infant feeding, wheezing, and allergy: A prospective study. Arch Dis Child, **68**(6): 724–728.

Butte W & Heinzow B (2002) Pollutants in house dust as indicators of indoor contamination. Rev Environ Contam Toxicol, **175**: 1–46.

Calderón J, Navarro ME, Jiménez-Capdeville ME, Santos-Díaz MA, Golden A, Rodríguez-Leyva I, Borja-Aburto VH, & Díaz-Barriga F (2001) Exposure to arsenic and lead and neuropsychological development in Mexican children. Environ Res, **85**: 69–76.

Canfield R, Henderson C, Cory-Slechta D, Cox C, Jusko T, & Lamphear B (2003) Intellectual impairment in children with blood lead concentrations below 10 µg per deciliter. N Engl J Med, **348**: 1517–1526.

Carmeliet P (2000) Mechanisms of angiogenesis and arteriogenesis. Nat Med, **4**: 389–395.

Carrizales L, Razo I, Téllez-Hernández JI, Torres-Nerio R, Torres A, Batres LE, Cubillas AC, & Díaz-Barriga F (2006) Exposure to arsenic and lead of children living near a copper-smelter in San Luis Potosi, Mexico. Importance of soil contamination for exposure of children. Environ Res, **101**(1): 1–10.

Carter RC, Jacobson SW, Molteno CD, Chiodo LM, Viljoen D, & Jacobson JL (2005) Effects of prenatal alcohol exposure on infant visual acuity. J Paediatr, **147**(4): 473–479.

Casey BJ, Tottenham N, Liston C, & Durston S (2005) Imaging the developing brain: what have we learned about cognitive development? Trends Cogn Sci, **9**(3): 104–110.

References

Cayler GG, Rudolph AM, & Nadas AS (1963) Systemic blood flow in infants and children with and without heart disease. Paediatrics, **32**: 186–201.

CDC (2003a) Surveillance summaries, September 12, 2003. Centers for Disease Control and Prevention. Morbid Mortal Wkly Rep, **52**(SS-10).

CDC (2003b) Second national report on human exposure to environmental chemicals. Atlanta, GA, United States Department of Health and Human Services, Centers for Disease Control and Prevention.

CDC (2005) Third national report on human exposure to environmental chemicals. Atlanta, GA, United States Department of Health and Human Services, Centers for Disease Control and Prevention (http://www.cdc.gov/exposurereport/3rd/).

Chang MH, Shau WY, Chen CJ, Wu TC, Kong MS, Liang DC, Hsu HM, Chen HL, Hsu HY, & Chen DS (2000) Hepatitis B vaccination and hepatocellular carcinoma rates in boys and girls. J Am Med Assoc, **284**: 3040–3042.

Chapin R (2002) The use of the rat in developmental immunotoxicology studies. Hum Exp Toxicol, **21**: 521–523.

Chapin R, Harris M, Davis B, Ward S, Wilson R, Mauney M, Lockhard A, Smialowicz R, Moser V, Burka L, & Collins B (1997) The effects of perinatal/juvenile methoxychlor exposure on adult rat nervous, immune and reproductive system function. Fundam Appl Toxicol, **40**: 138–157.

Chapin RE, Robbins WA, Schieve LA, Sweeney AM, Tabacova SA, & Tomashek KM (2004) Off to a good start: the influence of pre- and periconceptional exposures, parental fertility, and nutrition on children's health. Environ Health Perspect, **112**(1): 69–78.

Cheek AO, Kow K, Chen J, & McLachlan JA (1999) Potential mechanisms of action of thyroid disruption in humans: Interaction of organochlorine compounds with thyroid receptor, transthyretin, and thyroid-binding globulin. Environ Health Perspect, **107**(4): 273–278.

Chiron C, Raynaud C, Maziere B, Zilbovicius M, Laflamme L, Masure M-C, Dulac O, Bourguignon M, & Syrota A (1992) Changes in regional cerebral blood flow during brain maturation in children and adolescents. J Nucl Med, **33**: 696–703.

Chow WH, Linet MS, Liff JM, & Greenberg RS (1996) Cancers in children. In: Schottenfeld D & Fraumeni JF Jr eds. Cancer epidemiology and prevention, 2nd ed. New York, Oxford University Press, pp 1331–1369.

Christiani DC, Sharp RR, Collman GW, & Suk WA (2001) Applying genomic technologies in environmental health research: challenges and opportunities. J Occup Environ Med, **43**(6): 526–533.

Cicognani A, Pasini A, Pession A, Pirazzoli P, Burnelli R, Barbieri E, Mazzanti L, & Cacciari E (2003) Gonadal function and pubertal development after treatment of a childhood malignancy. J Paediatr Endocrinol Metab, **16**(Suppl 2): 321–326.

Clewell HJ, Teeguarden J, McDonald T, Sarangapani R, Lawrence G, Covington T, Gentry R, & Shipp A (2002) Review and evaluation of the potential impact of age- and gender-specific pharmacokinetic differences on tissue dosimetry. Crit Rev Toxicol, **32**: 329–389.

Coccini T, Randine G, Castoldi AF, Grandjean P, Ostendorp G, Heinzow B, & Manzo L (2006) Effects of developmental co-exposure to methylmercury and 2,2',4,4',5,5'-hexachlorobiphenyl (PCB153) on cholinergic muscarinic receptors in rat brain. Neurotoxicology, **27**(4): 468–477.

Cohen Hubal EA, Sheldon LS, Zufall MJ, Burke JM, & Thomas K (2000a) The challenge of assessing children's residential exposure to pesticides. J Expo Anal Environ Epidemiol, **10**: 638–649.

Cohen Hubal EA, Sheldon LS, Burke JM, McCurdy TR, Berry MR, Rigas ML, Zartarian VG, & Freeman NC (2000b) Children's exposure assessment: A review of factors influencing children's exposure, and the data available to characterize and assess that exposure. Environ Health Perspect, **108**(6): 475–486.

Cohn HE, Sacks EJ, Heymann MA, & Rudolph AM (1974) Cardiovascular responses to hypoxemia and acidemia in fetal lambs. Am J Obstet Gynecol, **120**(6): 817–824.

Collaer ML & Hines M (1995) Human behavioral sex differences: A role for gonadal hormones during early development. Psychol Bull, **118**: 55–107.

Collins MH, Moessinger AC, Kleinerman J, Bassi J, Rosso P, Collins AM, James LS, & Blanc WA (1985) Fetal lung hypoplasia associated with maternal smoking: A morphometric analysis. Paediatr Res, **19**: 408–412.

Colon I, Caro D, Bourdony CJ, & Rosario O (2000) Identification of phthalate esters in the serum of young Puerto Rican girls with premature breast development. Environ Health Perspect, **108**(9): 895–900.

Cook D (1976) Paediatric anaesthesia: Pharmacological considerations. Drugs, **12**: 212–221.

Cook DG & Strachan DP (1999) The health effects of passive smoking. 10: Summary of the effects of parental smoking on the respiratory health of children and implications for research. Thorax, **4**: 357–366.

Cook DG, Strachan DP, & Carey IM (1998) Parental smoking and spirometric indices in children. Thorax, **53**: 884–893.

Cooney MA, Buck Louis GM, Sun W, Rice MM, & Klebanoff MA (2006) Is conception delay a risk factor for reduced gestation or birthweight? Paediatr Perinat Epidemiol, **20**: 201–209.

Cooper C, Fall C, Egger P, Hobbs R, Eastell R, & Barker D (1997) Growth in infancy and bone mass later in life. Ann Rheumatol Dis, **56**: 17–21.

Cooper C, Javaid MK, Taylor P, Walker-Bone K, Dennison E, & Arden N (2002) The fetal origins of osteoporotic fracture. Calcif Tissue Int, **70**: 391–394.

Cooper RL, Stoker TE, Tyrey L, Goldman JM, & McElroy WK (2000) Atrazine disrupts the hypothalamic control of pituitary–ovarian function. Toxicol Sci, **53**: 297–307.

Corda S, Samuel SL, & Rappaport L (2000) Extracellular matrix and growth factors during heart growth. Heart Fail Rev, **5**: 119–130.

Corley RA, Mast TJ, Carney EW, Rogers JM, & Daston GP (2003) Evaluation of physiologically based models of pregnancy and lactation for their application in children's health risk assessments. Crit Rev Toxicol, **32**: 137–211.

Cory-Slechta DA, Thiruchelvam MT, Richfield EK, Barlow BK, & Brooks AI (2005) Developmental pesticide exposures and the Parkinson's disease phenotype. Birth Defects Res A Clin Mol Teratol, **73**: 136–139.

Costa LG, Cole TB, & Furlong CB (2003) Polymorphisms of paraoxonase (PON1) and their significance in clinical toxicology of organophosphates. J Toxicol Clin Toxicol, **41**: 37–45.

Costa LG, Cole TB, Vitalone A, & Furlong CE (2005) Measurement of paraoxonase (PON1) status as a potential biomarker of susceptibility to organophosphate toxicity. Clin Chim Acta, **352**: 37–47.

Counter SA, Vahter M, Laurell G, Buchanan LH, Ortega F, & Skerfving S (1997) High lead exposure and auditory sensory-neural function in Andean children. Environ Health Perspect, **105**(5): 522–526.

Couse JF & Korach KS (1999) Estrogen receptor null mice: what have we learned and where will they lead us? Endocr Rev, **20**: 358–417.

Couture-Haws L, Harris MW, McDonald MM, Lockhart AC, & Birnbaum LS (1991) Hydronephrosis in mice exposed to TCDD-contaminated breast milk: Identification of the peak period of sensitivity and assessment of potential recovery. Toxicol Appl Pharmacol, **107**(3): 413–428.

Cremonini F & Gasbarrini A (2003) Atopy, *Helicobacter pylori* and the hygiene hypothesis. Eur J Gastroenterol Hepatol, **15**: 635–636.

Cresteil T (1998) Onset of xenobiotic metabolism in children: toxicological implications. Food Addit Contam, **15**(Suppl): 45–51.

Cresteil T, Beaune P, Kremers P, Flinois JP, & Leroux JP (1982) Drug-metabolizing enzymes in human foetal liver: Partial resolution of multiple cytochrome P450. Paediatr Pharmacol, **2**: 199–207.

Crom WR (1994) Pharmacokinetics in the child. Environ Health Perspect, **102**(Suppl 11): 111–118.

Cummings AM & Kavlock RJ (2004) Gene–environment interactions: A review of effects on reproduction and development. Crit Rev Toxicol, **34**: 461–485.

Dallaire F, Dewailly E, Muckle G, Jacobson SW, Jacobson JL, & Ayotte P (2004) Acute infections and environmental exposure to organochlorines in Inuit infants from Nunavik. Environ Health Perspect, **112**(14): 1359–1365.

Damstra T (2002) Potential effects of certain persistent organic pollutants and endocrine disrupting chemicals on the health of children. Clin Toxicol, **40**: 459–466.

Damstra T, Barlow S, Bergman A, Kavlock R, & Van Der Kraak G (2002) Global assessment of the state-of-the-science of endocrine disruptors. Geneva, World Health Organization (WHO/PCS/EDC/02.2).

Danielsson BR & Webster WS (1997) Cardiovascular active drugs. In: Kavlock RJ & Daston GP eds. Drug toxicity in embryonic development. II. Advances in understanding mechanisms of birth defects: Mechanistic understanding of human developmental toxicants. Berlin, Springer-Verlag, pp 161–190.

Daston G, Faustman E, Ginsberg G, Fenner-Crisp P, Olin S, Sonawane B, Bruckner J, & Breslin W (2004) A framework for assessing risks to children from exposure to environmental agents. Environ Health Perspect, **112**(2): 238–256.

Davidson PW, Myers GJ, & Weiss B (2004) Mercury exposure and child development outcomes. Paediatrics, **113**(Suppl 4): 1023–1029.

Davies P, Reid L, Lister G, & Pitt B (1988) Postnatal growth of the sheep lung: A morphometric study. Anat Rec, **220**: 281–286.

Davies RJ & Devalia JL (1993) Air pollution and airway epithelial cells. Agents Actions Suppl, **43**: 87–96.

Davis DL, Gottlieb MB, & Stampnitzky JR (1998) Reduced ratio of male to female births in several industrial countries: A sentinel health indicator. J Am Med Assoc, **279**: 1018–1023.

Debes F, Budtz-Jorgensen E, Weihe P, White RF, & Grandjean P (2006) Impact of prenatal methylmercury exposure on neurobehavioral function at age 14 years. Neurotoxicol Teratol, **28**(3): 363–375.

Dees WL, Hiney JK, & Srivastava V (1998) Alcohol's effects on female puberty: The role of insulin-like growth factor 1. Alcohol Health Res World, **22**(3): 165–169.

Dejmek J, Selevan SG, Benes I, Solansky I, & Srám RJ (1999) Fetal growth and maternal exposure to particulate matter during pregnancy. Environ Health Perspect, **107**(6): 475–480.

Dejmek J, Solansky I, Benes I, Lenicek J, & Srám RJ (2000) The impact of polycyclic aromatic hydrocarbons and fine particles on pregnancy outcome. Environ Health Perspect, **108**(12): 1159–1164.

del Rio Gomez I, Marshall T, Tsai P, Shao YS, & Guo YL (2002) Number of boys born to men exposed to polychlorinated biphenyls. Lancet, **360**: 143–144.

Den Hond E & Schoeters G (2006) Endocrine disrupters and human puberty. Int J Androl, **29**(1): 264–271.

Denning DW, Allen R, Wilkinson AP, & Morgan MR (1990) Transplacental transfer of aflatoxin in humans. Carcinogenesis, **11**(6): 1033–1035.

Dennison E, Hindmarsh P, Fall C, Kellingray S, Barker D, Phillips D, & Cooper C (1999) Profiles of endogenous circulating cortisol and bone mineral density in healthy elderly men. J Clin Endocrinol Metabol, **84**: 3058–3063.

de Onis M & Blössner M (2000) Prevalence and trends of overweight among preschool children in developing countries. Am J Clin Nutr, **72**(4): 1032–1039.

de Onis M & Blössner M (2003) The World Health Organization global database on child growth and malnutrition: Methodology and applications. Int J Epidemiol, **32**(4): 518–526.

de Onis M, Blössner M, Borghi E, Frongillo EA, & Morris R (2004) Estimates of global prevalence of childhood underweight in 1990 and 2015. J Am Med Assoc, **291**: 2600–2606.

Devalia JL, Rusznak C, & Davies RJ (1999) Allergen/irritant interaction — Its role in sensitization and allergic disease. Allergy, **53**(4): 335–345.

Dewailly E, Ayotte P, Bruneau S, Gingras S, Belles-Isles M, & Roy R (2000) Susceptibility to infections and immune status in Inuit infants exposed to organochlorines. Environ Health Perspect, **108**(3): 205–211.

De Zwart LL, Haenen HEMG, Versantvoort CHNM, Wolterink G, Van Engelen JGM, & Sips AJAM (2004) Role of biokinetics in risk assessment of drugs and chemicals in children. Regul Toxicol Pharmacol, **39**: 282–309.

DHUD (2003) First national environmental health survey of child care centers. Final report. Washington, DC, United States Department of Housing and Urban Development, Office of Healthy Homes and Lead Hazard Control.

Díaz-Barriga F, Santos MA, Mejía JJ, Batres L, Yáñez L, Carrizales L, Vera E, Del Razo LM, & Cebrian ME (1993) Arsenic and cadmium absorption in children living near a smelter complex in San Luis Potosí, Mexico. Environ Res, **62**: 242–250.

Díaz-Barriga F, Navarro-Quezada A, Grijalva M, Grimaldo M, Loyola-Rodríguez JP, & Ortíz MD (1997a) Endemic fluorosis in México. Fluoride, **30**: 233–239.

Díaz-Barriga F, Batres L, Calderón J, Lugo A, Galvao L, Lara I, Rizo P, Arroyave ME, & McConnell R (1997b) The El Paso smelter twenty years later: residual impact on Mexican children. Environ Res, **74**: 11–16.

Díaz-Barriga F, Borja-Aburto V, Waliszewski S, & Yáñez L (2003) DDT in Mexico. In: Fiedler H ed. The handbook of environmental chemistry. Vol. 3. Part O. Persistent organic pollutants. Berlin, Springer-Verlag, pp 371–388.

Dibley MJ, Staehling N, Newburg P, & Trowbridge FL (1987) Development of normalized curves for the international growth reference: Historical and technical considerations. Am J Clin Nutr, **46**: 736–748.

Dickerson JWT & Widdowson EM (1960) Chemical changes in skeletal muscle during development. Biochem J, **74**: 247–257.

Dietert R & Lee J-E (2004) Toxicity of lead to the developing immune system. In: Holladay S ed. Developmental immunotoxicology. Boca Raton, FL, CRC Press.

Dietert RR & Piepenbrink MS (2005) Perinatal immunotoxicity: Why adult-exposure assessment fails to predict risk. Environ Health Perspect, **114**(4): 477–483.

Dietert RR, Etzel RA, Chen D, Halonen M, Holladay SD, Jarabek AM, Landreth K, Peden DB, Pinkerton K, Smialowicz RJ, & Zoetis T (2000) Workshop to identify critical windows of exposure for children's health: Immune and respiratory systems work group summary. Environ Health Perspect, **108**(Suppl 3): 483–490.

Dietert RR, Lee J-E, & Bunn TL (2002) Developmental immunotoxicology: Emerging issues. Hum Exp Toxicol, **21**: 479–485.

Dietert RR, Lee J-E, Olsen J, Fitch K, & Marsh JA (2003) Developmental immunotoxicity of dexamethasone: Comparison of fetal vs. adult exposures. Toxicology, **194**: 163–176.

Dietert RR, Lee J-E, Hussain I, & Piepenbrink M (2004) Developmental immunotoxicology of lead. Toxicol Appl Pharmacol, **198**(2): 86–94.

Dietrich KN, Ris MD, Succop PA, Berger OG, & Bornschein RL (2001) Early exposure to lead and juvenile delinquency. Neurotoxicol Teratol, **23**(6): 511–518.

DiFranza JR, Aligne A, & Weitzman M (2004) Prenatal and postnatal environmental tobacco smoke exposure and children's health. Paediatrics, **113**: 1007–1015.

Dockery DW, Speizer FE, Stram DO, Ware JH, Spengler JD, & Ferris BG Jr (1989) Effects of inhalable particles on respiratory health of children. Am Rev Respir Dis, **139**(3): 587–594.

Dodge R (1982) The effects of indoor pollution on Arizona children. Arch Environ Health, **37**: 151–155.

Dorne JL, Walton K, & Renwick AG (2005) Human variability in xenobiotics metabolism and pathway-related uncertainty factors for chemical risk assessment: A review. Food Chem Toxicol, **43**(2): 203–216.

Dutton GJ (1978) Developmental aspects of drug conjugation, with special reference to glucuronidation. Annu Rev Pharmacol Toxicol, **18**: 17–35.

Eastern Research Group (1998) Summary of the U.S. EPA workshop on the relationship between exposure duration and toxicity. Prepared for the Risk Assessment Forum, United States Environmental Protection Agency, Washington, DC.

Ebner K, Brewster DW, & Matsumura F (1988) Effects of 2,3,7,8-tetrachlorodibenzo-p-dioxin on serum insulin and glucose levels in the rabbit. J Environ Sci Health B, **23**: 427–438.

ECETOC (2005) Trends in children's health and the role of chemicals: state of the science review. Brussels, European Centre for Ecotoxicology and Toxicology of Chemicals, June (Technical Report No. 96).

Edmonds LD, Layde PM, James LM, Flynt JW, Erickson JD, & Oakley GP Jr (1981) Congenital malformations surveillance: Two American systems. Int J Epidemiol, **10**: 247–252.

Egal S, Hounsa A, Gong YY, Turner PC, Wild CP, Hall AJ, Hell K, & Cardwell KF (2005) Dietary exposure to aflatoxin from maize and groundnut in young children from Benin and Togo, West Africa. Int J Food Microbiol, **104**(2): 215–224.

Eisler R (2004) Mercury hazards from gold mining to humans, plants, and animals. Rev Environ Contam Toxicol, **181**: 139–198.

Elwood JM, Whitehead SM, Davison J, Stewart M, & Galt M (1990) Malignant melanoma in England: Risk associated with naevi, freckles, social class, hair colour, and sunburn. Int J Epidemiol, **19**: 801–810.

Ema M, Miyawaki E, & Kawashima K (2000) Critical period for adverse effects on development of reproductive system in male offspring of rats given di-*n*-butyl phthalate during late pregnancy. Toxicol Lett, **111**: 271–278.

Emery JL & Mithal A (1960) The number of alveoli in the terminal respiratory unit of man during late intrauterine life and childhood. Arch Dis Child, **35**: 544–547.

Emmen JM, McLuskey A, Adham IM, Engel W, Verhoef-Post M, Themmen AP, Grootegoed JA, & Brinkmann AO (2000) Involvement of insulin-like factor 3 (Insl3) in diethylstilbestrol-induced cryptorchidism. Endocrinology, **141**: 846–849.

Etzel RA ed (2003) Pediatric environmental health, 2nd ed. Elk Grove Village, IL, American Academy of Pediatrics, Committee on Environmental Health.

Ezzati M & Kammen DM (2001) Quantifying the effects of exposure to indoor air pollution from biomass combustion on acute respiratory infections in developing countries. Environ Health Perspect, **109**(5): 481–488.

Faith R & Moore J (1977) Impairment of thymus-dependent immune functions by exposure of the developing immune system to 2,3,7,8-tetrachlorodibenzo-*p*-dioxin (TCDD). J Toxicol Environ Health, **3**: 451–464.

Fall C, Hindmarsh P, Dennison E, Kellingray S, Barker D, & Cooper C (1998) Programming of growth hormone secretion and bone mineral density in elderly men: A hypothesis. J Clin Endocrinol Metab, **83**: 135–139.

Famy C, Streissguth AP, & Unis AS (1998) Mental illness in adults with fetal alcohol syndrome or fetal alcohol effects. Am J Psychiatry, **155**(4): 552–554.

Fan F, Wierda D, & Rozman K (1996) Effects of 2,3,7,8-tetrachlorodibenzo-*p*-dioxin on humoral and cell-mediated immunity in Sprague-Dawley rats. Toxicology, **106**: 221–228.

Fanucchi MV, Buckpitt AR, Murphy ME, & Plopper CG (1997) Naphthalene cytotoxicity of differentiating Clara cells in neonatal mice. Toxicol Appl Pharmacol, **144**: 96–110.

Faulk C, Hanrahan L, Anderson HA, Kanarek MS, Draheim L, Needham L, & Patterson D Jr (1999) Body burden levels of dioxins, furans, and PCBs among frequent consumers of Great Lakes sport fish. The Great Lakes Consortium. Environ Res, **80**: S19–S25.

Faustman EM, Silbernagel SM, Fenske RA, Burbacher TM, & Ponce RA (2000) Mechanisms underlying children's susceptibility to environmental toxicants. Environ Health Perspect, **108**(Suppl 1): 13–21.

Fenske RA, Lu C, Barr D, & Needham L (2002) Children's exposure to chlorpyrifos and parathion in an agricultural community in central Washington State. Environ Health Perspect, **110**(5): 549–553.

Fine J, Gasiewicz T, & Silverstone A (1989) Lymphocyte stem cell alterations following perinatal exposure to 2,3,7,8-tetrachlorodibenzo-p-dioxin. Mol Pharmacol, **35**: 18–25.

Fisher JS, Macpherson S, Marchetti N, & Sharpe RM (2003) Human "testicular dysgenesis syndrome": A possible model using in-utero exposure of the rat to dibutyl phthalate. Hum Reprod, **18**: 1383–1394.

Fleishaker JC (2003) Models and methods for predicting drug transfer into human milk. Adv Drug Deliv Rev, **55**: 643–652.

Fomon SJ (1966) Body composition of the infant. Part I: The male "reference infant". In: Falkner F ed. Human development. Philadelphia, PA, W.B. Saunders Company, pp 239–246.

Franklin P, Dingle P, & Stick S (2000) Raised exhaled nitric oxide in healthy children is associated with domestic formaldehyde levels. Am J Respir Crit Care Med, **161**: 1757–1759.

Friedman JM & Polifka JE (2000) Teratogenic effects of drugs: A resource for clinicians, 2nd ed. Baltimore, MD, The John Hopkins University Press.

Friis-Hansen B (1971) Body composition during growth. In vivo measurements and biochemical data correlated to differential anatomical growth. Paediatrics, **47**(Suppl 2): 264–274.

Gallagher TM & Black GW (1985) Uptake of volatile anaesthetics in children. Anaesthesia, **40**: 1073–1077.

García Vargas GG, Rubio Andrade M, Del Razo LM, Borja Aburto V, Vera Aguilar E, & Cebrian ME (2001) Lead exposure in children living in a smelter community in region Lagunera, Mexico. J Toxicol Environ Health A, **62**: 417–429.

Garrett MH, Hooper MA, Hooper BM, Rayment PR, & Abramson MJ (1999) Increased risk of allergy in children due to formaldehyde exposure in homes. Allergy, **54**(4): 330–337.

References

Gauderman WJ, Gilliland F, Vora H, Avol E, Stram D, McConnell R, Thomas D, Lurmann F, Margolis HG, Rappaport EB, Berhane K, & Peters JM (2002) Association between air pollution and lung function growth in Southern Californian children. Results from a second cohort. Am J Respir Crit Care Med, **166**(1): 76–84.

Gehring U, Cyrys J, Sedlmeir G, Brunekreef B, Bellander T, Fischer P, Bauer CP, Reinhardt D, Wichmann HE, & Heinrich J (2002) Traffic-related air pollution and respiratory health during the first 2 years of life. Eur Respir J, **19**: 690–698.

Gehrs B & Smialowicz R (1997) Alterations in the developing immune system of the F344 rat after perinatal exposure to 2,3,7,8-tetrachlorodibenzo-p-dioxin. I. Effects on the fetus and the neonate. Toxicology, **122**: 219–228.

Gehrs B & Smialowicz R (1999) Persistent suppression of the delayed hypersensitivity in adult F344 rats after perinatal exposure to 2,3,7,8-tetrachlorodibenzo-p-dioxin. Toxicology, **134**: 79–88.

Gehrs B, Riddle M, Williams C, & Smialowicz R (1997) Alterations in the developing immune system of the F344 rat after perinatal exposure to 2,3,7,8-tetrachlorodibenzo-p-dioxin. II. Effects on the pup and the adult. Toxicology, **122**: 229–240.

Gereda JE, Leung DY, & Liu AH (2000a) Levels of environmental endotoxin and prevalence of atopic disease. J Am Med Assoc, **284**(13): 1652–1653.

Gereda JE, Leung DY, Thatayatikom A, Streib JE, Price MR, Klinnert MD, & Liu AH (2000b) Relation between house-dust endotoxin exposure, type 1 T-cell development, and allergen sensitisation in infants at high risk of asthma. Lancet, **355**: 1680–1683.

Gilbert SF (2005) Mechanisms for the environmental regulation of gene expression. Birth Defects Res C Embryo Today, **72**: 291–299.

Gilbert T, Lelievre-Pegorier M, Malienou R, Meulemans A, & Merlet-Benichou C (1987) Effects of prenatal and postnatal exposure to gentamicin on renal differentiation in the rat. Toxicology, **43**(3): 301–313.

Gill WB, Schumacher GF, & Bibbo M (1977) Pathological semen and anatomical abnormalities of the genital tract in human male subjects exposed to diethylstilbestrol in utero. J Urol, **117**: 477–480.

Gill WB, Schumacher GF, Bibbo M, Straus FH 2nd, & Schoenberg HW (1979) Association of diethylstilbestrol exposure in utero with cryptorchidism, testicular hypoplasia and semen abnormalities. J Urol, **122**: 36–39.

Gilmour MI (1995) Interaction of air pollutants and pulmonary allergic responses in experimental animals. Toxicology, **105**(2–3): 335–342.

Ginsberg G, Hattis D, Sonawane B, Russ A, Banati P, Kozlak M, Smolenski S, & Goble R (2002) Evaluation of child/adult pharmacokinetic differences from a database derived from the therapeutic drug literature. Toxicol Sci, **66**: 185–200.

Ginsberg G, Hattis D, Miller R, & Sonawane B (2004a) Paediatric pharmacokinetic data: Implications for environmental risk assessment for children. Paediatrics, 113(4): 973–983.

Ginsberg G, Slikker W Jr, Bruckner J, & Sonawane B (2004b) Incorporating children's toxicokinetics into a risk framework. Environ Health Perspect, 112(2): 272–283.

Ginsberg G, Hattis D, Russ A, & Sonawane B (2004c) Physiologically based pharmacokinetic (PBPK) modeling of caffeine and theophylline in neonates and adults: Implications for assessing children's risks from environmental agents. J Toxicol Environ Health A, 67(4): 297–329.

Ginsberg GL, Foos BP, & Firestone MP (2005) Review and analysis of inhalation dosimetry methods for application to children's risk assessment. J Toxicol Environ Health A, 68(8): 573–615.

Gladen BC & Rogan WJ (1991) Effects of perinatal polychlorinated biphenyls and dichlorodiphenyl dichloroethene on later development. J Paediatr, 119(1 Pt 1): 58–63.

Gladtke E (1973) Pharmacokinetics in relation to age. Boll Chim Farm, 112: 333–341.

Glinianaia S, Rankin J, Bell R, Pless-Mulloli T, & Howel D (2004) Does particulate air pollution contribute to infant death? Environ Health Perspect, 112(14): 1365–1370.

Gluckman PD & Pinal CS (2003) Regulation of fetal growth by the somatotrophic axis. J Nutr, 133: 1741S–1746S.

Goetzova I, Skovranek I, & Samanek M (1977) Muscle blood flow in children, measured by ^{133}Xe clearance method. Cor Vasa, 19(2): 161–164.

Gohlke JM, Griffith WC, Bartell SM, Lewandowski TA, & Faustman EM (2002) A computational model for neocortical neuronogenesis predicts ethanol-induced neocortical neuron number deficits. Dev Neurosci, 24(6): 467–477.

Goldey ES & Crofton KM (1998) Thyroxine replacement attenuates hypothyroxinemia, hearing loss, and motor deficits following developmental exposure to Aroclor 1254. Toxicol Sci, 45: 94–105.

Goldman JM, Laws SC, Balchak SK, Cooper RL, & Kavlock RJ (2000) Endocrine-disrupting chemicals: prepubertal exposures and effects on sexual maturation and thyroid activity in the female rat. A focus on the EDSTAC recommendations. Crit Rev Toxicol, 30: 135–196.

Gomez RA, Sequeira Lopez ML, Fernandez L, Chernavvsky DR, & Norwood VF (1999) The maturing kidney: development and susceptibility. Ren Fail, 21(3–4): 283–291.

Gordon B, Mackay R, & Rehfuess E (2004) Inheriting the world: The atlas of children's health and the environment. Geneva, World Health Organization.

Gorski JR & Rozman K (1987) Dose–response and time course of hypothyroxemia and hypoinsulinemia and characterization of insulin hypersensitivity in 2,3,7,8-tetrachloro-dibenzo-p-dioxin (TCDD)-treated rats. Toxicology, 44: 297–307.

Grandjean P (1992) Individual susceptibility to toxicity. Toxicol Lett, **64–65**: 43–51.

Grandjean P, Weihe P, White RF, Debes F, Araki S, Yokoyama K, Murata K, Sorensen N, Dahl R, & Jorgensen PJ (1997) Cognitive deficit in 7-year-old children with prenatal exposure to methylmercury. Neurotoxicol Teratol, **19**(6): 417–428.

Grandjean P, Murata K, Budtz-Jørgensen E, & Wihe P (2004) Cardiac autonomic activity in methylmercury neurotoxicity: 14-year follow-up of a Faroese birth cohort. J Paediatr, **144**: 169–176.

Gray JA & Kavlock RJ (1991) Physiological consequences of early neonatal growth retardation: Effects of alpha-difluoromethylornithine on renal growth and function in the rat. Teratology, **43**(1): 19–26.

Gray KA, Klebanoff MA, Brock JW, Zhou H, Darden R, Needham L, & Longnecker MP (2005) In utero exposure to background levels of polychlorinated biphenyls and cognitive functioning among school-age children. Am J Epidemiol, **162**(1): 17–26.

Gray LE Jr & Ostby JS (1995) In utero 2,3,7,8-tetrachlorodibenzo-*p*-dioxin (TCDD) alters reproductive morphology and function in female rat offspring. Toxicol Appl Pharmacol, **133**(2): 285–294.

Gray LE Jr, Ostby J, Monosson E, & Kelce WR (1999) Environmental antiandrogens: low doses of the fungicide vinclozolin alter sexual differentiation of the male rat. Toxicol Environ Health, **15**(1–2): 48–64.

Gray LE Jr, Ostby J, Furr J, Price M, Veeramachaneni DN, & Parks L (2000) Perinatal exposure to the phthalates DEHP, BBP, and DINP, but not DEP, DMP, or DOTP, alters sexual differentiation of the male rat. Toxicol Sci, **58**: 350–365.

Greaves SJ, Ferry DG, McQueen EG, Malcolm DS, & Buckfield PM (1975) Serial hexachlorophene blood levels in the premature infant. N Z Med J, **81**: 334–336.

Gregory GA, Eger EI II, & Munson ES (1969) The relationship between age and halothane requirement in man. Anaesthesiology, **30**: 488–491.

Grijalva-Haro MI, Barba-Leyva ME, & Laborin-Alvarez A (2001) [Fluoride intake and excretion in children of Hermosillo, Sonora, Mexico.] Salud Publica Mex, **43**: 127–134 (in Spanish).

Groeneveld CN, Hakkert BC, Bos PMJ, & De Heer C (2004) Extrapolation for exposure duration in oral toxicity: A quantitative analysis of historical toxicity data. Hum Ecol Risk Assess, **10**(4): 709–716.

Grunert D, Schöning M, & Rosendahl W (1990) Renal blood flow and flow velocity in children and adolescents: duplex Doppler evaluation. Eur J Paediatr, **149**: 287–292.

Guignard JP & Gouyon JB (1988) Adverse effects of drugs on the immature kidney. Biol Neonate, **53**(4): 243–252.

Gulson BL, Mahaffey KR, Jameson CW, Patison N, Law AJ, Mizon KJ, Korsch MJ, & Pederson D (1999) Impact of diet on lead in blood and urine in female adults and relevance to mobilization of lead from bone stores. Environ Health Perspect, **107**(4): 257–263.

Gundert-Remy U, Sonich-Mullin C, & IPCS Uncertainty and Variability Planning Workgroup and Drafting Group (2002) The use of toxicokinetic and toxicodynamic data in risk assessment: an international perspective. Sci Total Environ, **288**(1–2): 3–11.

Gundert-Remy U, Dahl SG, Boobis A, Kremers P, Kopp-Schneider A, Oberemm A, Renwick A, & Pelkonen O (2003) Molecular approaches to the identification of biomarkers of exposure and effect — report of an expert meeting organized by COST Action B15. Toxicol Lett, **156**(2): 227–240.

Guo YL, Lambert GH, & Hsu CC (1995) Growth abnormalities in the population exposed in utero and early postnatally to polychlorinated biphenyls and dibenzofurans. Environ Health Perspect, **103**(Suppl 6): 117–122.

Guo YL, Lambert GH, Hsu C-C, & Hsu MM (2004) Yucheng: Health effects of prenatal exposure to polychlorinated biphenyls and dibenzofurans. Int Arch Occup Environ Health, **77**: 153–158.

Guo Z (2002) Development of a Windows-based indoor air quality simulation package. Environ Model Softw, **15**: 403–410 [models and information available at http://www.epa.gov/appcdwww/iemb/model.htm].

Guron G & Friberg P (2000) An intact renin–angiotensin system is a prerequisite for normal renal development. J Hypertens, **18**: 123–137.

Ha EH, Lee JT, Kim H, Hong YC, Lee BE, Park HS, & Christiani DC (2003) Infant susceptibility of mortality to air pollution in Seoul, South Korea. Pediatrics, **111**: 284–290.

Habener JF, Kemp DM, & Thomas MK (2005) Minireview: Transcriptional regulation in pancreatic development. Endocrinology, **146**(3): 1025–1034.

Haddad S, Restieri C, & Krishnan K (2001) Characterization of age-related changes in body weight and organ weights from birth to adolescence in humans. J Toxicol Environ Health A, **64**: 453–464.

Haddow JE, Palomaki GE, Allan WC, Williams JR, Knight GJ, Gagnon J, O'Heir CE, Mitchell ML, Hermos RJ, Waisbren SE, Faix JD, & Klein RZ (1999) Maternal thyroid deficiency during pregnancy and subsequent neuropsychological development of the child. N Engl J Med, **341**: 549–555.

Hammer GD, Parker KL, & Schimmer BP (2005) Minireview: Transcriptional regulation of adrenocortical development. Endocrinology, **146**(3): 1018–1024.

Hanley NA, Hagan DM, Clement-Jones M, Ball SG, Strachan T, Salas-Cortes L, McElreavey K, Lindsay S, Robson S, Bullen P, Ostrer H, & Wilson DI (2000) SRY, SOX9, and DAX1 expression patterns during human sex determination and gonadal development. Mech Dev, **91**: 403–407.

Hanrahan JP, Tager IB, Segal MR, Tosteson TD, Castile RG, Van Vunakis H, Weiss ST, & Speizer FE (1992) The effect of maternal smoking during pregnancy on early infant lung function. Am Rev Respir Dis, **145**: 1129–1135.

Harada M (1978) Congenital Minamata disease: intrauterine methylmercury poisoning. Teratology, **18**(2): 285–288.

Harrison MJ, Wolfe DE, Lau TS, Mitnick RJ, & Sachdev DP (1991) Radiation-induced meningiomas: Experience at the Mount Sinai Hospital and review of the literature. J Neurosurg, **75**: 564–574.

Hass U, Lund SP, & Elsner J (1994) Effects of prenatal exposure to N-methylpyrrolidone on postnatal development and behavior in rats. Neurotoxicol Teratol, **16**: 241–249.

Hass U, Lund SP, Simonsen L, & Fries AS (1995) Effects of prenatal exposure to xylene on postnatal development and behavior in rats. Neurotoxicol Teratol, **17**: 341–349.

Hass U, Dalgaard M, Jarfelt K, & Kledal TSA (2004) OECD conceptual framework for testing and assessment of endocrine disrupters as a basis for regulation of substances with endocrine disrupting properties. Tema Nord, **555**: 1–100.

Hasselblad V, Eddy DM, & Kotchmar DJ (1992) Synthesis of environmental evidence: Nitrogen dioxide epidemiology studies. J Air Waste Manage Assoc, **42**: 662–671.

Hatch MC, Warburton D, & Santella RM (1990) Polycyclic aromatic hydrocarbon–DNA adducts in spontaneously aborted fetal tissue. Carcinogenesis, **11**(9): 1673–1675.

Hattis D, Ginsberg G, Sonawane B, Smolenski S, Russ A, Kozlak M, & Goble R (2003) Differences in pharmacokinetics between children and adults — II. Children's variability in drug elimination half-lives and in some parameters needed for physiologically-based pharmacokinetic modeling. Risk Anal, **23**: 117–142.

Health Canada (2003) Canadian Arctic contaminants assessment report — Phase II. Ottawa, Ontario, Minister of Indian Affairs and Northern Development.

Heinrich J (2003) Nonallergic respiratory morbidity improved along with a decline of traditional air pollution levels: A review. Eur Respir J, **21**(Suppl 40): 64–69.

Hellerstrom C & Swenne I (1991) Functional maturation and proliferation of fetal pancreatic beta-cells. Diabetes, **40**(Suppl 2): 89–93.

Hellstrom M, Kalen M, Lindahl P, Abramsson A, & Betsholtz C (1999) Role of PDGF-B and PDGFR-beta in recruitment of vascular smooth muscle cells and pericytes during embryonic blood vessel formation in the mouse. Development, **126**(14): 3047–3055.

Henderson BE, Benton B, Cosgrove M, Baptista J, Aldrich J, Townsend D, Hart W, & Mack TM (1976) Urogenital tract abnormalities in sons of women treated with diethylstilbestrol. Pediatrics, **58**: 505–507.

Henriksen GL, Ketchum NS, Michalek JE, & Swaby JA (1997) Serum dioxin and diabetes mellitus in veterans of Operation Ranch Hand. Epidemiology, **8**(3): 252–258.

Henriksen TB, Baird DD, Olsen J, Hedegaard M, Secher NJ, & Wilcox AJ (1999) Time to pregnancy and preterm delivery. Obstet Gynecol, **89**: 595–599.

Heo Y, Lee W, & Lawrence D (1997) In vivo the environmental pollutants lead and mercury induce oligoclonal T-cell responses skewed toward type-2 reactivities. Cell Immunol, **179**: 185–195.

Herbst AL (1999) Diethylstilbestrol and adenocarcinoma of the vagina. Am J Obstet Gynecol, **181**: 1576–1578.

Herbst AL, Ulfelder H, & Poskanzer DC (1971) Adenocarcinoma of the vagina. Association of maternal stilbestrol therapy with tumor appearance in young women. N Engl J Med, **284**: 879–881.

Herrera-Portugal C, Ochoa H, Franco-Sanchez G, Yáñez L, & Díaz-Barriga F (2005) Environmental pathways of exposure to DDT for children living in a malarious area of Chiapas, Mexico. Environ Res, **99**(2): 158–163.

Hesselmar B, Aberg N, Aberg B, Eriksson B, & Bjorksten B (1999) Does early exposure to cat or dog protect against later allergy development? Clin Exp Allergy, **29**(5): 611–617.

Hicks SP (1954) The effects of ionizing radiation, certain hormones, and radiomimetic drugs on the developing nervous system. J Cell Physiol, **43**(Suppl 1): 151–178.

Hirsch T, Weiland SK, Von Mutius E, Safeca AF, Grafe H, Csaplovics E, Duhme K, Keil U, & Leupold W (1999) Inner city air pollution and respiratory health and atopy in children. Eur Respir J, **14**: 669–677.

Hirshfield AN (1994) Relationship between the supply of primordial follicles and the onset of follicular growth in rats. Biol Reprod, **50**: 421–428.

Hoar RM & Monie IW (1981) Comparative development of specific organ systems. In: Kimmel CA & Buelke-Sam J eds. Developmental toxicology. New York, Raven Press, pp 13–33.

Hoei-Hansen CE, Holm M, Rajpert-De Meyts E, & Skakkebaek NE (2003) Histological evidence of testicular dysgenesis in contralateral biopsies from 218 patients with testicular germ cell cancer. J Pathol, **200**: 370–374.

Holladay SD & Blaylock BL (2002) The mouse as a model for developmental immunotoxicology. Hum Exp Toxicol, **21**(9–10): 525–531.

Holladay SD & Luster MI (1994) Developmental immunotoxicology. In: Kimmel CA & Buelke-Sam J eds. Developmental toxicology, 2nd ed. New York, Raven Press, pp 93–118.

Holladay SD & Smialowicz R (2000) Development of the murine and human immune system: Differential effects of immunotoxicants depend on time of exposure. Environ Health Perspect, **108**(Suppl 3): 463–473.

Holladay SD, Lindstrom P, Blaylock BL, Comment CE, Germolec DR, Heindell JJ, & Luster MI (1991) Perinatal thymocyte antigen expression and postnatal immune development altered by gestational exposure to 2,3,7,8-tetrachlorodibenzo-*p*-dioxin (TCDD). Teratology, **44**: 385–393.

Holman CDJ & Armstrong BK (1984) Cutaneous malignant melanoma and indicators of total accumulated exposure to the sun: An analysis separating histogenetic types. J Natl Cancer Inst, **73**: 75–82.

Holsapple M (2002) Developmental immunotoxicology and risk assessment: A workshop summary. Hum Exp Toxicol, **21**: 472–478.

Holsapple M, West L, & Landreth K (2003) Species comparison of anatomical and functional immune system development. Birth Defects Res B Dev Reprod Toxicol, **68**: 321–334.

Holson JF, Hogue CJR, Kimmel CA, & Carlo G (1981) Suitability of experimental studies for predicting hazards to human development: criteria for evaluation study designs. In: Proceedings, The Toxicology Forum, 1981 Annual Winter Meeting, 16–18 February 1981, Arlington, VA. Washington, DC, The Toxicology Forum, pp 354–390.

Holson JF, DeSesso JM, Jacobson CF, & Farr CH (2000) Appropriate use of animal models in the assessment of risk during prenatal development: An illustration using inorganic arsenic. Teratology, **62**: 51–71.

Hook JB & Baillie MD (1979) Perinatal renal pharmacology. Annu Rev Pharmacol Toxicol, **19**: 491–509.

Horak F, Studnicka M, Gartner C, Spengler JD, Tauber E, Urbanek R, Veiter A, & Frischer T (2002) Particulate matter and lung function growth in children: A 3 year follow-up study in Austrian schoolchildren. Eur Respir J, **19**: 838–845.

Howell S & Shalet S (1998) Gonadal damage from chemotherapy and radiotherapy. Endocrinol Metab Clin North Am, **27**: 927–943.

Hsu ST, Ma CI, Hsu SK, Wu SS, Hsu NH, Yeh CC, & Wu SB (1985) Discovery and epidemiology of PCB poisoning in Taiwan: A four-year followup. Environ Health Perspect, **59**: 5–10.

Huisman M, Koopman-Esseboom C, Fidler V, Hadders-Algra M, van der Paauw CG, Tuinstra LG, Weisglas-Kuperus N, Sauer PJ, Touwen BC, & Boersma ER (1995) Perinatal exposure to polychlorinated biphenyls and dioxins and its effect on neonatal neurological development. Early Hum Dev, **41**(2): 111–127.

Hutchinson LJ, Amler RW, Lybarger JA, & Chappell W (1992) Neurobehavioral test batteries for use in environmental health field studies. Atlanta, GA, United States Department of Health and Human Services, Public Health Service, Agency for Toxic Substances and Disease Registry.

Hwang SJ, Beaty TH, Panny SR, Street NA, Joseph JM, Gordon S, McIntosh I, & Francomano CA (1995) Association study of transforming growth factor alpha (TGF alpha) TaqI polymerase and oral clefts: Indication of gene–environment interaction in a population-based sample of infants with birth defects. Am J Epidemiol, **141**(7): 629–636.

Hwang YH, Bornschein RL, Grote J, Menrath W, & Roda S (1997) Environmental arsenic exposure of children around a former copper smelter site. Environ Res, **72**: 72–81.

Hytten FE (1984) Physiological changes in the mother related to drug handling. In: Krauer B, Krauer F, Hytten FE, & del Pozo E eds. Drugs and pregnancy: Maternal drug handling: Fetal drug exposure. New York, Academic Press, pp 7–17.

IARC (1992) Solar and ultraviolet radiation. Lyon, International Agency for Research on Cancer (IARC Monographs on the Evaluation of Carcinogenic Risks to Humans, Vol. 55).

IARC (1997) Epstein-Barr virus and Kaposi's sarcoma herpesvirus/human herpesvirus 8. Lyon, International Agency for Research on Cancer (IARC Monographs on the Evaluation of Carcinogenic Risks to Humans, Vol. 70).

IARC (2000) Ionizing radiation, Part 1: X- and gamma (γ)-radiation, and neutrons. Lyon, International Agency for Research on Cancer (IARC Monographs on the Evaluation of Carcinogenic Risks to Humans, Vol. 75).

IARC (2001) Ionizing radiation, Part 2: Some internally deposited radionuclides. Lyon, International Agency for Research on Cancer (IARC Monographs on the Evaluation of Carcinogenic Risks to Humans, Vol. 78).

IARC (2002) Some traditional herbal medicines, some mycotoxins, naphthalene and styrene. Lyon, International Agency for Research on Cancer, pp 171–274 (IARC Monographs on the Evaluation of Carcinogenic Risks to Humans, Vol. 82).

IARC (2004) Some drinking-water disinfectants and contaminants, including arsenic. Lyon, International Agency for Research on Cancer (IARC Monographs on the Evaluation of Carcinogenic Risks to Humans, Vol. 84).

Ibanez L, Dimartino-Nardi J, Potau N, & Saenger P (2000) Premature adrenarche — normal variant or forerunner of adult disease? Endocr Rev, **21**: 671–696.

ICRP (1975) Report of the ICRP [International Commission on Radiological Protection] Task Group on Reference Man. Oxford, Pergamon Press.

IEH (1995) Indoor air quality in the home. Assessment A2. Leicester, Institute for Environment and Health.

Iliff A & Lee VA (1952) Pulse rate, respiratory rate, and body temperature of children between two months and eighteen years of age. Child Dev, **23**(4): 237–245.

ILSI (2003) Final report: Workshop to develop a framework for assessing risks to children from exposure to environmental agents. Washington, DC, International Life Sciences Institute, Risk Science Institute.

Infante-Rivard C, Gauvrin D, Malo JL, & Suissa S (1999) Maternal smoking and childhood asthma. Am J Epidemiol, **150**: 528–531.

References

IPCS (1983) Guidelines on studies in environmental epidemiology. Geneva, World Health Organization, International Programme on Chemical Safety (Environmental Health Criteria 27).

IPCS (1984) Principles for evaluating health risks to progeny associated with exposure to chemicals during pregnancy. Geneva, World Health Organization, International Programme on Chemical Safety (Environmental Health Criteria 30).

IPCS (1986a) Principles and methods for the assessment of neurotoxicity associated with exposure to chemicals. Geneva, World Health Organization, International Programme on Chemical Safety (Environmental Health Criteria 141).

IPCS (1986b) Principles for evaluating health risks from chemicals during infancy and early childhood: The need for a special approach. Geneva, World Health Organization, International Programme on Chemical Safety (Environmental Health Criteria 59).

IPCS (1993) Biomarkers and risk assessment: concepts and principles. Geneva, World Health Organization, International Programme on Chemical Safety (Environmental Health Criteria 155).

IPCS (1994) Assessing human health risks of chemicals: Derivation of guidance values for health-based exposure limits. Geneva, World Health Organization, International Programme on Chemical Safety (Environmental Health Criteria 170).

IPCS (1999a) Principles for the assessment of risks to human health from exposure to chemicals. Geneva, World Health Organization, International Programme on Chemical Safety (Environmental Health Criteria 210).

IPCS (1999b) Principles and methods for assessing allergic hypersensitization associated with exposure to chemicals. Geneva, World Health Organization, International Programme on Chemical Safety (Environmental Health Criteria 212).

IPCS (2000) Human exposure assessment. Geneva, World Health Organization, International Programme on Chemical Safety (Environmental Health Criteria 214).

IPCS (2001a) Biomarkers in risk assessment: Validity and validation. Geneva, World Health Organization, International Programme on Chemical Safety (Environmental Health Criteria 222).

IPCS (2001b) Neurotoxicity risk assessment for human health: Principles and approaches. Geneva, World Health Organization, International Programme on Chemical Safety (Environmental Health Criteria 223).

IPCS (2001c) Arsenic and arsenic compounds. Geneva, World Health Organization, International Programme on Chemical Safety (Environmental Health Criteria 224).

IPCS (2001d) Principles for evaluating health risks to reproduction associated with exposure to chemicals. Geneva, World Health Organization, International Programme on Chemical Safety (Environmental Health Criteria 225).

IPCS (2002) Global assessment of the state-of-the-science of endocrine disruptors. Geneva, World Health Organization, International Programme on Chemical Safety.

IPCS (2004a) IPCS risk assessment terminology. Part 1: IPCS/OECD key generic terms used in chemical hazard/risk assessment; Part 2: IPCS glossary of key exposure assessment terminology. Geneva, World Health Organization, International Programme on Chemical Safety (Harmonization Project Document No. 1).

IPCS (2004b) Principles for modelling dose–response for the risk assessment of chemicals (draft). Geneva, World Health Organization, International Programme on Chemical Safety (Environmental Health Criteria; available at http://www.who.int/ipcs/methods/harmonization/dose_response/en/).

IPCS (2005) Chemical-specific adjustment factors for interspecies differences and human variability: Guidance document for use of data in dose/concentration–response assessment. Geneva, World Health Organization, International Programme on Chemical Safety (Harmonization Project Document No. 2).

Jaakkola JJ, Paunio M, Virtanen M, & Heinonen OP (1991) Low-level air pollution and upper respiratory infections in children. Am J Public Health, **81**(8): 1060–1063.

Jacobson JL & Jacobson SW (2002a) Association of prenatal exposure to an environmental contaminant with intellectual function in childhood. J Toxicol Clin Toxicol, **40**(4): 467–475.

Jacobson JL & Jacobson SW (2002b) Effects of prenatal alcohol exposure on child development. Alcohol Res Health, **26**(4): 282–286.

Jacobson JL & Jacobson SW (2003) Prenatal exposure to polychlorinated biphenyls and attention at school age. J Pediatr, **143**: 780–788.

Jahnke GD, Choksi NY, Moore JA, & Shelby MD (2004) Thyroid toxicants: Assessing reproductive health effects. Environ Health Perspect, **112**(3): 363–368.

Jarabek AM (1995) Consideration of temporal toxicity challenges current default assumptions. Inhal Toxicol, **7**: 927–946.

Jarrell J (2002) Rationale for the study of the human sex ratio in population studies of polluted environments. Cad Saude Publica, **18**(2): 429–434.

Jarvis D, Chinn S, Sterne J, Luczynska C, & Burney P (1998) The association of respiratory symptoms and lung function with the use of gas cooking. Eur Respir J, **11**: 651–658.

Javaid MK & Cooper C (2002) Prenatal and childhood influences on osteoporosis. Best Pract Res Clin Endocrinol Metab, **16**: 349–367.

Jedrychowski W, Bendkowska I, Flak E, Penar A, Jacek R, Kaim I, Spengler JD, Camann D, & Perera FP (2004) Estimated risk for altered fetal growth resulting from exposure to fine particles during pregnancy: An epidemiologic prospective cohort study in Poland. Environ Health Perspect, **112**(14): 1398–1402.

Jenkins HS, Devalia JL, Mister RL, Bevan AM, Rusznak C, & Davies RJ (1999) The effect of exposure to ozone and nitrogen dioxide on the airway response of atopic asthmatics to inhaled allergen: dose- and time-dependent effects. Am J Respir Crit Care Med, **160**(1): 33–39.

References

Jensen TK, Henriksen TB, Hjollund NH, Scheike T, Kolstad H, Giwercman A, Ernst E, Bonde JP, Skakkebaek NE, & Olsen J (1998) Adult and prenatal exposures to tobacco smoke as risk indicators of fertility among 430 Danish couples. Am J Epidemiol, **148**: 992–997.

Jensen TK, Joffe M, Scheike T, Skytthe A, Gaist D, & Christensen K (2005) Time trends in waiting time to pregnancy among Danish twins. Hum Reprod, **20**(4): 955–964.

Jick H & Porter J (1977) Relation between smoking and age of natural menopause. Report from the Boston Collaborative Drug Surveillance Program, Boston University Medical Center. Lancet, **1**: 1354–1355.

JMPR (2004) Guidance on the establishment of acute reference doses. In: Pesticide residues in food — 2004. Report of the Joint WHO/FAO Meeting on Pesticide Residues 2004. Rome, Food and Agriculture Organization of the United Nations (FAO Plant Production and Protection Paper 178).

Joad JP, JI C, Kott KS, Bric JM, & Pinkerton KE (1995) In utero and postnatal effects of sidestream cigarette smoke exposure on lung function, hyperresponsiveness, and neuroendocrine cells in rats. Toxicol Appl Pharmacol, **132**(1): 63–71.

Joad JP, Bric JM, Peake JL, & Pinkerton KE (1999) Perinatal exposure to aged and diluted sidestream cigarette smoke produces airway hyperresponsiveness in older rats. Toxicol Appl Pharmacol, **155**(3): 253–260.

Joffe M & Li Z (1994) Association of time to pregnancy and the outcome of pregnancy. Fertil Steril, **62**(1): 71–75.

Jones KL (1988) Smith's recognizable patterns of human malformations, 4th ed. Philadelphia, PA, W.B. Saunders Company, pp 1–9.

Jones KL & Smith DW (1973) Recognition of the fetal alcohol syndrome in early infancy. Lancet, **2**: 999–1001.

Juchau MR (1981) Enzymatic bioactivation and inactivation of chemical teratogens and transplacental carcinogens/mutagens. In: Juchau MR ed. The biochemical basis of chemical teratogenesis. New York, Elsevier/North Holland, pp 63–94.

Juchau MR & Faustman-Watts EM (1983) Pharmacokinetic considerations in the maternal-placenta unit. Clin Obstet Gynecol, **26**: 379–390.

Kacew S (1992) General principles in pharmacology and toxicology applicable to children. In: Guzelian PS, Henry CJ, & Olin SS eds. Similarities and differences between children and adults: Implication for risk assessment. Washington, DC, ILSI Press.

Källén B (2006) Human studies — Epidemiologic techniques in developmental and reproductive toxicology. In: Hood RD ed. Developmental and reproductive toxicology, a practical approach. Boca Raton, FL, CRC Press, pp 799–840.

Karmaus W, Huang S, & Cameron L (2002) Parental concentration of dichlorodiphenyl dichloroethane and polychlorinated biphenyls in Michigan fish eaters and sex ratio in offspring. J Occup Med, **44**: 8–13.

Karpuzoglu-Sahin E, Hissong B, & Ahmed S (2001) Interferon-gamma levels are upregulated by 17-beta-estradiol and diethylstilbestrol. J Reprod Immunol, **52**: 113–127.

Karube T, Odagiri Y, Takemoto K, & Watanabe S (1989) Analyses of transplacentally induced sister chromatid exchanges and micronuclei in mouse fetal liver cells following maternal exposure to cigarette smoke. Cancer Res, **49**(13): 3550–3552.

Kaufman MH & Navaratnam V (1981) Early differentiation of the heart in mouse embryos. J Anat, **133**: 235–246.

Kavlock R, Boekelheide K, Chapin R, Cunningham M, Faustman E, Foster P, Golub M, Henderson R, Hinberg I, Little R, Seed J, Shea K, Tabacova S, Tyl R, Williams P, & Zacharewski T (2002a) NTP Center for the Evaluation of Risks to Human Reproduction: Phthalates expert panel report on the reproductive and developmental toxicity of di-*n*-octyl phthalate. Reprod Toxicol, **16**(5): 721–734.

Kavlock R, Boekelheide K, Chapin R, Cunningham M, Faustman E, Foster P, Golub M, Henderson R, Hinberg I, Little R, Seed J, Shea K, Tabacova S, Tyl R, Williams P, & Zacharewski T (2002b) NTP Center for the Evaluation of Risks to Human Reproduction: Phthalates expert panel report on the reproductive and developmental toxicity of di-isodecyl phthalate. Reprod Toxicol, **16**(5): 655–678.

Kavlock R, Boekelheide K, Chapin R, Cunningham M, Faustman E, Foster P, Golub M, Henderson R, Hinberg I, Little R, Seed J, Shea K, Tabacova S, Tyl R, Williams P, & Zacharewski T (2002c) NTP Center for the Evaluation of Risks to Human Reproduction: Phthalates expert panel report on the reproductive and developmental toxicity of di(2-ethylhexyl) phthalate. Reprod Toxicol, **16**(5): 529–653.

Kavlock R, Boekelheide K, Chapin R, Cunningham M, Faustman E, Foster P, Golub M, Henderson R, Hinberg I, Little R, Seed J, Shea K, Tabacova S, Tyl R, Williams P, & Zacharewski T (2002d) NTP Center for the Evaluation of Risks to Human Reproduction: Phthalates expert panel report on the reproductive and developmental toxicity of di-*n*-butyl phthalate. Reprod Toxicol, **16**(5): 489–527.

Kavlock R, Boekelheide K, Chapin R, Cunningham M, Faustman E, Foster P, Golub M, Henderson R, Hinberg I, Little R, Seed J, Shea K, Tabacova S, Tyl R, Williams P, & Zacharewski T (2002e) NTP Center for the Evaluation of Risks to Human Reproduction: Phthalates expert panel report on the reproductive and developmental toxicity of butyl benzyl phthalate. Reprod Toxicol, **16**(5): 453–487.

Kavlock RJ & Gray JA (1982) Evaluation of renal function in neonatal rats. Biol Neonate, **41**(5–6): 279–288.

Kearns GL, Abdel-Rahman SM, Alander SW, Blowey DL, Leeder JS, & Kauffman RE (2003) Developmental pharmacology — drug disposition, action, and therapy in infants and children. N Engl J Med, **349**: 1157–1167.

Keen R, Egger P, Fall C, Major P, Lanchbury J, Spector TD, & Cooper C (1997) Polymorphisms of the vitamin D receptor, infant growth, and adult bone mass. Calcif Tissue Int, **60**: 233–235.

References

Kelly SJ, Goodlett CR, Hulsether SA, & West JR (1988) Impaired spatial navigation in adult female but not adult male rats exposed to alcohol during the brain growth spurt. Behav Brain Res, **27**: 247–257.

Kelsh MA, Buffler PA, Daaboul JJ, Rutherford GW, Lau EC, Barnard JC, Exuzides AK, Madl AK, Palmer LG, & Lorey FW (2003) Primary congenital hypothyroidism, newborn thyroid function, and environmental perchlorate exposure among residents of a Southern California community. J Occup Environ Med, **45**: 1116–1127.

Khoury MJ & Flanders D (1996) Nontraditional epidemiologic approaches in the analysis of gene–environment interaction: case–control studies with no controls. Am J Epidemiol, **144**: 207–213.

Kimmel CA, Holson JF, Hogue CJ, & Carlo GL (1984) Reliability of experimental studies for predicting hazards to human development. Jefferson, AR, National Center for Toxicological Research (NCTR Technical Report for Experiment 6015).

Kimmel CA, Kimmel GL, & Euling SY (2006) Developmental and reproductive toxicity risk assessment for environmental agents. In: Hood RD ed. Developmental and reproductive toxicology, a practical approach. Boca Raton, FL, CRC Press.

Kimmel GL (1995) Exposure-duration relationships: The risk assessment process for health effects other than cancer. Inhal Toxicol, **7**: 873–880.

Kimmel GL, Williams PL, Claggett TW, & Kimmel CA (2002) Response-surface analysis of exposure-duration relationships: The effects of hyperthermia on embryonic development of the rat in vitro. Toxicol Sci, **69**: 391–399.

Kirby ML (1997) The heart. In: Thorogood P ed. Embryos, genes and birth defects. London, John Wiley and Sons, pp. 231–250.

Kirby RS (1993) The coding of underlying cause of death from fetal death certificates: Issues and policy considerations. Am J Public Health, **83**: 1088–1094.

Kjellstrom T, Kennedy P, Wallis S, & Mantell C (1986) Physical and mental development of children with prenatal exposure to mercury from fish. Stage 1. Preliminary tests at age 4. Solna, National Swedish Environmental Board (Report No. 3080).

Kjellstrom T, Kennedy P, Wallis S, Stewart A, Friberg L, Lind B, Wutherspoon P, & Mantell C (1989) Physical and mental development of children with prenatal exposure to mercury from fish. Stage 2. Interviews and psychological tests at age 6. Solna, National Swedish Environmental Board (Report No. 3642).

Klaassen CD ed. (1996) Casarett and Doull's toxicology: The basic science of poisons, 5th ed. New York, McGraw-Hill Companies.

Kleinschmidt D & Lillehei KO (1995) Radiation-induced meningioma with a 63 year latency period. Case report. J Neurosurg, **82**: 487–488.

Kodama K, Preston DI, Pierce DA, Shimizu Y, Suyama A, & Tahara E (2003) Radiation effects on cancer mortality among atomic bomb survivors. Proc Am Assoc Cancer Res, **44**: 1278 (Abstract No. 6394).

Koplan JP, Liverman CT, & Kraak VA eds (2005) Preventing childhood obesity: Health in the balance. Washington, DC, National Academies Press.

Koren G (2001) Maternal–fetal toxicology: A clinician's guide, 3rd ed. New York, Marcel Dekker.

Korenbrot CC, Huhtaniemi IT, & Weiner RI (1977) Preputial separation as an external sign of pubertal development in the male rat. Biol Reprod, **17**: 298–303.

Kovar J, Sly PD, & Willet KE (2002) Postnatal alveolar development of the rabbit. J Appl Physiol, **93**: 629–635.

Koyun M, Akman S, & Guven AG (2004) Mercury intoxication resulting from school barometers in three unrelated adolescents. Eur J Pediatr, **163**(3): 131–134.

Kramer MS (2003) The epidemiology of adverse pregnancy outcomes: An overview. J Nutr, **133**(5 Suppl 2): 1592S–1596S.

Krasnegor NA, Otto DA, Bernstein JH, Burke R, Chappell W, Eckerman DA, Needleman HL, Oakley G, Rogan W, & Terracciano G (1992) Pediatric neurobehavioral testing for environmental health studies. In: Hutchinson LJ, Amler RW, Lybarger JA, & Chappell W eds. Neurobehavioral test batteries for use in environmental health field studies. Atlanta, GA, United States Department of Health and Human Services, Agency for Toxic Substances and Disease Registry.

Krauer B (1987) Physiological changes and drug disposition during pregnancy. In: Nau H & Scott WJ eds. Pharmacokinetics in teratogenesis. Vol. 1. Boca Raton, FL, CRC Press, pp 3–12.

Krovetz LJ, Grumbar PA, Hardin S, Morgan AV, & Schiebler GL (1969) Complications following use of four angiocardiographic contrast media in infants and children. Invest Radiol, **4**(1): 13–18.

Krzyzanowski M, Quackenboss JJ, & Lebowitz MD (1990) Chronic respiratory effects of indoor formaldehyde exposure. Environ Res, **52**(2): 117–125.

Kumar VH, Lakshinrushimha S, Abiad MT, Chess PR, & Ryan RM (2005) Growth factors in lung development. Adv Clin Chem, **40**: 261–316.

Kunzli N, Lurmann F, Segal M, Ngo L, Balmes J, & Tager IB (1997) Association between lifetime ambient ozone exposure and pulmonary function in college freshmen — results of a pilot study. Environ Res, **72**: 8–23.

Kuratsune M, Yoshimura T, Matsuzaka J, & Yamaguchi A (1971) Yusho, a poisoning caused by rice oil contaminated with polychlorinated biphenyls. HSMHA Health Rep, **86**(12): 1083–1091.

Lamm SH & Doemland M (1999) Has perchlorate in drinking water increased the rate of congenital hypothyroidism? J Occup Environ Med, **41**: 409–411.

Lammer EJ, Brown LE, Anderha MT, & Guyer B (1989) Classification and analysis of fetal deaths in Massachusetts. J Am Med Assoc, **261**: 1757–1762.

Landreth K (2002) Critical windows in development of the rodent immune system. Hum Exp Toxicol, **21**: 493–498.

Landrigan PJ, Kimmel CA, Correa A, & Eskenazi B (2004) Children's health and the environment: Public health issues and challenges for risk assessment. Environ Health Perspect, **112**(2): 257–265.

Langston C (1983) Normal and abnormal structural development of the human lung. In: Kavlock RJ & Grabowski CT eds. Abnormal functional development of the heart, lungs, and kidneys: Approaches to functional teratology. New York, A.R. Liss, pp 75–91.

Lanphear BP, Hornung R, Khoury J, Yolton K, Baghurst P, Bellinger DC, Canfield RL, Dietrich KN, Bornschein R, Greene T, Rothenberg SJ, Needleman HL, Schnaas L, Wasserman G, Graziano J, & Roberts R (2005) Low-level environmental lead exposure and children's intellectual function: An international pooled analysis. Environ Health Perspect, **113**(7): 894–899.

Lau C & Kavlock RJ (1994) Functional toxicity in the developing heart, lung, and kidney. In: Kimmel CA & Buelke-Sam J eds. Developmental toxicology, 2nd ed. New York, Raven Press, pp 119–188.

Lau C & Rogers JM (2005) Embryonic and fetal programming of physiological disorders in adulthood. Birth Defects Res C Embryo Today, **72**: 300–312.

Lau S, Illi S, Sommerfeld C, Niggemann B, Bergmann R, von Mutius E, & Wahn U (2000) Early exposure to house-dust mite and cat allergens and development of childhood asthma: A cohort study. Multicentre Allergy Study Group. Lancet, **356**(9239): 1392–1397.

Lawrence RA (1989) Breast-feeding and medical disease. Med Clin North Am, **73**: 583–603.

Laws SC, Ferrell JM, Stoker TE, Schmid J, & Cooper RL (2000) The effects of atrazine on female Wistar rats: An evaluation of the protocol for assessing pubertal development and thyroid function. Toxicol Sci, **58**: 366–376.

Lee J-E, Chen S, Golemboski K, Parson P, & Dietert R (2001) Developmental windows of differential lead-induced immunotoxicity in chickens. Toxicology, **156**: 161–170.

Lee J-E, Naqi S, Kao E, & Dietert R (2002) Embryonic exposure to lead: Comparison of immune and cellular responses in unchallenged and virally stressed chickens. Arch Toxicol, **75**: 717–724.

Lee KT, Mattson SN, & Riley EP (2004) Classifying children with heavy prenatal alcohol exposure using measures of attention. J Int Neuropsychol Soc, **10**(2): 271–277.

Leech JA, Wilby K, & McMullen E (1999) Environmental tobacco smoke exposure patterns: A subanalysis of the Canadian Human Time–Activity Pattern Survey. Can J Public Health, **90**: 244–249.

Lehmann I, Thoelke A, Rehwagen M, Rolle-Kampczyk U, Schlink U, Schulz R, Borte M, Diez U, & Herbarth O (2002) The influence of maternal exposure to volatile organic compounds on the cytokine secretion profile of neonatal T cells. Environ Toxicol, **17**(3): 203–210.

Lehmann KP, Phillips S, Sar M, Foster PM, & Gaido KW (2004) Dose-dependent alterations in gene expression and testosterone synthesis in the fetal testes of male rats exposed to di (*n*-butyl) phthalate. Toxicol Sci, **81**: 60–68.

Leviton A, Kirby C, Guild-Wilson M, & Neff RK (1993) The Boston Teacher Questionnaire. 2. Assessments of validity. J Child Neurol, **8**: 54–63.

Levy G, Khanna NN, Soda DM, Tsuzuki O, & Stern L (1975) Pharmacokinetics of acetaminophen in the human neonate: Formation of acetaminophen glucuronide and sulphate in relation to plasma bilirubin concentration and d-glucaric acid excretion. Pediatrics, **55**: 818–825.

LifeLine Group (2005) Aggregate and Cumulative Exposure and Risk Assessment Software, Version 4.3. Annandale, VA, The LifeLine Group, Inc. (http://www.thelifelinegroup.org/index.htm#software; accessed 5 May 2005).

Lindbjerg IF (1966) Leg muscle blood-flow measured with 133-xenon after ischaemia periods and after muscular exercise performed during ischaemia. Clin Sci, **30**(3): 399–408.

Lindbohm M-L, Taskinen H, Sallmén M, & Hemminki K (1990) Spontaneous abortions among women exposed to organic solvent. Am J Ind Med, **17**: 449–463.

Lipscomb JA, Fenster L, Wrensch M, Shusterman D, & Swan S (1991) Pregnancy outcomes in women potentially exposed to occupational solvents and women working in the electronics industry. J Occup Med, **33**(5): 597–604.

Lochry EA, Hoberman AM, & Christian MS (1985) Detection of prenatal effects on learning as a function of differential criteria. Neurobehav Toxicol Teratol, **7**(6): 697–701.

Longnecker MP, Wolff MS, Gladen BC, Brock JW, Grandjean P, Jacobson JL, Korrick SA, Rogan WJ, Weisglas-Kuperus N, Hertz-Picciotto I, Ayotte P, Stewart P, Winneke G, Charles MJ, Jacobson SW, Dewailly E, Boersma ER, Altshul LM, Heinzow B, Pagano JJ, & Jensen AA (2003) Comparison of polychlorinated biphenyl levels across studies of human neurodevelopment. Environ Health Perspect, **111**(1): 65–70.

Longnecker MP, Klebanoff MA, Dunson DB, Guo X, Chen Z, Zhou H, & Brock JN (2005) Maternal serum levels of DDT metabolite DDE in relation to fetal loss in previous pregnancy. Environ Res, **97**(2): 127–133.

López-Carrillo L, Torres-Sanchez L, Garrido F, Papaqui-Hernandez J, Palazuelos-Rendon E, & Lopez-Cervantes M (1996) Prevalence and determinants of lead intoxication in Mexican children of low socioeconomic status. Environ Health Perspect, **104**(11): 1208–1211.

Lottrup G, Andersson AM, Leffers H, Mortensen GK, Toppari J, Skakkebaek NE, & Main KM (2006) Possible impact of phthalates on infant reproductive health. Int J Androl, **29**(1): 172–180.

Lowrey GH (1973) Growth and development of children, 6th ed. Chicago, IL, Yearbook Medical Publishers.

Luebke R, Chen D, Dietert R, Yang Y, King M, & Luster M (2004) Increased sensitivity of the developing immune system to xenobiotics: evidence supporting the concept of developmental immunotoxicity testing guidelines. Report to the United States Environmental Protection Agency, Washington, DC.

Luebke RW, Chen DH, Dietert R, Yang Y, King M, & Luster MI (2006) The comparative immunotoxicity of five selected compounds following developmental or adult exposure. J Toxicol Environ Health B Crit Rev, **9**: 1–26.

Luster M, Dean J, & Germolec D (2003) Consensus workshop on methods to evaluate developmental immunotoxicity. Environ Health Perspect, **111**(4): 575–583.

Lynberg MC & Edmonds LD (1996) State use of birth defects surveillance. In: LS Wilcox & JS Marks eds. From data to action: CDC's public health surveillance for women, infants, and children. Atlanta, GA, United States Department of Health and Human Services, Centers for Disease Control and Prevention, pp 217–230.

Lynberg MC & Khoury MJ (1990) Contribution of birth defects to infant mortality among racial/ethnic minority groups, United States, 1983. MMWR CDC Surveill Summ, **39**: 1–12.

Mahaffey KR (1995) Nutrition and lead: strategies for public health. Environ Health Perspect, **103**(Suppl 6): 191–196.

Maltoni C, Lefemine G, Ciliberti A, Cotti G, & Carretti D (1981) Carcinogenicity bioassays of vinyl chloride monomer: A model of risk assessment on an experimental basis. Environ Health Perspect, **41**: 3–29.

Manchester DK, Weston A, Choi JS, Trivers GE, Fennessey PV, Quintana E, Farmer PB, Mann DL, & Harris CC (1988) Detection of benzo[a]pyrene diol epoxide–DNA adducts in human placenta. Proc Natl Acad Sci U S A, **85**(23): 9243–9247.

Marcoux R (1994) [Activity and work of children in urban Mali.] Pop Sahel, **21**: 39–43 (in French).

Markwald R, Trusk T, Gittenberger-De Groot A, & Poelmann R (1997) Cardiac morphogenesis: Formation and septation of the primary heart tube. In: Kavlock RJ & Daston GP eds. Drug toxicity in embryonic development. I. Advances in understanding mechanisms of birth defects: Morphogenesis and processes at risk. Berlin, Springer-Verlag, pp 11–40.

Marshall EG, Gensburg LJ, Deres DA, Geary NS, & Cayo MR (1997) Maternal residential exposure to hazardous wastes and risk of central nervous system and musculoskeletal birth defects. Arch Environ Health, **52**: 416–425.

Marshall WA & Tanner JM (1969) Variations in pattern of pubertal changes in girls. Arch Dis Child, **45**: 13–23.

Martinez FD, Cline M, & Burrows B (1992) Increased incidence of asthma in children of smoking mothers. Pediatrics, **89**: 21–26.

Martinez-Frias ML, Bermejo E, & Frias JL (2000) Pathogenetic classification of a series of 27,145 consecutive infants with congenital defects. Am J Med Genet, **90**: 246–249.

Marty MS, Chapin R, Parks L, & Thorsrud BA (2003) Development and maturation of the male reproductive system. Birth Defects Res B Dev Reprod Toxicol, **68**: 125–136.

Massaro G & Massaro D (1986) Development of bronchiolar epithelium in rats. Am J Physiol, **250**(5 Pt 2): R783–R788.

Massaro G, Davis L, & Massaro D (1984) Postnatal development of the bronchiolar Clara cells in rats. Am J Physiol, **247**: C197–C203.

Matikainen T, Perez GI, Jurisicova A, Pru JK, Schlezinger JJ, Ryu HY, Laine J, Sakai T, Korsmeyer SJ, Casper RF, Sherr DH, & Tilly JL (2001) Aromatic hydrocarbon receptor-driven Bax gene expression is required for premature ovarian failure caused by biohazardous environmental chemicals. Nat Genet, **28**: 355–360.

Matikainen TM, Moriyama T, Morita Y, Perez GI, Korsmeyer SJ, Sherr DH, & Tilly JL (2002) Ligand activation of the aromatic hydrocarbon receptor transcription factor drives Bax-dependent apoptosis in developing fetal ovarian germ cells. Endocrinology, **143**: 615–620.

Matt N, Ghyselinck NB, Wendling O, Chambon P, & Mark M (2003) Retinoic acid–induced developmental defects are mediated by RARb/RXR heterodimers in the pharyngeal endoderm. Development, **130**: 2083–2093.

Mattison DR & Thorgeirsson SS (1979) Ovarian aryl hydrocarbon hydroxylase activity and primordial oocyte toxicity of polycyclic aromatic hydrocarbons in mice. Cancer Res, **39**: 3471–3475.

Mattison DR, Blann E, & Malek A (1991) Physiological alterations during pregnancy: impact on toxicokinetics. Fundam Appl Toxicol, **16**: 215–218.

Mattson SN, Schoenfeld AM, & Riley EP (2001) Teratogenic effects of alcohol on brain and behavior. Alcohol Res Health, **25**(3): 185–191.

Maxwell SM, Apeagyei F, de Vries HR, Mwanmut DD, & Hendrickse RG (1989) Aflatoxins in breast milk, neonatal cord blood and sera of pregnant women. J Toxicol, **8**(1,2): 19–29.

Mayani A, Barel S, Soback S, & Almagor M (1997) Dioxin concentrations in women with endometriosis. Hum Reprod, **12**: 373–375.

McGee R, Reeder A, Williams S, Bandaranayake M, & Tan AH (2002) Observations of summer sun protection among children in New Zealand: 1998–2000. N Z Med J, **115**: 103–106.

McMartin KI, Chu M, Kopecky E, Einarson TR, & Koren G (1998) Pregnancy outcome following maternal organic solvent exposure: A meta-analysis of epidemiologic studies. Am J Ind Med, **34**: 288–292.

Meek ME, Renwick A, Ohanian E, Dourson M, Lake B, Naumann BD, & Vu V (2002) Guidelines for application of chemical-specific adjustment factors in dose/concentration response assessment. Toxicology, **181–182**: 115–120.

Meistrich ML, Wilson G, Brown BW, da Cunha MF, & Lipshultz LI (1992) Impact of cyclophosphamide on long-term reduction in sperm count in men treated with combination chemotherapy for Ewing and soft tissue sarcomas. Cancer, **70**: 2703–2712.

Melnick S, Cole P, Anderson D, & Herbst AI (1987) Rates and risks of diethylstilbestrol-related clear-cell adenocarcinoma of the vagina and cervix. An update. N Engl J Med, **316**: 514–516.

Mendola P, Robinson LK, Buck Louis GM, Druschel CM, Fitzgerald EF, Sever LE, & Vena JE (2005) Birth defects risk associated with maternal fish consumption: Potential effect modification by sex of offspring. Environ Res, **97**: 133–140.

Merchant H (1975) Rat gonadal and ovarian organogenesis with and without germ cells. An ultrastructural study. Dev Biol, **44**: 1–21.

Merchant JA, Naleway AL, Svendsen ER, Kelly KM, Burmeister LF, Stromquist AM, Taylor CD, Thorne PS, Reynolds SJ, Sanderson WT, & Chrischilles EA (2005) Asthma and farm exposures in a cohort of rural Iowa children. Environ Health Perspect, **113**(3): 350–356.

Mesrogli M & Dieterle S (1993) Embryonic losses after in vitro fertilization and embryo transfer. Acta Obstet Gynecol Scand, **72**(1): 36–38.

Meyer A, Seidler FJ, & Slotkin TA (2004) Developmental effects of chlorpyrifos extend beyond neurotoxicity: Critical periods for immediate and delayed onset effects on cardiac and hepatic cell signaling. Environ Health Perspect, **112**(2): 170–178.

Michalek AM, Buck GM, Nasca PC, Freedman AN, Baptiste MS, & Mahoney MC (1996) Gravid health status and medication use and risk of neuroblastoma. Am J Epidemiol, **143**: 996–1001.

Michalek JE, Akhtar FZ, & Kiel JL (1999) Serum dioxin, insulin, fasting glucose, and sex hormone–binding globulin in veterans of Operation Ranch Hand. J Clin Endocrinol Metab, **84**: 1540–1543.

Migliaccio G, Migliaccio A, Petti S, Mavilio F, Russo G, Lazzaro D, Testa U, Marinucci M, & Peschle C (1986) Human embryonic hemopoiesis — kinetics of progenitors and precursors underlying the yolk sac–liver transition. J Clin Invest, **78**: 51–60.

Miller T, Golemboski K, Ha R, Bunn T, Sanders F, & Dietert R (1998) Developmental exposure to Pb causes persistent immunotoxicity in Fischer 344 rats. Toxicol Sci, **42**: 129–135.

Ministry of Public Health (1954) Mortality and morbidity during the London fog of December 1952. London, Her Majesty's Stationary Office (Reports on Public Health and Medical Subjects No. 95).

Mocarelli P, Gerthoux PM, Ferrari E, Patterson DG, Kieszak SM, Brambilla P, Vincoli N, Signorini S, Tramacere P, Carreri V, Sampson EJ, Turner WE, & Needham LL (2000) Paternal concentrations of dioxin and sex ratio of offspring. Lancet, **355**(9218): 1858–1863.

Montgomery SM & Ekbom A (2002) Smoking during pregnancy and diabetes mellitus in a British longitudinal birth cohort. Br Med J, **324**: 26–27.

Moore KL (1988) The developing human. Philadelphia, PA, W.B. Saunders Company.

Morford LL, Henck JW, Breslin WJ, & DeSesso JM (2004) Hazard identification and predictability of children's health risk from animal data. Environ Health Perspect, **112**(2): 266–271.

Morgan MK, Sheldon LS, Croghan CW, Jones PA, Robertson GL, Chuang JC, Wilson NK, & Lyu CW (2005) Exposures of preschool children to chlorpyrifos and its degradation product 3,5,6-trichloro-2-pyridinol in their everyday environments. J Expo Anal Environ Epidemiol, **15**: 297–309.

Morishima A, Grumbach MM, Simpson ER, Fisher C, & Qin K (1995) Aromatase deficiency in male and female siblings caused by a novel mutation and the physiological role of estrogens. J Clin Endocrinol Metab, **80**: 3689–3698.

Mowat DL, Wang F, Pickett W, & Brison RJ (1998) A case–control study of risk factors for playground injuries among children in Kingston and area. Inj Prev, **4**: 39–43.

Msall ME (1996) Functional assessment in neurodevelopmental disabilities. In: Capute AJ & Accardo PJ eds. Developmental disabilities in infancy and childhood, 2nd ed. Vol. 1. Neurodevelopmental diagnosis and treatment. Baltimore, MD, Paul H. Brooks Publishing, pp 371–392.

Msall ME, Rogers BT, Buck GM, Mallen S, Catanzaro NL, & Duffy LC (1993) Functional status of extremely premature infants at kindergarten entry. Dev Med Child Neurol, **35**: 312–320.

Murata K, Weihe P, Araki S, Budtz-Jorgensen E, & Grandjean P (1999) Evoked potentials in Faroese children prenatally exposed to methylmercury. Neurotoxicol Teratol, **21**(4): 471–472.

Murata K, Weihe P, Budtz-Jorgensen E, Jorgensen PJ, & Grandjean P (2004) Delayed brainstem auditory evoked potential latencies in 14-year-old children exposed to methylmercury. J Pediatr, **144**(2): 177–183.

Murgueytio AM, Evans RG, Sterling DA, Clardy SA, Shadel BN, & Clements BW (1998) Relationship between lead mining and blood lead levels in children. Arch Environ Health, **53**: 414–423.

Murtaugh LC & Melton DA (2003) Genes, signals, and lineages in pancreas development. Annu Rev Cell Dev Biol, **19**: 71–89.

Myers GJ, Marsh DO, Davidson PW, Cox C, Shamlaye CF, Tanner M, Choi A, Cernichiari E, Choisy O, & Clarkson TW (1995) Main neurodevelopmental study of Seychellois children following in utero exposure to methylmercury from a maternal fish diet: Outcome at six months. Neurotoxicology, **16**(4): 653–664.

Myers GJ, Davidson PW, Cox C, Shamlaye CF, Palumbo D, Cernichiari E, Sloane-Reeves J, Wilding GE, Kost J, Huang LS, & Clarkson TW (2003) Prenatal methylmercury exposure from ocean fish consumption in the Seychelles child development study. Lancet, 361(9370): 1686–1692.

Mylchreest E, Cattley RC, & Foster PM (1998) Male reproductive tract malformations in rats following gestational and lactational exposure to di(n-butyl) phthalate: an antiandrogenic mechanism? Toxicol Sci, 43: 47–60.

Mylchreest E, Sar M, Cattley RC, & Foster PM (1999) Disruption of androgen-regulated male reproductive development by di(n-butyl) phthalate during late gestation in rats is different from flutamide. Toxicol Appl Pharmacol, 156: 81–95.

Mylchreest E, Wallace DG, Cattley RC, & Foster PM (2000) Dose-dependent alterations in androgen-regulated male reproductive development in rats exposed to di(n-butyl) phthalate during late gestation. Toxicol Sci, 55: 143–151.

Mylchreest E, Sar M, Wallace DG, & Foster PM (2002) Fetal testosterone insufficiency and abnormal proliferation of Leydig cells and gonocytes in rats exposed to di(n-butyl) phthalate. Reprod Toxicol, 16: 19–28.

Nakatsuka H, Watanabe T, Ikeda M, Hisamichi S, Shimizu H, Fujisaku S, Ichinowatari Y, Konno J, Kuroda S, Ida Y, Suda S, & Kato K (1991) Comparison of the health effects between indoor and outdoor air pollution in north-eastern Japan. Environ Int, 17: 51–59.

Napalkov NP, Rice JM, Tomatis L, & Yamasaki H eds (1989) Perinatal and multigeneration carcinogenesis. Lyon, International Agency for Research on Cancer (IARC Scientific Publications No. 96).

NCHS (1997) Fertility, family planning, and women's health: New data from the 1995 National Survey of Family Growth. Hyattsville, MD, United States Department of Health and Human Services, Centers for Disease Control and Prevention, National Center for Health Statistics (Vital and Health Statistics Series 23, No. 19).

NCHS (1998) NHANES III household youth data file documentation. National Health and Nutrition Examination Survey III, 1988–1994. Hyattsville, MD, United States Department of Health and Human Services, Centers for Disease Control and Prevention, National Center for Health Statistics (CD-ROM Series 11).

NCHS (2003) 2000 CDC growth charts: United States. Hyattsville, MD, United States Department of Health and Human Services, Centers for Disease Control and Prevention, National Center for Health Statistics (http://www.cdc.gov/growthcharts).

Nebert DW (2005) Inter-individual susceptibility to environmental toxicants — A current assessment. Toxicol Appl Pharmacol, 207: S34–S42.

Needham LL, Özkaynak H, Whyatt RM, Barr DB, Wang RY, Naeher L, Akland G, Bahadori T, Bradman A, Fortmann R, Liu L-JS, Morandi M, O'Rourke MK, Thomas K, Quackenboss J, Ryan PB, & Zartarian V (2005) Exposure assessment in the national children's study: introduction. Environ Health Perspect, 113(8): 1076–1082.

Needleman HL (2004) Lead poisoning. Annu Rev Med, 55: 209–222.

Needleman HL, Gunnoe C, Leviton A, Reed R, Peresie H, Maher C, & Barrett P (1979) Deficits in psychologic and classroom performance of children with elevated dentine lead levels. N Engl J Med, **300**(13): 689–695.

Needleman HL, Riess JA, Tobin MJ, Biesecker GE, & Greenhouse JB (1996) Bone lead levels and delinquent behavior. JAMA, **275**(5): 363–369.

Nef S, Shipman T, & Parada LF (2000) A molecular basis for estrogen-induced cryptorchidism. Dev Biol, **224**: 354–361.

Neri M, Ugolini D, Bonassi S, Fucic A, Holland N, Knudsen L, Srám R, Ceppi M, Bocchini V, & Merlo DF (2006) Children's exposure to environmental pollutants and biomarkers of genetic damage. II. Results of a comprehensive literature search and meta-analysis. Mutat Res, **612**(1): 14–39.

Neslon E, Goubet-Wiemers C, Guo Y, & Jodscheit K (1999) Maternal passive smoking during pregnancy and fetal developmental toxicity: Part 2. Histological changes. Hum Exp Toxicol, **18**: 257–264.

Newschaffer CJ, Falb MD, & Gurney JG (2005) National autism prevalence trends from United States special education. Pediatrics, **115**(3): e277–282.

Ng TP, Seet CSR, Tan WC, & Foo SC (2001) Nitrogen dioxide exposure from domestic gas cooking and airway response in asthmatic women. Thorax, **56**: 596–601.

NHMRC (1997) The health effects of passive smoking. A scientific information paper. Australian Government, National Health and Medical Research Council, November.

Niimura F, Okubo S, Fogo A, & Ichikawa I (1997) Temporal and spatial expression pattern of the angiotensinogen gene in mice and rats. Am J Physiol, **272**(1 Pt 2): R142–R147.

Nitta H, Sato T, Nakai S, Maeda K, Aoki S, & Ono M (1993) Respiratory health associated with exposure to automobile exhaust. I. Results of cross-sectional studies in 1979, 1982 and 1983. Arch Environ Health, **48**: 53–58.

Nong A, McCarver DG, Hines RN, & Krishnan K (2006) Modelling interchild differences in pharmacokinetics on the basis of subject-specific data on physiology and hepatic CYP2E1 levels: A case study with toluene. Toxicol Appl Pharmacol, **214**(1): 78–87.

NRC (1983) Risk assessment in the federal government: Managing the process. Report of the Committee on the Institutional Means for the Assessment of Risks to Public Health, Commission on Life Sciences, National Research Council. Washington, DC, National Academy Press.

NRC (1993) Pesticides in the diets of infants and children. Report of the Committee on Pesticides in the Diets of Infants and Children, Board on Agriculture and Board on Environmental Studies and Toxicology, Commission on Life Sciences, National Research Council. Washington, DC, National Academy Press.

NRC (1994) Science and judgment in risk assessment. Washington, DC, National Research Council, Commission on Life Sciences, Committee on Risk Assessment of Hazardous Air Pollutants.

NRC (1999) Hormonally active agents in the environment. Report of the Committee on Hormonally Active Agents in the Environment, Board on Environmental Studies and Toxicology, Commission on Life Sciences, National Research Council. Washington, DC, National Academy Press, pp 1–430.

NRC (2000a) Scientific frontiers in developmental toxicology and risk assessment. Report of the Committee on Developmental Toxicology, Board on Environmental Studies and Toxicology, Commission on Life Sciences, National Research Council. Washington, DC, National Academy Press, pp 1–327.

NRC (2000b) Toxicological effects of methylmercury. Report of the Committee on the Toxicological Effects of Methylmercury, Board on Environmental Studies and Toxicology, Commission on Life Sciences, National Research Council. Washington, DC, National Academy Press.

NRC (2001) Evaluating chemical and other agent exposures for reproductive and developmental toxicity. Report of the Subcommittee on Reproductive and Developmental Toxicology, Committee on Toxicology, Board on Environmental Studies and Toxicology, Commission on Life Sciences, National Research Council. Washington, DC, National Academy Press.

Nriagu JO & Pacyna JM (1988) Quantitative assessment of worldwide contamination of air, water, and soils by trace metals. Nature, **333**: 134–139.

NTP (1998) Report on the workshop on "Scientific issues relevant to the assessment of health effects from exposure to methylmercury". Research Triangle Park, NC, United States Department of Health and Human Services, National Institute of Environmental Health Sciences, National Toxicology Progam (http://ntp.niehs.nih.gov/index.cfm?objectid=03614B65-BC68-D231-4E915F93AF9A6872#execsumm).

Oakley GP Jr (2004) Oral synthetic folic acid and vitamin B12 supplements work — if one consumes them. Nutr Rev, **62**(6 Pt 2): S22–S26; discussion S27–S28.

OECD (1981) OECD Guideline for Testing of Chemicals 414: Prenatal developmental toxicity study. Paris, Organisation for Economic Co-operation and Development.

OECD (1983) OECD Guideline for Testing of Chemicals 415: One-generation reproduction toxicity study. Paris, Organisation for Economic Co-operation and Development (http://www.oecd.org/dataoecd/18/12/1948458.pdf).

OECD (1995) OECD Guideline for Testing of Chemicals 421: Reproduction/developmental toxicity screening test. Paris, Organisation for Economic Co-operation and Development (http://www.oecd.org/dataoecd/18/14/1948474.pdf).

OECD (1996) OECD Guideline for Testing of Chemicals 422: Combined repeated dose toxicity study with the reproduction/developmental toxicity screening test. Paris, Organisation for Economic Co-operation and Development (http://www.oecd.org/dataoecd/18/30/1948410.pdf).

OECD (1999) Environmental exposure assessment strategies for existing industrial chemicals in OECD Member Countries. Paris, Organisation for Economic Co-operation and Development (Series on Testing and Assessment No. 17).

OECD (2001a) OECD Guideline for Testing of Chemicals 414: Prenatal developmental toxicity study. Paris, Organisation for Economic Co-operation and Development.

OECD (2001b) OECD Guideline for Testing of Chemicals 416: Two-generation reproduction toxicity study. Paris, Organisation for Economic Co-operation and Development.

OECD (2003a) OECD Guideline for Testing of Chemicals. Proposal for a new guideline 426. Developmental neurotoxicity study. Paris, Organisation for Economic Co-operation and Development.

OECD (2003b) OECD draft report of the validation of the rat uterotrophic bioassay: Phase 2. Testing of potent and weak oestrogen agonist by multiple laboratories. Paris, Organisation for Economic Co-operation and Development (ENV/JM/TG/EDTA(2003)1; http://www.epa.gov/scipoly/oscpendo/pubs/edmvac/uterotrophic_oecd_rodent_validation_p2_3_5_2003.pdf).

OECD (2003c) OECD draft report of the validation of the rodent Hershberger bioassay: Phase 2. Testing of androgen agonist, androgen antagonist and 5 alpha-reductase inhibitor in dose response studies by multiple laboratories. Paris, Organisation for Economic Co-operation and Development (ENV/JM/TG/EDTA(2003)5).

OECD (2004) Draft guidance document on reproductive toxicity testing and assessment. Paris, Organisation for Economic Co-operation and Development (Series on Testing and Assessment No. 43).

Ogawa A, Sakurai Y, Kayama T, & Yoshimoto T (1989) Regional cerebral blood flow with age: changes in rCBF in childhood. Neurol Res, **11**: 173–176.

Olin SS & Sonawane BR (2003) Workshop to develop a framework for assessing risks to children from exposure to environmental agents. Environ Health Perspect, **111**(12): 1524–1526.

Olney JW, Farber NB, Wozniak DF, Jevtovic-Todorovic V, & Ikonomidou C (2000) Environmental agents that have the potential to trigger massive apoptotic neurodegeneration in the developing brain. Environ Health Perspect, **108**(Suppl 3): 383–388.

Olsen J, Rachootin P, & Schiodt AV (1983) Alcohol use, conception time, and birthweight. J Epidemiol Commun Health, **37**: 63–65.

Olshan AF, Smith J, Cook MN, Grufferman S, Pollock BH, Stram DO, Seeger RC, Look AT, Cohn SL, Castleberry RP, & Bondy ML (1999) Hormone and fertility drug use and the risk of neuroblastoma: A report from the Children's Cancer Group and the Pediatric Oncology Group. Am J Epidemiol, **150**: 930–938.

Oosterlee A, Drijver M, Lebret E, & Brunekreef B (1996) Chronic respiratory symptoms of children and adults living along streets with high traffic density. Occup Environ Med, **53**: 241–247.

O'Rahilly R & Muller F eds (1992) Human embryology and teratology. New York, Wiley-Liss.

Ostby J, Kelce WR, Lambright C, Wolf CJ, Mann P, & Gray LE Jr (1999) The fungicide procymidone alters sexual differentiation in the male rat by acting as an androgen-receptor antagonist in vivo and in vitro. Toxicol Ind Health, 15(1–2): 80–93.

Osterloh JD (1991) Observations on the effect of parathyroid hormone on environmental blood lead concentrations in humans. Environ Res, 54: 8–16.

Ostro BD, Eskeland GS, Sanchez JM, & Feyzioglu T (1999) Air pollution and health effects: A study of medical visits among children in Santiago, Chile. Environ Health Perspect, 107(1): 69–73.

Ottman R (1996) Gene–environment interaction: Definitions and study designs. Prev Med, 25(6): 764–770.

Ozanne SE (2001) Metabolic programming in animals. Br Med Bull, 60: 143–152.

Pacini F, Vorontsova T, Demidchik EP, Molinaro E, Agate L, Romei C, Shavrova E, Cherstvoy ED, Ivashkevitch Y, Kuchinskaya E, Schlumberger M, Ronga G, Filesi M, & Pinchera A (1997) Post-Chernobyl thyroid carcinoma in Belarus children and adolescents: Comparison with naturally-occurring thyroid carcinoma in Italy and France. J Clin Endocrinol Metab, 82: 3563–3569.

Palma T, Riley M, & Capel JE (1996) Development and evaluation of enhancements to the Hazardous Air Pollutant Exposure Model (HAPEM-MS3). Cary, NC, International Technology Corporation.

Palmer AK (1981) Regulatory requirements for reproductive toxicology: Theory and practice. In: Kimmel CA & Buelke-Sam J eds. Developmental toxicology. New York, Raven Press, pp 259–288.

Pande JN, Bhatta N, Biswas D, Pandey RM, Ahluwalia G, Siddaramaia NH, & Khilnani GC (2002) Outdoor air pollution and emergency room visits at a hospital in Delhi. Indian J Chest Dis Allied Sci, 44: 13–19.

Park JH, Gold DR, Spiegelman DL, Burge HA, & Milton DK (2001) House dust endotoxin and wheeze in the first year of life. Am J Respir Crit Care Med, 163(2): 322–328.

Park SY & Jameson JL (2005) Minireview: Transcriptional regulation of gonadal development and differentiation. Endocrinology, 146(3): 1035–1042.

Parnia S, Brown JL, & Frew AJ (2002) The role of pollutants in allergic sensitization and the development of asthma. Allergy, 57(12): 1111–1117.

Pastides H, Calabrese EJ, Hosmer DW Jr, & Harris DR Jr (1988) Spontaneous abortion and general illness symptoms among semiconductor manufacturers. J Occup Med, 30(7): 543–551.

Peden D (2000) Development of atopy and asthma: Candidate environmental influences and important periods of exposure. Environ Health Perspect, 108(Suppl 3): 475–482.

Pekkanen J, Timonen KL, Ruuskanen J, Reponen A, & Mirme A (1999) Effects of ultrafine and fine particles in urban air on peak expiratory flow in children. Lancet, **353**: 874–878.

Perera FP, Whyatt RM, Jedrychowski W, Rauh V, Manchester D, Santella RM, & Ottman R (1998) Recent developments in molecular epidemiology. Am J Epidemiol, **147**: 309–314.

Perera FP, Jedrychowski W, Rauh V, & Whyatt RM (1999) Molecular epidemiologic research on the effect of environmental pollutants on the fetus. Environ Health Perspect, **107**(Suppl 3): 451–460.

Perera FP, Rauh V, Tsai WY, Kinney P, Camann D, Barr D, Bernert T, Garfinkel R, Tu YH, Diaz D, Dietrich J, & Whyatt RM (2003) Effects of transplacental exposure to environmental pollutants on birth outcomes in a multiethnic population. Environ Health Perspect, **111**(2): 201–205.

Pershagen G, Rylander E, Norberg S, Eriksson M, & Nordvall S (1995) Air pollution involving nitrogen dioxide exposure and wheezing bronchitis in children. Int J Epidemiol, **24**(6): 1147–1153.

Philips DIW, Barker DJP, Fall CHD, Seckl JR, Whorwood CB, & Wood PJ (1998) Elevated plasma cortisol concentrations: An expression for the relationship between low birth weight and adult cardiovascular risk factors. J Clin Endocrinol Metab, **83**: 757–760.

Piegorsch WW, Weinberg CR, & Taylor JA (1994) Non-hierarchical logistic models and case-only designs for assessing susceptibility in population-based case–control studies. Stat Med, **13**: 153–162.

Pierano WB, Mattie D, & Smith P (1995) Proceedings of the Conference on Temporal Aspects in Risk Assessment for Noncancer Endpoints. Inhal Toxicol, **7**: 837–1029.

Pineda-Zavaleta AP, Garcia-Vargas G, Borja-Aburto VH, Acosta-Saavedra LC, Vera Aguilar E, Gomez-Munoz A, Cebrian ME, & Calderon-Aranda ES (2004) Nitric oxide and superoxide anion production in monocytes from children exposed to arsenic and lead in region Lagunera, Mexico. Toxicol Appl Pharmacol, **198**: 283–290.

Pinkerton KE & Joad JP (2000) The mammalian respiratory system and critical windows of exposure for children's health. Environ Health Perspect, **108**(Suppl 3): 457–462.

Platt RW, Joseph KS, Ananth CV, Grondines J, Abrahamowicz M, & Kramer MS (2004) A proportional hazards model with time-dependent covariates and time-varying effects for analysis of fetal and infant death. Am J Epidemiol, **160**(3): 199–206.

Plopper CG, Weir AJ, Chang A, Voit M, Philpot RM, & Buckpitt AR (1994) Elevated susceptibility to 4-ipomeanol cytotoxicity in immature Clara cells of neonatal rabbits. J Pharmacol Exp Ther, **269**: 867–880.

Plowchalk DR & Mattison DR (1991) Phosphoramide mustard is responsible for the ovarian toxicity of cyclophosphamide. Toxicol Appl Pharmacol, **107**: 472–481.

Pongracz JE & Stockley RA (2006) Wnt signalling in lung development and diseases. Respir Res, **7**: 15 (http://respiratory-research.com/content/7/1/15).

Porterfield SP & Hendry LB (1998) Impact of PCBs on thyroid hormone directed brain development. Toxicol Ind Health, **14**: 103–120.

Poulsen P, Vaag AA, Kyvik KO, Moller Jensen D, & Beck-Nielsen H (1997) Low birth weight is associated with NIDDM in discordant monozygotic and dizygotic twin pairs. Diabetologia, **40**: 439–446.

Prescott S, Taylor A, King B, Dunstan J, Upham J, Thorton C, & Holt P (2003) Neonatal interleukin-12 capacity is associated with variations in allergen-specific immune responses in the neonatal and postnatal periods. Clin Exp Allergy, **33**: 566–572.

Preston RJ & Williams GM (2005) DNA-reactive carcinogens: mode of action and human cancer hazard. Crit Rev Toxicol, **35**(8–9): 673–683.

Price K, Haddad S, & Krishnan K (2003) Physiological modeling of age-specific changes in the pharmacokinetics of organic chemicals in children. J Toxicol Environ Health A, **66**(5): 417–433.

Price PS, Conolly RB, Chaisson CF, Gross EA, Young JS, Mathis ET, & Tedder DR (2003) Modeling interindividual variation in physiological factors used in PBPK models of humans. Crit Rev Toxicol, **33**(5): 469–503.

Pronczuk J, Moy G, & Vallenas C (2004) Breast milk: An optimal food. Environ Health Perspect, **112**(13): A722–A723.

Pronczuk de Garbino J (2002) The sentinel role of poisons centers in the protection of children's environmental health. J Toxicol Clin Toxicol, **40**(4): 493–497.

Pryor JL, Hughes C, Foster W, Hales BF, & Robaire B (2000) Critical windows of exposure for children's health: The reproductive system in animals and humans. Environ Health Perspect, **108**(Suppl 3): 491–503.

Pui CH (1991) Epipodophyllotoxin-related acute myeloid leukaemia. Lancet, **338**(8780): 1468.

Radde IC (1985) Mechanisms of drug absorption and their development. In: Macleod SM & Radde IC eds. Textbook of pediatric clinical pharmacology. Littleton, MA, PSG Publishing Company, pp 17–43.

Raimondo S & Draghetti MT (1990) Influence of length of intra-uterine life on the appearance of developmental markers and neuro-behavioral reflexes in rat. Teratology, **42**: 31A.

Raizenne M, Neas LM, Damokosh AI, Dockery DW, Spengler JD, Koutrakis P, Ware JH, & Speizer FE (1996) Health effects of acid aerosols on North American children: Pulmonary function. Environ Health Perspect, **104**(5): 506–514.

Ravelli AC, van der Meulen JHP, Michels RPJ, Osmond C, Barker DJP, Hales CN, & Bleker OP (1998) Glucose tolerance in adults after prenatal exposure to famine. Lancet, **351**(9097): 173–177.

Ravelli GP, Stein ZA, & Susser MW (1976) Obesity in young men after famine exposure in utero and early infancy. N Engl J Med, **295**(7): 349–353.

Rayner JL, Wood C, & Fenton SE (2004) Exposure parameters necessary for delayed puberty and mammary gland development in Long-Evans rats exposed in utero to atrazine. Toxicol Appl Pharmacol, **195**: 23–34.

Reif JS, Tsongas TA, Mitchell J, Keefe TJ, Tessari JD, Metzger L, & Amler R (1993) Risk factors for exposure to arsenic at a hazardous waste site. Expo Anal Environ Epidemiol, **3**: 73–86.

Reiss R, Anderson EL, & Lape J (2003) A framework and case study for exposure assessment in the Voluntary Children's Chemical Evaluation Program. Risk Anal, **23**(5): 1069–1084.

Renwick AG (1998) Toxicokinetics in infants and children in relation to the ADI and TDI. Food Addit Contam, **15**: 17–35.

Renwick AG, Dorne JL, & Walton K (2000) An analysis of the need for an additional uncertainty factor for infants and children. Regul Toxicol Pharmacol, **31**(3): 286–296.

Renwick AG, Barlow SM, Hertz-Picciotto I, Boobis AR, Dybing E, Edler L, Eisenbrand G, Greig JB, Kleiner J, Lambe J, Muller DJ, Smith MR, Tritscher A, Tuijtelaars S, van den Brandt PA, Walker R, & Kroes R (2003) Risk characterisation of chemicals in food and diet. Food Chem Toxicol, **41**(9): 1211–1271.

Rice D & Barone S Jr (2000) Critical periods of vulnerability for the developing nervous system: evidence from humans and animal models. Environ Health Perspect, **108**(Suppl 3): 511–533.

Rice DC (1996) Behavioral effects of lead: Commonalities between experimental and epidemiologic data. Environ Health Perspect, **104**(Suppl 2): 337–351.

Rice JM (2004) Causation of nervous system tumors in children: Insights from traditional and genetically engineered animal models. Toxicol Appl Pharmacol, **199**: 175–191.

Richter-Reichhelm HB, Althoff J, Schulte A, Ewe S, & Gundert Remy U (2002) Workshop report. Children as a special subpopulation: focus on immunotoxicity. Federal Institute for Health Protection of Consumers and Veterinary Medicine (BgVV), 15–16 November 2001, Berlin, Germany. Arch Toxicol, **76**(7): 377–382.

Riedel F, Hasenauer E, Barth PJ, Koziorowski A, & Rieger CH (1996) Formaldehyde exposure enhances inhalative allergic sensitization in the guinea pig. Allergy, **51**(2): 94–99.

Risau W (1998) Development and differentiation of endothelium. Kidney Int Suppl, **67**: S3–S6.

Ritz B, Yu F, Chapa G, & Fruin S (2000) Effect of air pollution on preterm birth among children born in Southern California between 1989 and 1993. Epidemiology, **11**: 502–511.

Ritz B, Yu F, Fruin S, Chapa G, Shaw GM, & Harris JA (2002) Ambient air pollution and risk of birth defects in Southern California. Am J Epidemiol, **155**: 17–25.

References

Robbiano L, Parodi A, Venturelli S, & Brambilla G (1989) Comparison of DNA alkylation, fragmentation, and repair in maternal and fetal tissues of pregnant rats treated with a single dose of ethyl methanesulfonate, ethyl-N-nitrosourea, N-nitrosodiethylamine, and methyl-N-nitrosourea. Teratog Carcinog Mutagen, **9**(3): 157–166.

Rockett JC, Lynch CD, & Buck GM (2004) Biomarkers for assessing reproductive development and health: Part 1 — Pubertal development. Environ Health Perspect, **112**(1): 105–112.

Rodier PM (1994) Vulnerable periods and processes during central nervous system development. Environ Health Perspect, **102**(Suppl 2): 121–124.

Rodier PM (1995) Developing brain as a target of toxicity. Environ Health Perspect, **103**(Suppl 6): 73–76.

Rodier PM (2004) Environmental causes of central nervous system maldevelopment. Pediatrics, **113**(4): 1076–1083.

Rodier PM, Ingram JL, Tisdale B, Nelson S, & Romano J (1996) Embryological origin for autism: developmental anomalies of the cranial nerve motor nuclei. J Comp Neurol, **370**(2): 247–261.

Roemer W, Clench-Aas J, Englert N, Hoek G, Katsouyanni K, Pekkanen J, & Brunekreef B (1999) Inhomogeneity in response to air pollution in European children (PEACE project). Occup Environ Med, **56**: 86–92.

Rogan WJ, Gladen BC, McKinney JD, Carreras N, Hardy P, Thullen J, Tinglestad J, & Tully M (1986) Neonatal effects of transplacental exposure to PCBs and DDE. J Pediatr, **109**(2): 335–341.

Rogan WJ, Gladen BC, Hung KL, Koong SL, Shih LY, Taylor JS, Wu YC, Yang D, Ragan NB, & Hsu CC (1988) Congenital poisoning by polychlorinated biphenyls and their contaminants in Taiwan. Science, **241**(4863): 334–336.

Ron E (1996) Thyroid cancer. In: Schottenfeld D & Fraumeni JF Jr eds. Cancer epidemiology and prevention, 2nd ed. New York, Oxford University Press, pp 1000–1021.

Ron E, Modan B, & Boice JD (1988a) Mortality after radiotherapy for ringworm of the scalp. Am J Epidemiol, **127**: 713–725.

Ron E, Modan B, Boice JD Jr, Alfandary E, Stovall M, Chetrit A, & Katz L (1988b) Tumors of the brain and nervous system after radiotherapy in childhood. N Engl J Med, **319**: 1033–1039.

Ronchetti R, Macri F, Ciofetta GE, Indinnimeo L, Cutrera R, Bonci E, Antognoni G, & Martinez FD (1990) Increased serum immunoglobulin E and increased prevalence of eosinophilia in 9 year old children of smoking parents. J Allergy Clin Immunol, **86**: 400–407.

Ronis MJ, Gandy J, & Badger T (1998) Endocrine mechanisms underlying reproductive toxicity in the developing rat chronically exposed to dietary lead. J Toxicol Environ Health A, **54**: 77–99.

Rooney A, Fournier M, Bernier J, & Cyr D (2003) Neonatal exposure to propylthiouracil induces a shift in lymphoid cell sub-populations in the developing postnatal male rat spleen and thymus. Cell Immunol, **223**: 91–102.

Ruan XZ, Varghese Z, Powis SH, & Moorhead JF (2005) Nuclear receptors and their coregulators in kidney. Kidney Int, **68**(6): 2444–2461.

Ruhle W, Graf Von Ballestrem CL, Pult HM, & Gnirs J (1995) [Correlation of cotinine levels in amniotic fluid, umbilical arterial blood and maternal blood.] Geburtshilfe Frauenheilkd, **55**: 156–159 (in German).

Rumchev K, Stick S, Spickett J, & Phillips M (2000) Childhood asthma and exposure to formaldehyde and volatile organic compounds. Respirology, 5(Suppl): A26.

Rumchev KB, Spickett JT, Bulsara MK, Phillips MR, & Stick SM (2002) Domestic exposure to formaldehyde significantly increases the risk of asthma in young children. Eur Respir J, **20**(2): 403–408.

Rutledge JC & Generoso WM (1998) Malformations in pregastrulation developmental toxicology. In: Korach KS ed. Reproductive and developmental toxicology. New York, Marcel Dekker, pp 73–86.

Ryan TJ, Hart EM, & Kappler LL (2002) VOC exposures in a mixed-use university art building. Am Ind Hyg Assoc J, **63**: 703–708.

Rylance GW (1988) Prescribing for infants and children. Br Med J, **296**: 984–986.

Rylander L, Stromberg U, & Hagmar L (1995) Decreased birthweight among infants born to women with a high dietary intake of fish contaminated with persistent organochlorine compounds. Scand J Work Environ Health, **21**: 368–375.

Sadler TW (2000) Susceptible periods during embryogenesis of the heart and endocrine glands. Environ Health Perspect, **108**(Suppl 3): 555–561.

Salanitre E & Rackow H (1969) The pulmonary exchange of nitrous oxide and halothane in infants and children. Anesthesiology, **30**(4): 388–394.

Saldiva PH, Lichtenfels AJ, Paiva PS, Barone IA, Martins MA, Massad E, Pereira JC, Xavier VP, Singer JM, & Bohm GM (1994) Association between air pollution and mortality due to respiratory disease in children in Sao Paulo, Brazil. Environ Res, **65**: 218–225.

Salle BL, Delvin EE, Lapillonne A, Bishop NJ, & Glorieux FH (2000) Perinatal metabolism of vitamin D. Am J Clin Nutr, **71**(Suppl 5): 1317S–1324S.

Salome CM, Brown NJ, Marks GB, Woolcock AJ, Johnson GM, Nancarrow PC, Quigley S, & Tiong J (1996) Effect of nitrogen dioxide and other combustion products on asthmatic subjects in a home-like environment. Eur Resp J, **9**(5): 910–918.

Sarangapani R, Gentry PR, Covington TR, Teeguarden JG, & Clewell HJ (2003) Evaluation of the potential impact of age- and gender-specific lung morphology and ventilation rate on the dosimetry of vapors. Inhal Toxicol, **15**: 987–1016.

References

Savage MO & Lowe DG (1990) Gonadal neoplasia and abnormal sexual differentiation. Clin Endocrinol (Oxf), **32**: 519–533.

Schantz SL, Widholm JJ, & Rice DC (2003) Effects of PCB exposure on neuropsychological function in children. Environ Health Perspect, **111**(3): 357–576.

Schenker MB, Gold EB, Beaumont JJ, Eskenazi B, Hammond K, Lasley BL, McCurdy SA, Samuels SJ, Saiki CL, & Swan SH (1995) Association of spontaneous abortion and other reproductive effects with work in the semiconductor industry. Am J Ind Med, **28**: 639–659.

Schwartz GJ, Haydock GB, Edelman CM, & Spitzer A (1976) A simple estimate of glomerular filtration rate in children derived from body length and plasma creatinine. Pediatrics, **51**: 875–878.

Schwela D (2000) Air pollution and health in urban areas. Rev Environ Health, **15**: 13–42.

Schwenk M, Gundert-Remy U, Heinemeyer G, Olejniczak K, Stahlmann R, Kaufmann W, Bolt HM, Greim H, von Keutz E, Gelbke HP, & DGPT (2003) Children as a sensitive subgroup and their role in regulatory toxicology: DGPT workshop report. Arch Toxicol, **77**(1): 2–6.

Scialli AR, Swan SH, Amler RW, Baird DD, Eskenazi B, Gist G, Hatch MC, Kesner S, Lemasters GK, Marcus M, Paul ME, Schulte P, Taylor Z, Wilcox AJ, & Zahniser C (1997) Assessment of reproductive disorders and birth defects in communities near hazardous chemical sites. II: Female reproductive disorders. Reprod Toxicol, **11**: 231–242.

Sciarillo WG, Alexander G, & Farrell KP (1992) Lead exposure and child behavior. Am J Public Health, **82**(10): 1356–1360.

Scully RE (1981) Neoplasia associated with anomalous sexual development and abnormal sex chromosomes. Pediatr Adolesc Endocrinol, **8**: 203–217.

Seed J, Carney EW, Corley RA, Crofton KM, DeSesso JM, Foster PMD, Kavlock R, Kimmel G, Klaunig J, Meek ME, Preston RJ, Slikker W Jr, Tabacova S, Williams GM, Wiltse J, Zoeller RT, Fenner-Crisp P, & Patton DE (2005) Overview: Using mode of action and life stage information to evaluate the human relevance of animal toxicity data. Crit Rev Toxicol, **35**(8–9): 664–672.

Sekhon HS, Keller JA, Benowitz VL, & Spindel ER (2001) Prenatal nicotine exposure alters pulmonary function in newborn rhesus monkeys. Am J Respir Crit Care Med, **1645**: 989–994.

Selevan SG, Kimmel CA, & Mendola P (2000) Identifying critical windows of exposure for children's health. Environ Health Perspect, **108**(Suppl 3): 451–455.

Selevan SG, Rice DC, Hogan KA, Euling SY, Pfahles-Hutchens A, & Bethel J (2003) Blood lead concentrations and delayed puberty in girls. N Engl J Med, **348**: 1527–1536.

Senn KM, McGuinness BM, Buck Louis GM, Vena JE, Anderson S, & Rogers BT (2005) Longitudinal study of babies born to mothers enrolled in a preconception prospective pregnancy study: Study design and methodology, New York State angler cohort study. Environ Res, **97**(2): 163–169.

Shahab M, Mastronardi C, Seminara SB, Crowley WF, Ojeda SR, & Plant TM (2005) Increased hypothalamic GPR54 signaling: A potential mechanism for initiation of puberty in primates. Proc Natl Acad Sci U S A, **102**(6): 2129–2134.

Sharpe RM (2003) The "oestrogen hypothesis" — where do we stand now? Int J Androl, **26**: 2–15.

Sharpe RM & Skakkebaek NE (1993) Are oestrogens involved in falling sperm counts and disorders of the male reproductive tract? Lancet, **341**: 1392–1395.

Sharpe RM, Fisher JS, Millar MM, Jobling S, & Sumpter JP (1995) Gestational and lactational exposure of rats to xenoestrogens results in reduced testicular size and sperm production. Environ Health Perspect, **103**(12): 1136–1143.

Shea KM & American Academy of Pediatrics Committee on Environmental Health (2003) Pediatric exposure and potential toxicity of phthalate plasticizers. Pediatrics, **111**: 1467–1474.

Shenefelt RE (1972) Morphogenesis of malformations in hamsters caused by retinoic acid: Relation to dose and stage at treatment. Teratology, **5**(1): 103–118.

Shepard TH (2004) Shepard's catalog of teratogenic agents. Baltimore, MD, Johns Hopkins University Press (http://depts.washington.edu/~terisweb/teris/).

Sher ES, Xu XM, Adams PM, Craft CM, & Stein SA (1998) The effects of thyroid hormone level and action in developing brain: Are these targets for the actions of polychlorinated biphenyls and dioxins? Toxicol Ind Health, **14**: 121–158.

Shiromizu K, Thorgeirsson SS, & Mattison DR (1984) Effect of cyclophosphamide on oocyte and follicle number in Sprague-Dawley rats, C57BL/6N and DBA/2N mice. Pediatr Pharmacol (New York), **4**(4): 213–221.

Shirota M, Soda S, Katoh C, Asai S, Sato M, Ohta R, Watanabe G, Taya K, & Shirota K (2003) Effects of reduction of the number of primordial follicles on follicular development to achieve puberty in female rats. Reproduction, **125**: 85–94.

Shock NW (1944) Basal blood pressure and pulse rate in adolescents. Am J Dis Child, **68**: 16–22.

Sholler GF, Celermajer JM, Whight CM, & Bauman AE (1987) Echo Doppler assessment of cardiac output and its relation to growth in normal infants. Am J Cardiol, **60**: 1112–1116.

Shu XO, Gao YT, Linet MS, Brinton LA, Gao RN, Jin F, & Fraumeni JF Jr (1987) Chloramphenicol use and childhood leukaemia in Shanghai. Lancet, **2**(8565): 934–937.

Shuey DL, Lau C, Logsdon TR, Zucker RM, Elstein KH, Narotsky MG, Setzer RW, Kavlock RJ, & Rogers JM (1994) Biologically-based dose–response modeling in developmental toxicology: Biochemical and cellular sequelae of 5-fluorouracil exposure in the developing rat. Toxicol Appl Pharmacol, **126**: 129–144.

Shyr SW, Crowley WR, & Grosvenor CE (1986) Effect of neonatal prolactin deficiency on prepubertal tuberoinfundibular and tuberohypophyseal dopaminergic neuronal activity. Endocrinology, **119**: 1217–1221.

Sin KW & Tsang HF (2003) Large-scale mercury exposure due to a cream cosmetic: Community-wide case series. Hong Kong Med J, **9**: 329–334.

Singer EJ, Wegmann PC, Lehman MD, Christensen MS, & Vinson LJ (1971) Barrier development, ultrastructure, and sulfhydryl content of the fetal epidermis. J Soc Cosmet Chem, **22**: 119–137.

Sjodin A, Carlsson H, Thuresson K, Sjolin S, Bergman A, & Ostman C (2001) Flame retardants in indoor air at an electronics recycling plant and at other work environments. Environ Sci Technol, **35**: 448–454.

Skakkebaek NE, Rajpert-De Meyts E, & Main KM (2001) Testicular dysgenesis syndrome: An increasingly common development disorder with environmental aspects. Hum Reprod, **16**: 972–978.

Skakkebaek NE, Holm M, Hoei-Hansen C, Jorgensen N, & Rajpert-De Meyts E (2003) Association between testicular dysgenesis syndrome (TDS) and testicular neoplasia: Evidence from 20 adult patients with signs of maldevelopment of the testis. APMIS, **111**: 1–9.

Skakkebaek NE, Jorgensen N, Main KM, Rajpert-De Meyts E, Leffers H, Andersson AM, Juul A, Carlsen E, Mortensen GK, Jensen TK, & Toppari J (2006) Is human fecundity declining? Int J Androl, **29**(1): 2–11.

Smedley PL & Kinniburgh DG (2002) A review of the source, behaviour and distribution of arsenic in natural waters. Appl Geochem, **17**: 517–568.

Smialowicz R (2002) The rat as a model in developmental immunotoxicology. Hum Exp Toxicol, **21**: 513–519.

Smialowicz, R, Riddle M, Rogers R, Luebke R, & Copeland C (1989) Immunotoxicity of tributyltin oxide in rats exposed as adults or pre-weanlings. Toxicology, **57**: 97–111.

Smialowicz R, Williams W, & Copeland C (2001) Effect of perinatal/juvenile heptachlor exposure on adult immune and reproductive system function in rats. Toxicol Sci, **61**: 164–175.

Smiley-Jewell S, Nishio S, Weir AJ, & Plopper CG (1998) Neonatal Clara cell toxicity by 4-ipomeanol alters bronchiolar organisation in adult rabbits. Am J Physiol, **274**(4 Pt 1): L485–L498.

Smith EP, Boyd J, Frank GR, Takahashi H, Cohen RM, Specker B, Williams TC, Lubahn DB, & Korach KS (1994) Estrogen resistance caused by a mutation in the estrogen-receptor gene in a man. N Engl J Med, **331**: 1056–1061.

Smith KR & Mehta S (2003) Burden of disease from indoor air pollution in developing countries: Comparison of estimates. Int J Hyg Environ Health, **206**: 279–289.

Smith KR, Samet JM, Romieu I, & Bruce N (2000) Indoor air pollution in developing countries and acute lower respiratory infections in children. Thorax, **55**: 518–532.

Snyder J, Filipov N, Parsons P, & Lawrence D (2000) The efficiency of maternal transfer of lead and its influence on plasma IgE and splenic cellularity of mice. Toxicol Sci, **57**: 87–94.

Sohval AR (1954) Testicular dysgenesis as an etiologic factor in cryptorchidism. J Urol, **72**: 693–702.

Sohval AR (1956) Testicular dysgenesis in relation to neoplasm of the testicle. J Urol, **75**: 285–291.

Solecki R, Davies L, Dellarco V, Dewhurst I, Raaij M, & Tritscher A (2005) Guidance on setting of acute reference dose (ARfD) for pesticides. Food Chem Toxicol, **43**(11): 1569–1593.

Song X, Seidler FJ, Saleh JL, Zhang J, Padilla S, & Slotkin TA (1997) Cellular mechanisms for developmental toxicity of chlorpyrifos: targeting the adenylyl cyclase signaling cascade. Toxicol Appl Pharmacol, **145**: 158–174.

Sonich-Mullin C, Fielder R, Wiltse J, Baetcke K, Dempsey J, Fenner-Crisp P, Grant D, Hartley M, Knaap A, Kroese D, Mangelsdorf I, Meek E, Rice JM, & Younes M (2001) IPCS conceptual framework for evaluating a mode of action for chemical carcinogenesis. Regul Toxicol Pharmacol, **34**: 146–152.

Spielberg SP (1992) Anticonvulsant adverse drug reactions: Age dependent and age independent. In: Guzelian PS, Henry CJ, & Olin SS eds. Similarities and differences between children and adults: Implication for risk assessment. Washington, DC, International Life Sciences Institute, ILSI Press, pp 104–106.

Sporik R & Platts-Mills TA (2001) Allergen exposure and the development of asthma. Thorax, **56**(Suppl 2): 58–63.

Sporik R, Ingram JM, Price W, Sussman JH, Honsinger RW, & Platts-Mills TA (1995) Association of asthma with serum IgE and skin test reactivity to allergens among children living at high altitude. Tickling the dragon's breath. Am J Respir Crit Care Med, **151**(5): 1388–1392.

Srám RJ, Binkova B, Dejmek J, & Bobak M (2005) Ambient air pollution and pregnancy outcomes: A review of the literature. Environ Health Perspect, **113**(4): 375–382.

Stennard FA & Harvey RP (2005) T-box transcription factors and their roles in regulatory hierarchies in the developing heart. Development, **132**: 4897–4910.

Steuerwald U, Weihe P, Jorgensen PJ, Bjerve K, Brock J, Heinzow B, Budtz-Jorgensen E, & Grandjean P (2000) Maternal seafood diet, methylmercury exposure, and neonatal neurologic function. J Pediatr, **136**(5): 599–605.

Stewart CF & Hampton EM (1987) Effect of maturation on drug disposition in pediatric patients. Clin Pharm, **6**: 548–564.

Stieb DM, Judek S, & Burnett RT (2002) Meta-analysis of time-series studies of air pollution and mortality: Effects of gases and particles and the influence of causes of death, age, and season. J Air Waste Manage Assoc, **52**: 470–484.

Stillman RJ (1982) In utero exposure to diethylstilbestrol: Adverse effects on the reproductive tract and reproductive performance and male and female offspring. Am J Obstet Gynecol, **142**: 905–921.

Stoker TE, Robinette CL, & Cooper RL (1999) Maternal exposure to atrazine during lactation suppresses suckling-induced prolactin release and results in prostatitis in the adult offspring. Toxicol Sci, **52**: 68–79.

Stoker TE, Parks LG, Gray LE, & Cooper RL (2000) Endocrine-disrupting chemicals: Prepubertal exposures and effects on sexual maturation and thyroid function in the male rat. A focus on the EDSTAC recommendations. Endocrine Disrupter Screening and Testing Advisory Committee. Crit Rev Toxicol, **30**(2): 197–252.

Stoltzfus RJ, Kvalsvig JD, Chwaya HM, Montresor A, Albonico M, Tielsch JM, Savioli L, & Pollitt E (2001) Effects of iron supplementation and anthelmintic treatment on motor and language development of preschool children in Zanzibar: Double blind, placebo controlled study. BMJ, **323**(7326): 1389–1393.

Strachan DP (1989) Hay fever, hygiene, and household size. Br Med J, **299**: 1259–1260.

Strachan DP (1999) Family size, infection and atopy: the first decade of the "hygiene hypothesis". J Allergy Clin Immunol, **104**: 554–558.

Strachan DP & Cook DG (1998a) Parental smoking, middle ear disease and adenotonsillectomy in children. Thorax, **53**: 50–56.

Strachan DP & Cook DG (1998b) Parental smoking and childhood asthma: Longitudinal and case–control studies. Thorax, **53**: 204–212.

Strange RC, Howie AF, Hume R, Matharoo B, Bell J, Hiley C, Jones P, & Beckett GJ (1989) The developmental expression of alpha-, mu- and pi-class glutathione S-transferases in human liver. Biochem Biophys Acta, **993**: 186–190.

Stratton K, Howe C, & Battaglia F (1996) Fetal alcohol syndrome: Diagnosis, epidemiology, prevention and treatment. Washington, DC, National Academy Press.

Streissguth AP (1993) Fetal alcohol syndrome in older patients. Alcohol Alcohol Suppl, **2**: 209–212.

Streissguth AP, Barr HM, Sampson PD, & Bookstein FL (1994) Prenatal alcohol and offspring development: The first fourteen years. Drug Alcohol Depend, **36**(2): 89–99.

Streissguth AP, Bookstein FL, Barr HM, Sampson PD, O'Malley K, & Young JK (2004) Risk factors for adverse life outcomes in fetal alcohol syndrome and fetal alcohol effects. J Dev Behav Pediatr, **25**(4): 228–238.

Strohsnitter WC, Noller KL, Hoover RN, Robboy SJ, Palmer JR, Titus-Ernstoff L, Kaufman RH, Adam E, Herbst AL, & Hatch EE (2001) Cancer risk in men exposed In utero to diethylstilbestrol. J Natl Cancer Inst, **93**: 545–551.

Sturmer T, Thurigen D, Spiegelman D, Blettner M, & Brenner H (2002) The performance of methods for correcting measurement error in case–control studies. Epidemiology, **13**: 507–516.

Styne DM (2003) The regulation of pubertal growth. Horm Res, **60**(Suppl 1): 22–26.

Suk WA (2002) Beyond the Bangkok Statement: research needs to address environmental threats to children. Environ Health Perspect, **110**(6): A284–286.

Suk WA, Ruchirawat KM, Balakrishnan K, Berger M, Carpenter D, Damstra T, de Garbino JP, Koh D, Landrigan PJ, Makalinao I, Sly PD, Xu Y, & Zheng BS (2003) Environmental threats to children's health in Southeast Asia and the Western Pacific. Environ Health Perspect, **111**(10): 1340–1347.

Susheela AK (1998) Scientific evidence on adverse effects of fluoride on human tissues due to fluoride contaminated drinking water, due to fluoridated dental products, due to fluoride therapy. Document presented to Members of Parliament, House of Lords and House of Commons, Westminster, London.

Suter GW, Vermeire T, Munns WR Jr, & Sekizawa J (2003) Framework for the integration of health and ecological risk assessment. Hum Ecol Risk Assess, **9**: 281–301.

Szantay V, Tamas S, Marian L, & Bochis G (1974) [Changes of hepatic blood flow in children as a function of age.] Rev Roum Med Intern, **11**: 91–93 (in French).

Tabacova S, Little R, Tsong Y, Vega A, & Kimmel CA (2003) Adverse pregnancy outcomes associated with maternal enalapril antihypertensive treatment. Pharmacoepidemiol Drug Saf, **12**: 633–646.

Tager IB, Weiss ST, Munoz A, Rosner B, & Speizer FE (1983) Longitudinal study of the effects of maternal smoking on pulmonary function in children. N Engl J Med, **309**: 699–703.

Tager IB, Ngo L, & Hanrahan JP (1995) Maternal smoking during pregnancy. Effects on lung function during the first 18 months of life. Am J Respir Crit Care Med, **152**: 977–983.

Tamburlini G, von Ehrenstein OS, & Bertollini R eds (2002) Children's health and environment: A review of the evidence. A joint report from the European Environment Agency and the WHO Regional Office for Europe. Copenhagen, European Environment Agency (Environmental Issue Report No. 29).

Tangbanluekal L & Robinette CL (1993) Prolactin mediates estradiol-induced inflammation in the lateral prostate of Wistar rats. Endocrinology, **132**: 2407–2416.

Taskinen H, Anttila A, Lindbohm M-L, Salimen M, & Himminki K (1989) Spontaneous abortions and congenital malformations among the wives of men occupationally exposed to organic solvents. Scand J Work Environ Health, **15**: 345–352.

Taylor K, Jackson L, Lynch C, Kostyniak P, & Buck Louis G (2006) Preconception maternal polychlorinated biphenyl concentrations and the secondary sex ratio. Environ Res, in press [Epub ahead of print 13 June].

Theus S, Lau K, Tabor D, Soderberg L, & Barnett J (1992) In vivo prenatal chlordane exposure induces development of endogenous inflammatory macrophages. J Leukoc Biol, **51**: 366–372.

Thurigen D, Spiegelman D, Blettner M, Heuer C, & Brenner H (2000) Measurement error correction using validation data: A review of methods and their applicability in case–control studies. Stat Methods Med Res, **9**: 447–474.

Tomatis L & Mohr U eds (1973) Transplacental carcinogenesis. Lyon, International Agency for Research on Cancer (IARC Scientific Publications No. 4).

Treluyer JM, Cheron G, Sonnier M, & Cresteil T (1996) Cytochrome P450 expression in sudden infant death syndrome. Biochem Pharmacol, **52**: 497–504.

Tucker MA, D'Angio GJ, Boice JD, Strong LC, Li FP, Stovall M, Stone BJ, Green DM, Lombardi F, & Newton W (1987) Bone sarcomas linked to radiotherapy and chemotherapy in children. N Engl J Med, **317**: 588–593.

Tufro-McReddie A, Johns DW, Geary KM, Dagli H, Everett AD, Chevalier RL, Carey RM, & Gomez RA (1994) Angiotensin II type 1 receptor: Role in renal growth and gene expression during normal development. Am J Physiol, **266**(6 Pt 2): F911–F918.

Turner PC, Sylla A, Diallo MS, Castegnaro JJ, Hall AJ, & Wild CP (2002) The role of aflatoxins and hepatitis viruses in the etiopathogenesis of hepatocellular carcinoma: A basis for primary prevention in Guinea–Conakry, West Africa. J Gastroenterol Hepatol, **17**(Suppl): S441–S448.

Tyler WS, Tyler NK, Last JA, Gillespie MJ, & Barstow TJ (1988) Comparison of daily and seasonal exposures of young monkeys to ozone. Toxicology, **50**(2): 131–144.

Tzimas G, Thiel R, Chahoud I, & Nau H (1997) The area under the concentration–time curve of all-*trans*-retinoic acid is the most suitable pharmacokinetic correlate to the embryotoxicity of this retinoid in the rat. Toxicol Appl Pharmacol, **143**(2): 436–444.

Ueda Y, Stick SM, Hall G, & Sly PD (1999) Control of breathing in infants born to smoking mothers. J Pediatr, **135**(2 Pt 1): 226–232.

UN (2001a) Report of the United Nations Secretary-General Kofi A. Annan: We the children: End-decade review of the follow-up to the World Summit for Children. New York, UNICEF for the United Nations (A/S-27/3; http://www.unicef.org).

UN (2001b) United Nations synthesis report on arsenic in drinking water (draft). Developed on behalf of the United Nations Administrative Committee on Cooperation Sub-Committee on Water Resources, with active participation of UNICEF, UNIDO, IAEA, and the World Bank. Geneva, World Health Organization (http://www.who.int/water_sanitation_health/dwq/arsenic3/en/).

UNDP (1999) Artisanal mining for sustainable livelihoods. New York, United Nations Development Programme.

UNEP (2000) Mining — facts, figures and environment. In: Mining and sustainable development. II. Challenges and perspectives. Paris, United Nations Environment Programme, Division of Technology, Industry, and Economics, pp 4–8 (Industry and Environment Vol. 23 Special Issue).

UNEP (2002) Global mercury assessment. Geneva, United Nations Environment Programme.

UNEP (2004) Stockholm Convention on Persistent Organic Pollutants (POPS). Geneva, United Nations Environment Programme (http://www.pops.int/).

UNHCR (2001) Refugee operations and environmental management: Selected lessons learned. United Nations High Commissioner for Refugees, Engineering and Environmental Services Section.

UNHCR (2002) Global Consultations Ec/Gc/02/9 on International Protection 4th Meeting Original: Refugee children. United Nations High Commissioner for Refugees.

UNHCR (2003) Statistics. Geneva, United Nations High Commissioner for Refugees (http://www.unhcr.org/cgi-bin/texis/vtx/statistics).

UNICEF (1990) First call for children: World Declaration and Plan of Action from the World Summit for Children and the Convention on the Rights of the Child. New York, United Nations Children's Fund.

UNICEF (2001a) Progress since the World Summit for Children: A statistical review. New York, United Nations Children's Fund.

UNICEF (2001b) Fluoride in water: An overview. New York, United Nations Children's Fund (http://www.unicef.org/wes/fluoride.pdf).

UNICEF (2001c) Partnerships to create child-friendly cities: Programming for child rights with local authorities. Florence, International Union of Local Authorities and United Nations Children's Fund (http://www.childfriendlycities.org/pdf/brochure.pdf).

UNICEF (2004) Child labour. New York, United Nations Children's Fund (http://www.unicef.org/protection/index_childlabour.html).

UNICEF (2005a) The state of the world's children 2005. New York, United Nations Children's Fund.

UNICEF (2005b) A study on street children in Zimbabwe. New York, United Nations Children's Fund (http://www.unicef.org/evaldatabase/ZIM_01-805.pdf).

References

UNICEF (2006) The state of the world's children 2006. New York, United Nations Children's Fund (http://www.unicef.org/sowc06/index.php).

USEPA (1990) Exposure factors handbook. Washington, DC, United States Environmental Protection Agency, Office of Health and Environmental Assessment (EPA/600/8-98/043).

USEPA (1991) Guidelines for developmental toxicity risk assessment. Fed Regist, **56**: 63798.

USEPA (1992a) Guidelines for exposure assessment. Fed Regist, **57**(104): 22888–22938.

USEPA (1992b) Environmental equity: Reducing risks for all communities. Washington, DC, United States Environmental Protection Agency, Office of Policy, Planning and Evaluation (http://www.epa.gov/history/topics/justice/01.htm).

USEPA (1996) Guidelines for reproductive toxicity risk assessment. Fed Regist, **61**(212): 56274–56322.

USEPA (1998) Developmental neurotoxicity study. Health effects test guidelines. Washington, DC, United States Environmental Protection Agency, Office of Prevention, Pesticides and Toxic Substances (EPA Document 712-C-98-239; OPPTS 870.6300; http://www.epa.gov/opptsfrs/publications/OPPTS_Harmonized/870_Health_Effects_Test_Guidelines/Series/870-6300.pdf).

USEPA (2000) Benchmark dose technical guidance document (external review draft). Washington, DC, United States Environmental Protection Agency (EPA/630/R-00/001; http://cfpub.epa.gov/ncea/raf/recordisplay.cfm?deid=20871).

USEPA (2001) Draft protocol for measuring children's non-occupational exposure to pesticides by all relevant pathways. Research Triangle Park, NC, United States Environmental Protection Agency, Office of Research and Development (EPA/600/R-03/026).

USEPA (2002a) Child-specific exposure factors handbook (interim report). Washington, DC, United States Environmental Protection Agency, Office of Research and Development, National Center for Environmental Assessment (EPA-600-P-00-002B).

USEPA (2002b) A review of the reference dose and reference concentration processes. Washington, DC, United States Environmental Protection Agency, Risk Assessment Forum (EPA/630/P-02/002F).

USEPA (2003a) Dietary exposure potential model: A model using extant food databases to estimate dietary exposure to chemical residues. Latest version 5.0 released April 2003. Washington, DC, United States Environmental Protection Agency (http://www.epa.gov/nerlcwww/depm.htm).

USEPA (2003b) Framework for cumulative risk assessment. Washington, DC, United States Environmental Protection Agency, Risk Assessment Forum (EPA/630/P-02/001F).

USEPA (2003c) Chromated copper arsenate (CCA): Cancellation of residential uses of CCA-treated wood. Washington, DC, United States Environmental Protection Agency (http://www.epa.gov/oppad001/reregistration/cca/residential_use_cancellation.htm).

USEPA (2004a) Background information on mercury sources and regulations. Washington, DC, United States Environmental Protection Agency (http://www.epa.gov/grtlakes/bnsdocs/mercsrce).

USEPA (2004b) A pilot study of children's total exposure to persistent pesticides and other persistent organic pollutants (CTEPP). Washington, DC, United States Environmental Protection Agency (EPA/600/R-04/193).

USEPA (2004c) Lead in paint, dust, and soil: Protect your child from lead poisoning. Washington, DC, United States Environmental Protection Agency (http://www.epa.gov/opptintr/lead/index.html).

USEPA (2005a) A framework for assessing health risks of environmental exposures to children. Washington, DC, United States Environmental Protection Agency, Office of Research and Development (EPA/600/R-05/093A).

USEPA (2005b) Human exposure modeling — Air Pollutants Exposure Model (APEX/TRIM.Expo$_{Inhalation}$). Washington, DC, United States Environmental Protection Agency (http://www.epa.gov/ttnmain1/fera/human_apex.html).

USEPA (2005c) Indoor air quality — Mold. Mold resources. Washington, DC, United States Environmental Protection Agency (http://www.epa.gov/mold/moldresources.html).

USEPA (2005d) Supplemental guidance for assessing susceptibility from early-life exposure to carcinogens. Washington, DC, United States Environmental Protection Agency, Risk Assessment Forum (EPA/630/R-03/).

USEPA (2005e) Integrated Exposure Uptake Biokinetic Model for Lead in Children, Windows® version (IEUBKwin v1.0 build 263) (December 2005) 32-bit version. Washington, DC, United States Environmental Protection Agency (http://www.epa.gov/superfund/programs/lead/products.htm#software).

USEPA (2006a) Guidance on selecting age groups for monitoring and assessing childhood exposures to environmental contaminants (2005), final report. Washington, DC, United States Environmental Protection Agency, Risk Assessment Forum (http://cfpub.epa.gov/ncea/cfm/recordisplay.cfm?deid=146583).

USEPA (2006b) Organophosphorus cumulative risk assessment, 2006 update. Washington, DC, United States Environmental Protection Agency, Office of Pesticide Programs (EPA ID Docket No. EPA-HQ-OPP-2006-0618).

USFDA (1996) Food Quality Protection Act. Public Law 104-107. Washington, DC, United States Food and Drug Administration (http://www.fda.gov/opacom/laws/foodqual/fqpatoc.htm).

Vainio S, Heikkila M, Kispert A, Chin N, & McMahon AP (1999) Female development in mammals is regulated by Wnt-4 signalling. Nature, **397**: 405–409.

Valent F, Little D, Bertollini R, Nemer L, Barbone F, & Tamburlini G (2004) Burden of disease attributable to selected environmental factors and injury among children and adolescents in Europe. Lancet, **363**(9426): 2032–2039.

Van Vliet P, Knape M, de Hartog J, Janssen N, Harssema H, & Brunekreef B (1997) Motor vehicle exhaust and chronic respiratory symptoms in children living near freeways. Environ Res, **74**: 122–132.

Vaupotic J (2002) Search for radon sources in buildings — kindergartens. J Environ Radioact, **61**: 365–372.

Vedal S, Petkau J, White R, & Blair J (1998) Acute effects of ambient inhalable particles in asthmatic and nonasthmatic children. Am J Respir Crit Care Med, **157**: 1034–1043.

Veldhuis JD, Roemmich JN, Richmond EJ, Rogol AD, Lovejoy JC, Sheffield-Moore M, Mauras N, & Bowers CY (2005) Endocrine control of body composition in infancy, childhood, and puberty. Endocr Rev, **26**: 114–146.

Venners SA, Korrick S, Xu X, Chen C, Guang W, Huang A, Altshul L, Perry M, Fu L, & Wang X (2005) Preconception serum DDT and pregnancy loss: A prospective study using a biomarker of pregnancy. Am J Epidemiol, **162**(8): 726–728.

Vohr BR & Msall ME (1997) Neuropsychological and functional outcomes of very low birth weight infants. Semin Perinatal, **21**(3): 202–220.

Volkmer RE, Ruffin RE, Wigg NR, & Davies N (1995) The prevalence of respiratory symptoms in South Australian children. II. Factors associated with indoor air quality. J Paediatr Child Health, **31**: 116–120.

Von Hertzen L (2002) Maternal stress and T-cell differentiation of the developing immune system: Possible implications for the development of asthma and atopy. J Allergy Clin Immunol, **109**: 923–998.

von Mutius E (2002) Environmental factors influencing the development and progression of pediatric asthma. J Allergy Clin Immunol, **109**(Suppl 6): S525–S532.

Vos J & Moore J (1974) Suppression of cellular immunity in rats and mice by maternal treatment with 2,3,7,8-tetrachlorodibenzo-*p*-dioxin. Int Arch Allergy Appl Immunol, **47**: 777–794.

Vreugdenhil HJ, Mulder PG, Emmen HH, & Weisglas-Kuperus N (2004) Effects of perinatal exposure to PCBs on neuropsychological functions in the Rotterdam cohort at 9 years of age. Neuropsychology, **18**(1): 185–189.

Waalkes MP, Ward JM, Liu J, & Diwan B (2003) Transplacental carcinogenicity of inorganic arsenic in the drinking water: Induction of hepatic, ovarian, pulmonary and adrenal tumors in mice. Toxicol Appl Pharmacol, **186**: 7–17.

Wacholder S (1991) Practical considerations in choosing between the case–cohort and nested case–control designs. Epidemiology, **2**: 155–158.

Wakeford R & Little MP (2003) Risk coefficients for childhood cancer after intrauterine irradiation: A review. Int J Radiat Biol, **79**: 293–309.

Walker C, Amed SA, Brown T, Ho SM, Hodges L, Lucier G, Russo J, Weigel N, Weise T, & Vandenbergh J (1999) Species, interindividual, and tissue specificity in endocrine signaling. Environ Health Perspect, **107**(Suppl 4): 619–624.

Walker JT & Walker OA (2000) A multiphasic approach for describing serial height data of Fels children: A hexaphasic-logistic-additive growth model. Growth Dev Aging, **64**(1–2): 33–49.

Walthall K, Cappon G, Hurtt M, & Zoetis T (2005) Postnatal development of the gastrointestinal system: A species comparison. Birth Defects Res B Dev Reprod Toxicol, **74**: 132–156.

Wang X, Zuckerman B, Pearson C, Kaufman G, Wang G, Niu T, Wise PH, Bauchner H, & Xu X (2002) Maternal cigarette smoking, metabolic gene polymorphism, and infant birth weight. JAMA, **287**: 195–202.

Wang X, Chen C, Wang L, Chen D, Guang W, & French J (2003) Conception, early pregnancy loss, and time to clinical pregnancy: A population-based prospective study. Fertil Steril, **79**: 577–584.

Wantke F, Demmer CM, Tappler P, Gotz M, & Jarisch R (1996) Exposure to gaseous formaldehyde induces IgE-mediated sensitization to formaldehyde in school-children. Clin Exp Allergy, **26**(3): 276–280.

Ware JH, Spengler JD, Neas LM, Samet JM, Wagner GR, Coultas D, Ozkaynak H, & Schwab M (1993) Respiratory and irritant health effects of ambient volatile organic compounds. The Kanawha County Health Study. Am J Epidemiol, **137**(12): 1287–1301.

Wasserman GA, Staghezza-Jaramillo B, Shrout P, Popovac D, & Graziano J (1998) The effect of lead exposure on behavior problems in preschool children. Am J Public Health, **88**(3): 481–486.

Wasserman GA, Liu X, Parvez F, Ahsan H, Factor-Litvak P, van Geen A, Slavkovich V, Lolacono NJ, Cheng Z, Hussain I, Momotaj H, & Graziano JH (2004) Water arsenic exposure and children's intellectual function in Araihazar, Bangladesh. Environ Health Perspect, **112**(13): 1329–1333.

Wasserman GA, Liu X, Parvez F, Ahsan H, Levy D, Factor-Litvak P, Kline J, van Geen A, Slavkovich V, Lolacono NJ, Cheng Z, Zheng Y, & Graziano JH (2006) Water manganese exposure and children's intellectual function in Araihazar, Bangladesh. Environ Health Perspect, **114**(1): 124–129.

Weinberg CR, Wilcox AJ, & Baird DD (1989) Reduced fecundability in women with prenatal exposure to cigarette smoke. Am J Epidemiol, **129**: 1072–1078.

Weisbach V, Koch HM, Angerer J, & Eckstein R (2006) Di(2-ethylhexyl)phthalate exposure of apheresis donors is procedure-related. Transfusion, **46**(8): 1457–1458.

Weiss B & Landrigan PJ (2000) The developing brain and the environment: An introduction. Environ Health Perspect, **108**(Suppl 3): 373–374.

References

Weisskopf MG, Anderson HA, & Hanrahan LP (2003) Decreased sex ratio following maternal exposure to polychlorinated biphenyls from contaminated Great Lakes sport-caught fish: A retrospective cohort study. Environ Health Global Access Sci Source, **2**: 2 (http://www.ehjournal.net/content/2/1/2).

Weller E, Long N, Smith A, Williams P, Ravi S, Gill J, Henessey R, Skornik W, Brain J, Kimmel C, Kimmel G, Holmes L, & Ryan L (1999) Dose-rate effects of ethylene oxide exposure on developmental toxicity. Toxicol Sci, **50**(2): 259–270.

Wessels D, Barr DB, & Mendola P (2003) Use of biomarkers to indicate exposure of children to organophosphate pesticides: Implications for a longitudinal study of children's environmental health. Environ Health Perspect, **111**(16): 1939–1946.

West L (2002) Defining critical windows in the development of the human immune system. Hum Exp Toxicol, **21**: 499–505.

WHO (1980) International classification of impairments, disabilities and handicaps: A manual of classification relating to the consequences of disease. Geneva, World Health Organization.

WHO (1983) Temporal relationships between indices of the fertile period. Fertil Steril, **39**: 647–655.

WHO (1997) Health and environment in sustainable development: Five years after the Earth Summit. Geneva, World Health Organization.

WHO (1999) Food safety — an essential public health issue for the new millennium. Geneva, World Health Organization (http://www.who.int/foodsafety/publications/general/brochure_1999/en/).

WHO (2001) Water for health: Taking charge. Geneva, World Health Organization.

WHO (2002a) Healthy environments for children. Geneva, World Health Organization (WHO/SDE/PHE/02.05).

WHO (2002b) The world health report: Reducing risks, promoting healthy life. Geneva, World Health Organization.

WHO (2002c) Children in the new millennium: Environmental impact on health. Geneva, World Health Organization, United Nations Environment Programme, and United Nations Children's Fund (http://www.unep.org/ceh/).

WHO (2003a) The world health report: Shaping the future. Geneva, World Health Organization.

WHO (2003b) Guidelines for safe recreational waters. Volume 1. Coastal and fresh waters. Geneva, World Health Organization.

WHO (2004a) Nutrition: Nutrition for health and development. Geneva, World Health Organization (http://www.who.int/nutrition/en/).

WHO (2004b) Burden of disease attributable to selected environmental factors and injuries among Europe's children and adolescents. Copenhagen, World Health Organization Regional Office for Europe (EUR/04/5046267/BD/10).

WHO (2004C) Inheriting the World. The Atlas of Children's Health and the Environment. Geneva, World Health Organization (http://www.who.int).

WHO (2005a) The world health report: Make every mother and child count. Redesigning child care: Survival, growth and development. Geneva, World Health Organization (http://www.who.int/whr/2005/en/).

WHO (2005b) Mayo report on addressing the worldwide tobacco epidemic through effective, evidence-based treatment. Geneva, World Health Organization (http://www.who.int/tobacco/resources/publications/mayo/en/index1.html).

WHO (2006) Guidelines for safe recreational waters. Volume 2. Swimming pools and similar environments. Geneva, World Health Organization.

Widdowson EM & Dickerson JWT (1964) Chemical composition of the body. In: Comar CL & Bronner F eds. Mineral metabolism. New York, Academic Press, pp 1–247.

Wieslander G, Norback D, Bjornsson E, Janson C, & Boman G (1997) Asthma and the indoor environment: The significance of emission of formaldehyde and volatile organic compounds from newly painted indoor surfaces. Int Arch Occup Environ Health, **69**(2): 115–124.

Wijeyaratne P (1993) Control of disease vectors: A current perspective. In: Forget G, Goodman T, & de Villiers A eds. Impact of pesticide use on health in developing countries. Ottawa, Ontario, International Development Research Centre, pp 263–279.

Wilcox AJ, Weinberg CR, O'Connor JF, Baird DD, Schlatterer JP, Canfield RE, Armstrong EG, & Nisula BC (1988) Incidence of early loss of pregnancy. N Engl J Med, **319**: 189–194.

Wild CP, Jiang YZ, Allen SJ, Jansen LA, Hall AJ, & Montesano R (1990) Aflatoxin-albumin adducts in human sera from different regions of the world. Carcinogenesis, **11**(12): 2271–2274.

Wilhelm M & Ritz B (2003) Residential proximity to traffic and adverse birth outcomes in Los Angeles county, California, 1994–1996. Environ Health Perspect, **111**(2): 207–216.

Williams M, Goldman MB, Mittendorf R, & Monson R (1991) Subfertility and the risk of low birthweight. Fertil Steril, **56**: 668–671.

Wilson JD, Griffin JE, & Russell DW (1993) Steroid 5 alpha-reductase 2 deficiency. Endocr Rev, **14**: 577–593.

Wilson JG (1965) Embryological considerations in teratology. In: Wilson JG & Warkany J eds. Teratology: Principles and techniques. Chicago, IL, University of Chicago Press.

Windham GC, Shusterman D, Swan S, Fenster L, & Eskenazi B (1991) Exposure to organic solvents and adverse pregnancy outcome. Am J Ind Med, **20**: 214–259.

References

Windham GC, Eaton A, & Hopkins B (1999) Evidence for an association between environmental tobacco smoke exposure and birthweight: A meta-analysis and new data. Paediatr Perinat Epidemiol, **13**: 35–57.

Winneke G, Walkowiak J, & Lilienthal H (2002) PCB-induced neurodevelopmental toxicity in human infants and its potential mediation by endocrine dysfunction. Toxicology, **181–182**: 161–165.

Wise LD, Beck SL, Beltrame D, Beyer BK, Chahoud I, Clark RL, Clark R, Druga AM, Feuston MH, Guittin P, Henwood SM, Kimmel CA, Lindstrom P, Palmer AK, Petrere JA, Solomon HM, Yasuda M, & York RG (1997) Terminology of developmental abnormalities in common laboratory mammals (version 1). Teratology, **55**(4): 249–292.

Wittsiepe J, Schrey P, Hack A, Selenka F, & Wilhelm M (2001) Comparison of different digestive tract models for estimating bioaccessibility of polychlorinated dibenzo-p-dioxins and dibenzofurans (PCDD/F) from red slag "Kieselrot". Int J Hyg Environ Health, **203**: 263–273.

Wjst M, Reitmeir P, Dold S, Wulff A, Nicolai T, von Loeffelholz-Colberg EF, & von Mutius E (1993) Road traffic and adverse effects on respiratory health in children. Br Med J, **307**: 596–600.

Wood JW (1994) Dynamics of human reproduction: Biology, biometry, demography. New York, Aldine de Gruyer.

Woodcock A & Custovic A (1998) Avoiding exposure to indoor allergens. Br Med J, **316**: 1075–1082.

World Bank (2001) The state of the world's children — early childhood. Washington, DC, The World Bank (http://www.unicef.org/sowc/index_sowc.html).

World Bank (2005) World development indicators 2005. Washington, DC, The World Bank (http://www.worldbank.org/data/wdi2005/).

WRI (2002) Environmental health indicator. Developing countries: Potential exposure to polluted outdoor air. Washington, DC, World Resources Institute (http://pdf.wri.org/ehi_outairdev.pdf).

Wright RO, Amarasiriwardena C, Woolf JR, & Bellinger DC (2006) Neuropsychological correlates of hair arsenic, manganese, and cadmium levels in school-age children residing near a hazardous waste site. Neurotoxicology, **27**(2): 210–216.

Wu T, Buck GM, & Mendola P (2003) Blood lead levels and sexual maturation in U.S. girls: The Third National Health and Nutrition Examination Survey, 1988–94. Environ Health Perspect, **111**(5): 737–741.

Wyler C, Braun-Fahrlander C, Kunzli N, Schindler C, Ackermann-Liebrich U, Perruchoud AP, Leuenberger P, & Wuthrich B (2000) Exposure to motor vehicle traffic and allergic sensitization. The Swiss Study on Air Pollution and Lung Diseases in Adults (SAPALDIA) Team. Epidemiology, **11**(4): 450–456.

Yamashita F & Hayashi M (1985) Fetal PCB syndrome: Clinical features, intrauterine growth retardation and possible alteration in calcium metabolism. Environ Health Perspect, 59: 41–45.

Yáñez L, Batres L, Carrizales L, Santoyo M, Escalante V, & Díaz-Barriga F (1994) Toxicological assessment of azarcon, a lead salt used as a folk remedy in Mexico. I. Oral toxicity in rats. J Ethnopharmacol, 41: 91–97.

Yáñez L, Ortiz-Péres D, Batres LE, Borja-Aburto VH, & Díaz-Barriga F (2002a) Levels of dichlorodiphenyltrichloroethane and deltamethrin in humans and environmental samples in malarious areas of Mexico. Environ Res, 88: 174–181.

Yáñez L, Ortiz D, Calderón J, Batres L, Carrizales L, Mejía J, Martínez L, García-Nieto E, & Díaz-Barriga F (2002b) Overview of human health and chemical mixtures: Problems facing developing countries. Environ Health Perspect, 110(Suppl 6): 901–909.

Yáñez L, García-Nieto E, Rojas E, Carrizales L, Mejía J, Calderón J, Razo I, & Díaz-Barriga (2003) DNA damage in blood cells from children exposed to arsenic and lead in a mining area. Environ Res, 93: 231–240.

Yazdanbakhsh M, Kremsner P, & van Ree R (2002) Allergy, parasites and the hygiene hypothesis. Science, 296: 490–494.

Yiin LM, Rhoads GG, & Lioy PJ (2000) Seasonal influences on childhood lead exposure. Environ Health Perspect, 108(2): 177–182.

Yolton K, Dietrich K, Auinger P, Lanphear BP, & Hornung R (2005) Exposure to tobacco smoke and cognitive abilities among U.S. children and adolescents. Environ Health Perspect, 113(1): 98–103.

Yoshimura T, Kaneko S, & Hayabuchi H (2001) Sex ratio in offspring of those affected by dioxin and dioxin like compounds: The Yusho, Seveso, and Yucheng incidents. Occup Environ Med, 58: 540–541.

Young S, Le Souef PN, Geelhoed GC, Stick SM, Turner KJ, & Landau LI (1991) The influence of a family history of asthma and parental smoking on airway responsiveness in early infancy. N Engl J Med, 324: 1168–1173.

Zarba A, Wild CP, Hall AJ, Montesano R, Hudson GJ, & Groopman JD (1992) Aflatoxin M_1 in human breast milk from The Gambia, west Africa, quantified by combined monoclonal antibody immunoaffinity chromatography and HPLC. Carcinogenesis, 13(5): 891–894.

Zartarian VG, Ozkaynak H, Burke JM, Zufall MJ, Rigas ML, & Furtaw EJ Jr (2000) A modeling framework for estimating children's residential exposure and dose to chlorpyrifos via dermal residue contact and nondietary ingestion. Environ Health Perspect, 108(6): 505–514.

Zoetis T & Hurtt ME (2003a) Species comparison of lung development. Birth Defects Res B Dev Reprod Toxicol, 68(2): 121–124.

Zoetis T & Hurtt ME (2003b) Species comparison of anatomical and functional renal development. Birth Defects Res B Dev Reprod Toxicol, 68(2): 111–120.

References

Zoetis T & Walls I eds (2003) Principles & practices for direct dosing of pre-weaning mammals in toxicity testing and research. A report of the ILSI Risk Science Institute Expert Working Group on Direct Dosing of Pre-weaning Mammals in Toxicity Testing. Washington, DC, International Life Sciences Institute, ILSI Press.

Zoetis T, Tassinari M, Bagi C, Walthall K, & Hurtt M (2003) Species comparison of postnatal bone growth and development. Birth Defects Res B Dev Reprod Toxicol, **68**(2): 86–110.

ANNEX 1: WORKING DEFINITIONS OF KEY TERMS

Adolescence: The period of life beginning with the appearance of secondary sex characteristics and terminating with the achievement of full maturity (usually 12–18 years of age).

Adult: The time of life usually starting at 18 years (some systems such as skeleton and brain may continue to develop).

Adverse effect: A treatment-related alteration from baseline that diminishes an organism's ability to survive, reproduce, or adapt to the environment.

Aggregate risk assessment: The evaluation of risk from exposure to a given chemical from multiple routes of exposure.

Critical period: A specific phase during which a developing system is particularly susceptible.

Cumulative risk assessment: The evaluation of the risk of exposure to two or more chemicals. The USEPA defines cumulative exposure under the Food Quality Protection Act to be the evaluation of the risk of exposure to two or more pesticides that work through a common mechanism of action.

Developmental toxicity: Taken in its widest sense, includes any effect interfering with normal development both before and after birth. The occurrence of adverse effects in the developing organism may result from exposure of either parent prior to conception, exposure during prenatal development, or exposure postnatally to the time of full maturity. Adverse developmental effects may be detected at any point in the lifespan of the organism.

Dose (exposure)–response relationship: Characterization of the relationship between administered dose or exposure and the biological change in organisms. It may be expressed as the severity of an effect in one organism (or part of an organism) or as the proportion of an exposed population that shows a specific reaction.

Annex 1: Working Definitions of Key Terms

Embryonic period: The period from fertilization to the end of major organogenesis.

Endocrine disruptor: An exogenous substance or mixture that alters function(s) of the endocrine system and consequently causes adverse health effects in an intact organism or its progeny or (sub)populations.

Environment: Factors external to the human host, including physical, chemical, biological, social, cultural, and economic factors — any or all of which can influence health status of populations.

Environmental exposures and *Environmental factors*: For this document, these terms refer to specific environmental chemicals and environmental pollutants.

Exposure assessment: The qualitative and/or quantitative assessment of the chemical nature, form, and concentration of a chemical to which an identified population is exposed from all sources (e.g. air, water, soil, and diet).

Exposure pathway: The physical course taken by an agent as it moves from a source to a point of contact with a person. The substance present is quantified as its concentration.

Exposure route: Exposure route denotes the different ways a substance may enter the body. The route may be dermal, ingestion, or inhalation.

Fetal period: The period from the end of embryogenesis to the completion of pregnancy.

Fetus: The period from eight weeks of pregnancy to birth.

Gestation: Length of time between conception and birth.

Hazard characterization: Involves determining whether or not an agent poses a hazard, at what doses, and under what conditions of exposure.

Hazard identification: The identification of the inherent capability of a substance to cause adverse effects.

Infant: The period from 28 days of age to one year.

Integrated risk assessment: A science-based approach that combines the processes of risk estimation for humans, biota, and natural resources in one assessment.

Lowest-observed-adverse-effect level (LOAEL): The lowest concentration or amount of a substance, found by experiment or observation, that causes an adverse alteration of morphology, functional capacity, growth, development, or lifespan of the target organism distinguishable from normal (control) organisms of the same species and strain under the same defined conditions of exposure.

Margin of exposure (MOE): The ratio of the NOAEL to the estimated exposure dose.

Mechanism of action: The detailed molecular knowledge of the key events leading to an adverse effect in an organism.

Mode of action: The cascade of events that occur during the development of an adverse effect following exposure to a chemical.

Neonate: The period from birth to 28 days of age.

No-observed-adverse-effect level (NOAEL): Highest concentration or amount of a substance, found by experiment or observation, that causes no detectable adverse alteration of morphology, functional capacity, growth, development, or lifespan of the target organism under defined conditions of exposure. Alterations of morphology, functional capacity, growth, development, or lifespan of the target organism may be detected that are not judged to be adverse.

No-observed-effect level (NOEL): Highest concentration or amount of a substance, found by experiment or observation, that causes no alterations of morphology, functional capacity, growth, development, or lifespan of the target organism distinguishable from those observed in normal (control) organisms of the same species and strain under the same defined conditions of exposure.

Annex 1: Working Definitions of Key Terms

Normal-term birth: The period of 40 ± 2 weeks of pregnancy.

Perinatal stage: The period of 29 weeks of pregnancy to seven days after birth.

Pregnancy: The condition of having an implanted embryo or fetus in the body, after fusion of an ovum and spermatozoon.

Preterm birth: A birth occurring at 24–37 weeks of pregnancy.

Risk assessment: An empirically based paradigm that estimates the risk of adverse effect(s) from exposure of an individual or population to a chemical, physical, or biological agent. It includes the components of hazard identification, assessment of dose–response relationships, exposure assessment, and risk characterization.

Risk characterization: The synthesis of critically evaluated information and data from exposure assessment, hazard identification, and dose–response considerations into a summary that identifies clearly the strengths and weaknesses of the database, the criteria applied to evaluation and validation of all aspects of methodology, and the conclusions reached from the review of scientific information.

Sexual maturation: Achievement of full development of the reproductive system and sexual function.

Susceptibility: An individual's intrinsic or acquired traits that modify the risk of illness (e.g. high susceptibility to cancer). Sensitivity and susceptibility are often used interchangeably, but susceptibility is the preferred term, because sensitivity has several other usages (e.g. detection limits for analytical methods).

Tolerable intake: An estimate of the intake of a substance that can occur over a lifetime without appreciable health risk. It may have different units, depending on the route of administration.

Toxicodynamics: The process of interaction of chemical substances with target sites and the subsequent reactions leading to adverse effects.

Toxicokinetics: The process of the uptake of potentially toxic substances by the body, the biotransformation they undergo, the distribution of the substances and their metabolites in the tissues, and the elimination of the substances and their metabolites from the body. Both the amounts and the concentrations of the substances and their metabolites are studied. (Pharmacokinetics is the term used to study pharmaceutical substances.)

Vulnerability: A matrix of physical, chemical, biological, social, and cultural factors that result in certain communities and subpopulations being more susceptible to environmental factors because of greater exposure to such factors or a compromised ability to cope with and/or recover from such exposure. Four types of vulnerability are considered with regard to a life stage approach: susceptibility or sensitivity, differential exposure, differential preparedness, and differential ability to recover.

RESUME, CONCLUSIONS ET RECOMMANDATIONS

1. Résumé

Les facteurs environnementaux jouent un rôle important dans la santé et le bien-être des enfants.[1] On possède des indications de plus en plus nombreuses selon lesquelles les enfants, qui représentent plus d'un tiers des habitants de la planète, comptent parmi les plus vulnérables d'entre eux et ont un état de santé dont la dépendance vis-à-vis des facteurs environnementaux est tout à fait autre que chez l'adulte. Les plus exposés à la souffrance sont ceux qui vivent dans la pauvreté, manquent de soins et sont en proie à la malnutrition. Ces enfants vivent souvent dans des taudis, ne disposent ni d'eau propre, ni de services d'assainissement et n'ont qu'un accès limité aux soins et à l'enseignement. On estime que dans les régions les plus pauvres du monde, un enfant sur cinq n'atteint pas son cinquième anniversaire, principalement en raison de maladies liées à l'état de l'environnement. Selon les estimations de l'Organisation mondiale de la Santé (OMS), les facteurs environnementaux peuvent être tenus pour responsables, à hauteur de plus de 30 %, de l'ensemble des maladies dont souffrent les enfants dans le monde.

La santé est sous la dépendance d'un certain nombre de facteurs. Outre le milieu physique, la génétique, la biologie, de même que les facteurs sociaux, économiques et culturels jouent un rôle majeur. Il est certes capital de comprendre la nature des facteurs dont l'action, au cours de l'enfance, va déterminer l'état de santé et façonner les comportements tout au long de l'existence, toutefois, c'est plutôt sur l'exposition aux substances chimiques présentes dans l'environnement que porte ce document. Il s'agit en l'occurrence d'une étude des principes scientifiques à prendre en considération pour évaluer le risque couru par les enfants en cas d'exposition, à certains stades déterminés de leur développement, aux substances chimiques présentes dans l'environnement, le but étant d'informer à ce sujet les responsables de la santé publique, les scientifiques des organismes de recherche et de réglementation ainsi que les autres

---

[1] Dans le présent document, le terme « enfant » englobe tous les stades du développement, de la conception à l'adolescence.

spécialistes qui ont la responsabilité de protéger la santé de l'enfant. Cette étude concerne plus spécifiquement les stades de développement que tel ou tel produit chimique particulier présent dans l'environnement ou encore une conséquence ou une maladie déterminées. Les stades de développement ou les périodes particulières au cours desquels l'organisme de l'enfant est sensible aux influences environnementales sont qualifiées de « fenêtres critiques d'exposition » ou de « fenêtres critiques de développement ». Ces divers stades de la vie sont définis par un certain nombre de processus dynamiques importants qui se déroulent au niveau moléculaire et cellulaire, au niveau des organes et appareils ou encore de l'organisme dans son ensemble. Ce sont les différences qui existent entre ces divers stades qui, parallèlement à l'exposition, vont déterminer la nature et la gravité des influences environnementales.

La sensibilité de l'enfant aux influences environnementales varie en fonction des divers stades de croissance et de développement dynamiques par lesquels il passe et du fait des différences d'ordre physiologique, métabolique ou comportemental entre ceux-ci. De la conception à l'adolescence, croissance et développement se déroulent à un rythme rapide qui peut être perturbé par l'exposition à des substances chimiques présentes dans l'environnement. Les processus en cause sont de nature anatomique, physiologique, métabolique, fonctionnelle, toxicocinétique ou toxicodynamique. Les voies et les modalités de cette exposition peuvent également varier selon les différents stades de développement de l'enfant. Il peut ainsi y avoir exposition in utero par passage transplacentaire d'une substance chimique de la mère à l'enfant ou encore par l'intermédiaire du lait lorsque l'enfant est nourri au sein. Un enfant consomme davantage de nourriture et de boisson par unité de poids corporel qu'un adulte et son régime alimentaire, s'il est différent, est souvent plus constant au cours des divers stades de développement. L'enfant a un rythme respiratoire plus rapide et le rapport de son aire corporelle à son poids est également plus élevé, ce qui l'expose davantage aux substances présentes dans l'environnement. Le comportement naturel d'un enfant, par exemple le fait de ramper sur le sol ou de porter ses mains à sa bouche, peut entraîner un type d'exposition qui n'existe pas chez l'adulte. Par ailleurs, ses voies métaboliques peuvent également différer de celles de l'adulte. Un enfant a devant lui un plus grand nombre d'années à vivre et par conséquent plus de temps pour acquérir des maladies chroniques qui mettent des décennies à se manifester et sont susceptibles d'être déclenchées par une

Résumé, Conclusions et Recommandations

exposition environnementale précoce. Bien souvent, l'enfant n'a pas conscience des risques inhérents à l'environnement et n'a généralement pas voix au chapitre dans ce domaine.

Devant l'accumulation de données montrant que l'enfant peut être exposé à un risque plus important au cours des différents stades de son développement, en termes de sensibilité biologique ou d'exposition, on se rend compte qu'il faudrait sans doute envisager l'évaluation du risque sous un autre angle pour protéger sa santé. Traditionnellement, l'évaluation des risques et les politiques menées en matière d'hygiène de l'environnement sont essentiellement centrées sur la santé des adultes et leur mode d'exposition, les données dont il est fait usage étant tirées d'études sur des êtres humains ou des animaux adultes. Il est donc nécessaire d'élargir le cadre théorique de l'évaluation des risques afin de pouvoir étudier l'exposition environnementale propre à l'enfant, depuis la conception jusqu'à l'adolescence, en prenant en compte la sensibilité particulière qui caractérise chaque stade de développement. Les données relatives à l'adulte ne permettent pas de prévoir la totalité des effets susceptibles de découler d'expositions subies au cours de l'enfance. L'évaluation du risque environnemental chez l'enfant doit s'effectuer en fonction du stade de développement.

Il existe chez l'enfant un grand nombre de maladies dont on sait ou soupçonne qu'elles sont liées à l'insalubrité de l'environnement. Presque partout dans le monde, les dangers traditionnellement liés à l'environnement continuent d'être à l'origine de la plupart des pathologies. Il s'agit notamment d'une mauvaise nutrition, d'un assainissement insuffisant, de la contamination de l'eau, de la présence endémique de vecteurs de maladies (par exemple de moustiques qui transmettent le paludisme) ou encore du rejet des déchets dans de mauvaises conditions d'hygiène. En outre, la progression rapide de la mondialisation et de l'industrialisation, couplée à des modes de production et de consommation qui ne sont pas viables, sont à l'origine du déversement dans l'environnement de volumes importants de produits chimiques. Bien que l'expression « exposition environnementale » englobe une pluralité de facteurs, elle est prise dans le présent document dans le sens plus restrictif d'exposition aux substances chimiques présentes dans l'environnement. Dans la plupart des cas, on n'a pas évalué la toxicité potentielle de ces substances pour l'enfant et l'on ne sait pas non plus quelles sont les sous-populations d'enfants les plus vulnérables. Dans plusieurs régions du monde, on observe une augmentation du l'incidence d'un certain nombre de maladies et de troubles pédiatriques importants (par ex. l'asthme ou les troubles neurocomportementaux). S'il est vrai que divers facteurs sont probablement en cause, cet état de fait dépend peut être, en partie, de la qualité de l'environnement dans lequel les enfants vivent, se développent et s'amusent.

Etablir les relations de cause à effet entre telle ou telle exposition environnementale particulière et des issues sanitaires complexes et plurifactorielles est une tâche à la fois difficile et stimulante, notamment lorsqu'il s'agit d'enfants. Chez l'enfant, le stade de développement durant lequel se produit l'exposition est tout aussi important que son ampleur. Il y a très peu d'études dans lesquelles l'exposition est caractérisée par rapport aux différents stades de développement. Les exemples dont on dispose montrent qu'une exposition à la même substance chimique peut avoir des conséquences très différentes sur le plan sanitaire selon qu'il s'agit d'un enfant ou d'un adulte. On a pu montrer que certaines de ces conséquences sont irréversibles et subsistent pendant toute la vie. De plus, la maturation des divers systèmes ou appareils ne s'effectue pas au même rythme, de sorte que la même dose d'un agent donné peut avoir des conséquences très différentes selon le stade de développement au cours duquel elle est reçue. Il peut également y avoir une longue période de latence entre l'exposition et l'apparition de ses effets, certains d'entre eux ne se manifestant que plus tardivement dans l'existence. Parmi les effets sur la santé qui résultent d'une exposition au cours d'un stade de développement donné, on peut citer notamment ceux qui s'observent pendant la période prénatale ou à la naissance (par ex. les fausses couches, les mortinaissances, le faible poids de naissance ou les malformations congénitales), chez le jeune enfant (par ex. la mortalité infantile, l'asthme, les troubles neurocomportementaux ou les déficits immunitaires) ou encore chez l'adolescent (par ex. une puberté précoce ou tardive). On commence à recueillir certaines données qui incitent à penser que l'augmentation du risque de certaines maladies de l'adulte (par ex. les cancers et les cardiopathies) peut être due pour une part, à une exposition à certaines substances chimiques environnementales au cours de l'enfance.

La recherche s'intéresse aux effets, sur la santé de l'enfant, des substances chimiques présentes dans l'environnement, mais les

Résumé, Conclusions et Recommandations

chercheurs se concentrent généralement sur l'exposition à des substances déterminées, comme les métaux lourds ou les pesticides et à un organe cible ou point d'aboutissement donnés. Il est remarquable de constater que ces travaux ne comportent aucune étude prospective longitudinale portant sur l'exposition pendant les fenêtres de sensibilité des divers stades de développement ou les différentes périodes de l'existence. Il n'existe pratiquement aucune étude consacrée à des expositions survenant au cours de la période périconceptionnelle, soit uniquement à ce stade, soit s'ajoutant à des expositions à d'autres stades. Grâce aux progrès technologiques et à de nouvelles méthodes, on espère désormais pouvoir repérer les expositions survenant aux cours de ces périodes critiques. Les chercheurs vont être en mesure de mettre en évidence la conception à un stade précoce et de déterminer le risque possible de mortalité embryonnaire prématurée compte tenu des conséquences pour la santé de l'enfant qui sont subordonnées à sa survie au cours du stade embryonnaire et du stade fœtal.

Les politiques de protection de l'enfance et les méthodes d'évaluation des risques doivent être élaborées en prenant en compte ce point fondamental que constitue la vulnérabilité particulière de l'enfant. Ce n'est pas parce qu'on ne possède pas la preuve absolue de l'existence de relations de cause à effet qu'il ne faut pas s'efforcer de réduire l'exposition aux substances présentes dans l'environnement ou ne pas mettre en œuvre des stratégies d'intervention ou de prévention.

2. Conclusions et recommandations

La connaissance des effets, sur la santé de l'enfant, d'une exposition à des substances présentes dans l'environnement a sensiblement progressé mais nous avons encore beaucoup à apprendre. Une évaluation des risques dans un souci de protection de l'enfant doit se fonder sur une meilleure connaissance des interactions entre exposition, sensibilité biologique et facteurs socio-économiques ou culturels (y compris nutritionnels) à chaque stade du développement. Pour y parvenir, il sera nécessaire d'effectuer les travaux de recherche suivants :

- Concevoir et effectuer des études prospectives sur des cohortes de femmes enceintes, de nourrissons et d'enfants plus âgés en s'efforçant de repérer les expositions qui se produisent lors des périodes critiques du développement et de déterminer leurs points d'aboutissement tout au long du développement humain. A cet effet, il faut essayer de recruter des couples avant la conception afin de recueillir des données essentielles pour comprendre l'influence des expositions survenant au cours de la période périconceptionnelle sur la santé de l'enfant.

- Continuer à mettre en place ou à développer des systèmes de surveillance en population pour recueillir en temps réel des données sur les points d'aboutissement sentinelles de l'exposition. Il s'agit notamment de systèmes de surveillance tels que l'enregistrement de la taille de naissance ou la tenue de registres des anomalies ou malformations congénitales afin de repérer les plus importantes d'entre elles. Il faudrait également qu'on envisage d'étudier davantage certains points d'aboutissement sentinelles de l'exposition tels que la fertilité, en mesurant des variables telles que le temps nécessaire à l'obtention d'une grossesse et le rapport de masculinité.

- Renforcer encore la surveillance de l'exposition chez l'enfant au cours des différents stades de son développement en s'efforçant notamment d'évaluer l'exposition globale ou cumulée.

- Renforcer la surveillance de l'exposition dans les pays en développement.

- Recenser les sous-populations les plus exposées.

- Elaborer des marqueurs biologiques valables, sensibles et économiques de l'exposition, de la sensibilité et des effets sur la santé, notamment au cours des premiers stades du développement.

- Améliorer la caractérisation des différences entre les propriétés toxicocinétiques et toxicodynamiques des produits xénobiotiques au cours des divers stades du développement. Etablir des bases de données répertoriant les paramètres physiologiques et pharmacocinétiques spécifiques des divers stades du développement tant chez l'animal que chez l'Homme.

Résumé, Conclusions et Recommandations

- Effectuer des études visant tout particulièrement à déterminer par quels mécanismes l'exposition aux substances chimiques environnementales au cours des différents stades du développement peut conduire à des effets nocifs sur la santé.

- Définir des événements cibles qui puissent être utilisés pour évaluer la fonction des organes ou appareils chez l'Homme et l'animal et identifier, chez les différentes espèces, les stades de développement qui sont similaires.

- Examiner l'intérêt des nouvelles techniques moléculaires ou d'imagerie pour déterminer les relations de cause à effet entre l'exposition et les effets observés aux différents stades de développement.

- Mieux caractériser les fenêtres de sensibilité des différents organes ou appareils eu égard aux points d'aboutissement structuraux ou fonctionnels.

- Elaborer et valider des modèles biologiques et des principes directeurs pour l'expérimentation animale applicables aux effets qui se produisent aux divers stades du développement.

- Déterminer quel type d'exposition il faudrait réduire pour obtenir un effet global maximal sur la santé de l'enfant.

L'élaboration de stratégies d'évaluation des risques portant sur les stades de développement par lesquels toutes les générations futures doivent passer est un élément capital de toute politique de santé publique. La protection de l'enfant est essentielle à la perpétuation de l'espèce humaine. Tous les pays et toutes les organisations nationales et internationales doivent considérer qu'il est prioritaire d'assurer aux enfants un cadre de vie sain en encourageant les comportements favorables à la santé et la prise de conscience à tous les niveaux : communauté, famille et enfants eux-mêmes. Pour mieux y parvenir, il est nécessaire d'effectuer des recherches sur l'efficacité de la réduction des risques et des modes d'intervention, et notamment de déterminer quels sont les moyens les plus efficaces pour éduquer le public et faire comprendre qu'il est nécessaire d'élaborer des politiques de santé publique, une législation et des normes de sécurité propres à assurer la protection de l'enfant. Tous les secteurs de la société ont un rôle important à jouer en participant activement à la promotion d'un cadre de vie sain et salubre pour tous.

RESUMEN, CONCLUSIONES Y RECOMENDACIONES

1. Resumen

Los factores ambientales desempeñan una función importante en la determinación de la salud y el bienestar de los niños.[1] Cada vez son más numerosas las pruebas que indican que los niños, que constituyen más de un tercio de la población mundial, son uno de los grupos más vulnerables de dicha población y que algunos factores ambientales pueden afectar a su salud de manera bastante diferente de como lo hace en los adultos. Los niños pobres, abandonados y desnutridos son los que más sufren. Estos niños con frecuencia viven en alojamientos insalubres, que carecen de agua limpia y servicios de saneamiento, y tienen un acceso limitado a la atención sanitaria y la educación. En las zonas más pobres del planeta uno de cada cinco niños no llegará a cumplir cinco años, debido en gran parte a enfermedades relacionadas con el medio ambiente. La Organización Mundial de la Salud (OMS) estima que más del 30% de la carga mundial de enfermedades infantiles se puede atribuir a factores ambientales.

La salud depende de una serie de factores. Además del entorno físico, la genética y la biología, desempeñan una función destacada los factores sociales, económicos y culturales. Aunque es fundamental comprender los diversos factores que influyen en la infancia para perfilar la salud y el comportamiento a lo largo de la vida, el presente documento se concentra de manera específica en la exposición a sustancias químicas presentes en el medio ambiente. En él se valoran los principios científicos que se han de tener en cuenta a la hora de evaluar los riesgos para la salud infantil de la exposición a sustancias químicas en el medio ambiente durante las distintas etapas del desarrollo y proporciona información a las autoridades sanitarias, los investigadores y los científicos encargados de la labor normativa, así como a otros expertos que se ocupan de la protección de la salud infantil. Este documento se concentra fundamentalmente en la etapa

---

[1] Los términos "niños" y "niño" tal como se utilizan en el presente documento comprenden las etapas del desarrollo que van desde la concepción hasta el final de la adolescencia.

del desarrollo, más que en la presencia de una sustancia química específica en el medio ambiente o una enfermedad o un efecto determinados. Los periodos de susceptibilidad específicos de la etapa del desarrollo se han denominado "fases críticas de exposición" o "fases críticas del desarrollo". Estas etapas biológicas distintivas se definen por procesos dinámicos importantes que se producen en las moléculas, las células, los órganos y el organismo. Son las diferencias en estas etapas de la vida, junto con la exposición, lo que definirá el carácter y la gravedad de las repercusiones del medio ambiente.

Los niños tienen una susceptibilidad diferente durante las distintas etapas de su vida debido a sus procesos dinámicos de crecimiento y desarrollo, así como a diferencias fisiológicas, metabólicas y de comportamiento. Desde la concepción hasta el final de la adolescencia se producen procesos rápidos de crecimiento y desarrollo que pueden sufrir alteraciones por la exposición a sustancias químicas en el medio ambiente. Se puede tratar de procesos anatómicos, fisiológicos, metabólicos, funcionales, toxicocinéticos y toxicodinámicos. Las vías y las pautas de la exposición también pueden variar en las distintas etapas de la infancia. Se puede producir exposición en el útero, por transferencia de la madre al feto de agentes ambientales a través de la placenta, o en los lactantes por la leche materna. Los niños consumen más alimentos y bebidas por kg de peso corporal que los adultos y sus regímenes alimenticios son diferentes y con frecuencia menos variables durante las diversas etapas del desarrollo. Tienen una tasa de inhalación más alta y una proporción mayor de superficie corporal con respecto al peso, lo cual puede dar lugar a niveles de exposición más elevados. El comportamiento normal de los niños, como arrastrarse por el suelo y meterse la mano en la boca, puede llevar a exposiciones que no afrontan los adultos. Las vías metabólicas de los niños pueden ser diferentes de las de los adultos. Los niños tienen más años de vida por delante y, por consiguiente, más tiempo para favorecer la aparición de enfermedades crónicas que tardan decenios en ponerse de manifiesto y que se pueden ver potenciadas por exposiciones tempranas en el medio ambiente. Con frecuencia no son conscientes de los riesgos ambientales y en general no intervienen en la adopción de decisiones.

El conocimiento cada vez más claro de que los niños pueden sufrir un riesgo mayor en distintas etapas del desarrollo, tanto con respecto a la susceptibilidad biológica como a la exposición, ha aumentado la sensibilización en el sentido de que tal vez se necesiten nuevos enfoques para la evaluación del riesgo con objeto de protegerlos de manera adecuada. Los enfoques de la evaluación del riesgo y las políticas de higiene del medio tradicionales se han concentrado fundamentalmente en los adultos y sus modalidades de exposición, utilizándose datos obtenidos de personas o animales adultos. Es necesario ampliar los modelos de evaluación del riesgo para evaluar exposiciones pertinentes a los niños desde antes de la concepción hasta la adolescencia, teniendo en cuenta las susceptibilidades específicas de cada etapa del desarrollo. El espectro completo de los efectos debidos a la exposición infantil no se puede predecir a partir de datos obtenidos de adultos. Los enfoques de la evaluación del riesgo para la exposición en la infancia deben estar vinculados a las etapas de la vida.

Se sabe (o se sospecha) que un amplio espectro de las enfermedades infantiles está asociado con entornos insalubres. En gran parte del mundo, los peligros tradicionales derivados de la higiene del medio siguen siendo la principal fuente de enfermedad. Entre ellos cabe mencionar la falta de nutrición adecuada, el saneamiento deficiente, el agua contaminada, la amplia difusión de vectores de enfermedades (por ejemplo, los mosquitos y el paludismo) y la eliminación poco segura de desechos. Además, la rápida globalización e industrialización, junto con sistemas no sostenibles de producción y consumo, han liberado grandes cantidades de sustancias químicas en el medio ambiente. Aunque el término "exposición ambiental" puede incluir diversos factores, este documento se concentra de manera específica en la exposición a sustancias químicas en el medio ambiente. No se ha evaluado la posible toxicidad de la mayoría de estas sustancias para los niños ni tampoco se han identificado las subpoblaciones de niños más vulnerables. La incidencia de varias enfermedades y trastornos pediátricos importantes (por ejemplo, asma, trastornos de neurocomportamiento) está aumentando en varias partes del mundo. Aunque probablemente intervienen diversos factores, esto puede deberse en parte a la calidad del medio ambiente en el que viven, crecen y juegan los niños.

Es difícil y problemático, particularmente en los niños, establecer vínculos causales entre exposiciones ambientales específicas y efectos multifactoriales complejos en la salud. Para los niños, la etapa de su desarrollo en que se produce la exposición puede ser tan importante como la propia magnitud de ésta. Son muy pocos los estudios que han caracterizado la exposición durante diferentes etapas del desarrollo. Hay ejemplos que han puesto de manifiesto que la exposición a la misma sustancia en el medio ambiente puede dar lugar a efectos muy diferentes en la salud de los niños en comparación con los adultos. Se ha demostrado que algunos de estos efectos son irreversibles y persisten durante toda la vida. Además, los diferentes sistemas orgánicos maduran a ritmos distintos y la misma dosis de un agente durante periodos diferentes del desarrollo puede tener consecuencias muy distintas. También puede haber un largo periodo de latencia entre la exposición y los efectos, no apareciendo algunas consecuencias hasta bastante tiempo después. Como ejemplos de efectos en la salud derivados de la exposición en el desarrollo cabe mencionar los observados en la etapa prenatal y al nacer (por ejemplo, aborto, muerte prenatal, peso bajo al nacer, defectos congénitos), en niños pequeños (por ejemplo, mortalidad infantil, asma, trastornos de neurocomportamiento e inmunológicos) y en adolescentes (por ejemplo, pubertad precoz o retardada). Hay nuevas pruebas que parecen indicar que el mayor riesgo de ciertas enfermedades en los adultos (por ejemplo, cáncer, enfermedades cardíacas) pueden derivarse en parte de la exposición durante la infancia a ciertas sustancias químicas presentes en el medio ambiente.

Aunque en la investigación se han estudiado los efectos de las sustancias químicas presentes en el medio ambiente sobre la salud infantil, los investigadores normalmente se han concentrado en la exposición a una sustancia química particular en el medio ambiente, como los metales pesados o los plaguicidas, y a un sistema orgánico o un efecto final determinado. Es sorprendente la ausencia de estudios longitudinales prospectivos para captar las exposiciones en fases del desarrollo o las etapas de la vida fundamentales. Prácticamente en ningún estudio se ha determinado la exposición periconcepcional, ya sea aislada o bien en combinación con las experimentadas en otras etapas de la vida. Los avances de la tecnología y las nuevas metodologías permiten esperar ahora que se puedan determinar las exposiciones durante estas fases críticas. Esto permitirá a los investigadores detectar pronto las concepciones y estimar el posible riesgo de mortalidad embrionaria temprana al examinar los efectos en la salud infantil de los cuales depende la supervivencia durante los periodos embrionario y fetal.

La especial vulnerabilidad de los niños debería servir de base para elaborar políticas de protección de la infancia y enfoques de evaluación del riesgo. La falta de pruebas completas para demostrar asociaciones causales no debería impedir que se realicen esfuerzos orientados a reducir la exposición o se apliquen estrategias de intervención y prevención.

2. Conclusiones y recomendaciones

Si bien se han adquirido conocimientos sustanciales sobre los efectos de la exposición a agentes del medio ambiente en la salud infantil, todavía queda mucho que aprender. Los enfoques de la evaluación del riesgo para la protección de la infancia deben basarse en un mayor conocimiento de la interacción de las exposiciones, la susceptibilidad biológica y los factores socioeconómicos y culturales (incluidos los nutricionales) en cada etapa del desarrollo. A fin de obtener un mayor conocimiento, habría que realizar ulteriores investigaciones en las esferas siguientes:

- Formular y aplicar estudios prospectivos de cohortes de mujeres embarazadas, lactantes y niños pequeños, con la determinación longitudinal de las exposiciones en las fases críticas y los efectos finales sensibles en la salud a lo largo del desarrollo humano como proceso continuo. Hay que realizar esfuerzos para seleccionar parejas antes de la concepción, a fin de examinar datos esenciales relativos a la exposición periconcepcional y la salud infantil.

- Seguir organizando y mejorando sistemas de vigilancia basados en la población para la determinación en tiempo real de los efectos finales de alerta en la salud. Esto incluye los sistemas de vigilancia actuales, como el registro vital del tamaño al nacer y la gestación y el registro de defectos congénitos para conocer las malformaciones importantes. En la investigación habría que prestar mayor atención al examen de nuevos efectos finales de alerta, por ejemplo la capacidad de fecundación medida en función del tiempo transcurrido hasta el embarazo y la proporción entre los sexos.

- Intensificar los esfuerzos de vigilancia de la exposición infantil durante las diferentes etapas del desarrollo, en particular las actividades encaminadas a evaluar las exposiciones agregadas y acumulativas.

- Reforzar los esfuerzos de vigilancia de la exposición en los países en desarrollo.

- Identificar las subpoblaciones con los niveles más elevados de exposición.

- Elaborar biomarcadores validados, sensibles y rentables de la exposición, la susceptibilidad y los efectos, en particular durante las primeras etapas del desarrollo.

- Mejorar la caracterización de las diferencias en las propiedades toxicocinéticas y toxicodinámicas de las sustancias xenobióticas en distintas etapas del desarrollo. Elaborar bases de datos de parámetros fisiológicos y farmacocinéticos específicos de las etapas del desarrollo, tanto en estudios con personas como con animales.

- Realizar durante las distintas etapas del desarrollo estudios concentrados en los mecanismos de acción mediante los cuales las exposiciones puedan causar efectos adversos.

- Establecer los efectos finales que se pueden utilizar para evaluar las funciones del sistema orgánico, tanto en las personas como en las especies animales, y para identificar periodos análogos del desarrollo en las distintas especies.

- Examinar la utilidad de las tecnologías moleculares y de creación de imágenes más recientes para evaluar las asociaciones causales entre la exposición y los efectos en distintas etapas del desarrollo.

- Mejorar la caracterización de las fases de susceptibilidad de los distintos sistemas orgánicos en relación con los efectos finales estructurales y funcionales.

- Elaborar y validar modelos biológicos y directrices para las pruebas en animales que puedan abordar los efectos en la salud en diferentes etapas del desarrollo.

- Determinar qué reducciones de la exposición tendrán los mayores efectos globales en la salud infantil.

Para cualquier programa de salud pública es esencial la elaboración de estrategias de evaluación del riesgo que aborden las etapas biológicas del desarrollo por las que deben pasar todas las generaciones futuras. La protección de los niños es la base de la sostenibilidad de la especie humana. En todos los países y organizaciones internacionales y nacionales deben tener carácter prioritario el suministro de un entorno inocuo para todos los niños y la reducción de la exposición a los peligros ambientales mediante la promoción de comportamientos sanos, educación y aumento de la sensibilización a todos los niveles, incluidos la comunidad, la familia y el propio niño. A fin de de poder alcanzar este objetivo, es necesario investigar la efectividad de la reducción del riesgo y las prácticas de intervención, en particular los medios más eficaces para educar y transmitir la necesidad de políticas de salud pública, legislación y normas sobre inocuidad para la protección de la infancia. La participación activa de todos los sectores de la sociedad desempeña una función importante en la promoción de entornos inocuos y sanos para todos.

www.ingramcontent.com/pod-product-compliance
Ingram Content Group UK Ltd.
Pitfield, Milton Keynes, MK11 3LW, UK
UKHW021315180426
11947UKWH00015B/1232